Qualitative Research Methods for Medicine and Health Sciences

Qualitative research methods are essential for addressing central questions arising from clinical and organisational practice. In medicine and healthcare, knowing and scientific knowledge cannot be reduced to what is measurable alone. It also depends on subjectivity, interpretation, clinical reasoning, interaction and ethical judgement. This book develops a coherent methodological framework in which these dimensions are understood as integral to knowledge development rather than as residual or secondary concerns.

The opening chapters establish the philosophical foundations for a qualitative methodology grounded in healthcare practice and distinctly committed to the epistemic impact of subjectivity. Ontological assumptions about health and illness are made explicit and systematically linked to epistemological and methodological choices. Subsequent chapters guide the reader through the core stages of the research process—from design and data development to analysis and interpretation—consistently demonstrating how underlying assumptions shape methodological strategies and conclusions. Empirical examples illustrate methodological reasoning, critical decisions and common pitfalls. Unlike many introductory texts, this book treats subjectivity, clinical judgement and interpretation not as threats to scientific rigour, but as indispensable resources for knowledge development. Rather than offering a broad survey of qualitative traditions, it presents a coherent, practice-based approach that affirms the scientific legitimacy of qualitative research on its own terms.

Written primarily for students and researchers new to qualitative methods at bachelor's, master's and doctoral levels in medicine and healthcare, the book also invites more experienced scholars to reflect critically on established methodological practices.

Kirsti Malterud MD PhD is Professor Emerita in General Practice at the University of Bergen, Norway.

Qualitative Research Methods for Medicine and Health Sciences

First English translation of the fifth Norwegian edition

Kirsti Malterud

Routledge
Taylor & Francis Group
LONDON AND NEW YORK

Designed cover image: Ceramic glaze pattern by Nina Malterud. Photo: Øystein Klakegg

First published 2027
by Routledge
4 Park Square, Milton Park, Abingdon, Oxon OX14 4RN

and by Routledge
605 Third Avenue, New York, NY 10158

Routledge is an imprint of the Taylor & Francis Group, an informa business

This book is the author's translation of Kvalitative forskningsmetoder for medisin og helsefag 5th edition, first published by Universitetsforlaget, Oslo/Norway 2025.

Language tools (OpenAI GPT-5.5 and DeepL Translator) were used selectively to support fluency and idiomatic English phrasing. All content and final wording are the author's own.

For Product Safety Concerns and Information please contact our EU representative GPSR@taylorandfrancis.com. Taylor & Francis Verlag GmbH, Kaufingerstraße 24, 80331 München, Germany.

British Library Cataloguing-in-Publication Data
A catalogue record for this book is available from the British Library

Library of Congress Cataloging-in-Publication Data
Names: Malterud, Kirsti author
Title: Qualitative research methods for medicine and health sciences / Kirsti Malterud.
Description: Abingdon, Oxon; New York, NY: Routledge, 2027. |
Includes bibliographical references and index. |
Identifiers: LCCN 2026016900 (print) | LCCN 2026016901 (ebook) |
ISBN 9781041330806 hbk | ISBN 9781041330790 pbk | ISBN 9781003786016 ebk
Subjects: LCSH: Medicine—Research—Methodology | Medical sciences—
Research—Methodology | Qualitative research—Methodology
Classification: LCC R852 .M35 2026 (print) | LCC R852 (ebook)
LC record available at https://lccn.loc.gov/2026016900
LC ebook record available at https://lccn.loc.gov/2026016901

ISBN: 9781041330806 (hbk)
ISBN: 9781041330790 (pbk)
ISBN: 9781003786016 (ebk)

DOI: 10.4324/9781003786016

Typeset in Sabon
by codeMantra

Contents

Preface

This book is written for medical doctors and other health professionals who wish to develop an understanding of qualitative research methods as approaches to make sense of everyday clinical and organisational practice. I take medicine and healthcare not merely as domains of study, but as sources of fundamental questions about health and illness, life and death, calling for forms of knowing attuned to the subjectivity of human experience, judgement, complexity and values.

Knowing and knowledge in applied, practice-based disciplines consist of more than what can be measured or standardised, such as experiences of health and illness, encounters between patients and professionals, ethical deliberation and reflection on how services are organised and function. Knowledge-based practice draws on research evidence, clinical expertise and patient values. Yet in many contexts, what counts as scientific knowledge continues to be shaped primarily by quantitative research traditions rooted in biomedicine and epidemiology.

My starting point, informed by lifelong experience as a general practitioner, is that many questions arising from clinical and system practice cannot be addressed adequately within these traditions alone. Exploring phenomena such as meaning, interaction, coping, complexity, diagnostic reasoning and professional judgement calls for qualitative research methods that understand subjectivity, interpretation and reflexivity as integral to knowledge development. Such approaches can lead to new and valuable knowledge, but only when they are grounded in assumptions that support relevant and robust methods, rather than being adopted uncritically from other research traditions.

Earlier Norwegian editions of this book have been used for several decades in education and research within the Scandinavian language sphere. Colleagues from outside this context have encouraged an English edition, not only for teaching, supervision and references in international publications, but because the methodological approach is grounded in applied medical and healthcare practice, offering a coherent basis for scientific legitimacy on its own terms. This English edition is my translation of the fifth Norwegian edition. I do not introduce a new version of this book but make the current edition accessible to a wider readership. Readers encountering the text for the first time should therefore understand it as a coherent presentation of my approach to qualitative research methods in medicine and health sciences, maturing during decades of theoretical, empirical and clinical work.

When academic standards are met, qualitative studies should be regarded as evidence. Throughout this book, I argue that scientific knowledge cannot be reduced to what is observable and measurable. In medicine and healthcare, knowing also involves experience, meaning-making, ethical judgement and reflections on how context and systems shape practice and outcomes. Qualitative research methods offer systematic ways of engaging with these dimensions, insofar as their underlying assumptions are made explicit and carried through into relevant and robust approaches.

Without such clarity, qualitative studies risk being shaped by quantitative, humanistic or social science ideals by default. Procedures and criteria developed for other purposes may be applied unreflectively, narrowing what can be seen, analysed and communicated, thereby distorting scientific soundness and truly relevant knowledge. Earlier debates, including my own contributions, often focused on similarities between qualitative and quantitative research in order to secure legitimacy. Today, I see a greater need to articulate their differences clearly, to safeguard the distinctive and creative contributions from qualitative methods to subjectivity in medical and healthcare knowledge.

In this edition, I place stronger emphasis on scientific thinking and humanistic perspectives than in the outset. This is reflected both in the conceptual framing and in my terminology. I use the terms knowledge and knowing distinctively side by side, with different nuances of meaning. I write of data development and data interaction rather than data collection, and of interpretations, conclusions and results rather than findings. These choices signal an understanding of research in which the researcher's subjectivity and active engagement are treated as resources and responsibilities that call for reflexive attentiveness, rather than sources of error to be eliminated. A sound grasp of the epistemological assumptions is necessary to navigate methodological approaches appropriately and to apply relevant and robust methods in developing new and valuable knowledge.

Compared to previous Norwegian editions, several chapters have been revised, and some are entirely new in the 5th edition. Chapter 11, on Systematic Text Condensation, has undergone substantial revision and should be read carefully even by those already familiar with the method. These changes reflect developments in the field and my own ongoing engagement with epistemological questions raised through research, peer review and supervision.

I have written this book primarily for students and researchers who are new to qualitative research methods at bachelor's, master's, or doctoral level. At the same time, more experienced researchers will also find questions and arguments that invite reflection on established practices. This book may be read from beginning to end, but it can also be used selectively. I recommend starting with the introductory chapters, where I establish assumptions necessary to understand the practical approaches and guidance that follow. An abundance of references is intended to invite further reading and to illustrate the diversity of this methodological field.

Epistemological assumptions and methodological approaches are illustrated through empirical examples, many drawn from my own research. This reflects a long-standing engagement with practice-based inquiry, shaped by more than 35 years of work as a general practitioner. Over time, it has become increasingly clear to me that qualitative research methods cannot be employed uniformly across disciplines. They must be designed congruent with the type of knowledge sought. Research grounded in applied practice-based disciplines rests on assumptions, purposes and procedures that in many ways differ from those of research conducted within the social sciences and humanities alone.

I hope this book will be perceived as a consistent contribution to link methodological choices and approaches to the epistemological assumptions underpinning them, and to do so from within. Rather than offering a broad survey of qualitative traditions, I aim to provide a coherent framework for developing qualitative studies that are both scientifically rigorous and closely aligned with realities in clinical and organisational practice.

I warmly thank fellow researchers Aase Aamland, Anette Fosse, Ann Dorrit Guassora, Marit Hafting, Anne Marit Mengshoel, Margrethe Schaufel, and Susanne Reventlow, whose encouragement, dialogue and critical engagement have sustained the revision and translation of this edition. Thank you also to Lill Salole, Maria Westervoll and Kristin Harbø Buland (Universitetsforlaget, Oslo) and graphic designer Anders Sagdalen for steady guidance during the development of the 5th Norwegian edition and encouragement towards translation. I am grateful to my friends in Möckernkiez/Berlin, who hosted and inspired me during important periods of writing. Finally, I thank my sister, Nina Malterud—an ingenious artist and dear interlocutor—whose exquisite ceramic glazes provided the basis for the cover image.

Bergen, June 2026
Kirsti Malterud

PART 1

Knowing human life, health and illness

CHAPTER 1

A rich and diverse knowledge base for practice and inquiry

Clinical practice and the development of healthcare services are based on knowing and knowledge from various sources. Biomedicine is necessary to understand anatomical structures, physiological processes and chemical principles that affect health and disease. Epidemiology delivers tools to describe and explain the prevalence, risk and distribution of diseases. Humanistic perspectives provide insight into people's experiences, perceptions, expectations and existential challenges related to health and illness. Development of new and valuable knowledge requires a breadth of relevant and robust research methods that correspond to the research questions. Qualitative research methods unwrap knowledge about humanist aspects of life related to health and illness for patients, healthcare professionals and administrators.

Subjectivity

Subjectivity encompasses individuals' personal perception, experience and awareness of the world and themselves. The concept is understood in various ways in different disciplines (Smith 2010, Thorne 2025). Research with humanistic perspectives develops knowledge about human phenomena with subjectivity from the participants' expressions of experiences, perceptions and judgements and the researcher's interpretations, understandings and communication (Gatens-Robinson 1986, Sandelowski 1996, Varpio, Ajjawi, et al. 2017, Braun & Clarke 2022). Subjectivity is the prerequisite for developing, analysing and interpreting data with qualitative research methods. When using such research methods in medicine and health sciences, we recognise subjectivity as a creative added value for the development of insight about human life, health and disease that strengthens the foundation of theory and practice. As a consequence, in this book I use both *knowing* and *knowledge* to distinguish between the active, situated and interpretive processes through which we seek to understand human life and experience, and the more articulated and systematic forms of understanding that take shape through these processes.

DOI: 10.4324/9781003786016-2

However, a focus on subjectivity does not mean that everything is relative and fluid in a qualitative study. *Reflexivity* (see Chapter 3) is a methodological antidote to random or predetermined conclusions, in that the researcher recognises the reciprocal influences between themselves, the person or thing being researched, and the context for knowledge development (Malterud 2001b, Alvesson & Sköldberg 2018, Braun & Clarke 2019). With insight into their own role, the researcher can discipline the subjective. As readers, we assume that the researcher provides us with insight into contextual assumptions that are significant for the interpretation of issues, data and results. *Intersubjectivity* is about the importance of sharing processes and results with others (Malterud 1993).

From biomedicine and natural science research, we recognise *objectivity* as an overarching ideal for scientific practice—a clear opposite of subjectivity. But in research with humanistic perspectives and qualitative methods, subjectivity is not the dirty cousin of an exemplary objectivity. Leder argues that medical culture denies one of its founding missions—a scientific understanding of interpretation in clinical judgements and decisions—in a false awareness that objectivity is a universal basis of science (Leder 1990).

In qualitative studies, we are not supposed to downplay or excuse subjectivity. On the contrary, we must learn how to know and recognise subjectivity as a valuable and necessary platform from which we can benefit in a scientifically sound manner when we want to learn more about people's lives, health and illness.

Knowledge-based practice—everything for your use

In most countries, health personnel are supposed to perform their work in accordance with the requirements for professional responsibility and diligent care that can be expected based on the health personnel's qualifications, the nature of the work and the situation in general. *Knowledge-based practice* (Figure 1.1), adapted from

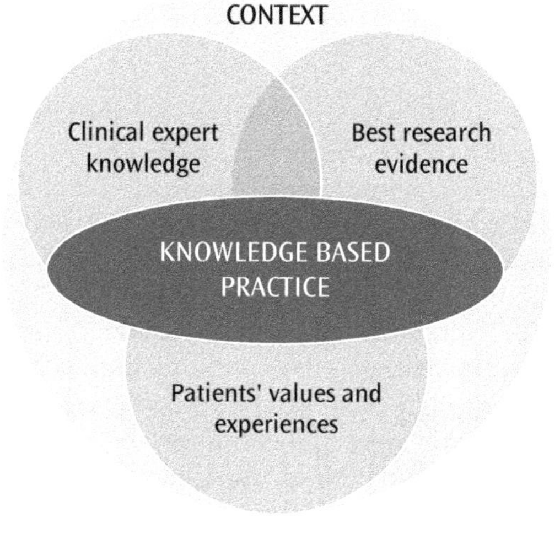

Figure 1.1 Knowledge-based practice

Source: Adapted from Sackett (1997) and Helsebiblioteket (2021)

evidence-based medicine (EBM) (see below), is based on the best evidence from research, patients' values and experiences as well as experience-based clinical expert knowledge (Sackett, Rosenberg, et al. 1996, Sackett 1997). Based on this knowledge base, the intended and unintended consequences of proposed measures in the health service must be assessed against values, use of resources, prioritisation criteria, laws and regulations.

EBM was developed on the basis of Sackett's model. However, over the years, the concept of EBM has taken on a more limited meaning, emphasising research-based knowledge—*evidence*. This book is about research methods, i.e. strategies that will lead to evidence—in this context, research-based knowledge developed using qualitative methods. In other words, evidence from qualitative studies entails the scientization of user knowledge and experience-based clinical knowledge (Eriksson & Martinsen 2012). For the purposes of this book, knowledge-based practice is therefore a more appropriate term than EBM.

People's view of the world determines what we perceive as current, relevant and valid ways of investigating the world. *Ontology* addresses the way we perceive the world and reality, while *epistemology* addresses how we consider knowledge about the world and reality (Lock & Strong 2010, Varpio, Ajjawi, et al. 2017, Pope & Mays 2020, Creswell & Poth 2024). Ontology and epistemology are sometimes informally referred to together as *O&E*, indicating that the two concepts are two sides of the same coin. Consistency between the two is a logical prerequisite for scientific knowledge (Chamberlain 2000, Carter and Little 2007). In research supposed to lead to valid knowledge, there must be correspondence between ontology and epistemology—*epistemological congruence*. We cannot use a screwdriver to hammer in a nail.

When we aim to develop knowledge about people's experiences, we need more research tools than laboratory experiments, statistics and epidemiology. Not everything can be counted and measured, and p-values do not tell us much about existential dilemmas or grief. As researchers, we need to develop ontological awareness. Only then can we choose and familiarise ourselves with research methods that respect our research questions and can accommodate the uniquely human in a scientific way (Pope & Mays 2020).

This is not a question of either-or, but of both-and. In medical and healthcare research and practice, we must have the ability to keep several balls in the air, so that we can make the best methodological choices and practice these with proper consistency. We also need to be familiar with methods we are not going to use ourselves, to be able to choose and develop a design with solid epistemological consistency.

Humanism frames the human subject as the primary point of reference, grounding knowledge in reflective judgement and lived practice while treating personal worth and dignity as non-negotiable starting points rather than derived properties. Humanistic perspectives are necessary when we want to contribute to increased insight into people's lives. The human aspects of clinical practice are not limited to doctor-patient communication—it can also be about the knowledge and experiences of healthcare professionals or administrators, or the relationship between people and systems. We can also explore existential questions, interaction, clinical procedures, or decision management. At all levels of healthcare, subjectivity can provide a meaningful basis for the knowledge we develop and use.

To be human

The sociologist of religion Christian S. Smith (1960-) describes the phenomenon of *emergence* (2010), which is a process in which simple units (such as cells) combine, interact and transform into something that is larger and different (such as organs or people) than what was the starting point. The opposite is *reductionism*, where the whole is explained by the individual parts, which can make sense in many technical-mechanical contexts. In medicine, for example, we sometimes talk about the machine failure model.

Complexity develops when the totality becomes something new—something more than the sum of its parts, which may in turn influence and change the simple units. The emergent forces stem from relationships and interactions between the individual elements. Smith points out that emergence encompasses not only scientific contexts such as biology, physics and chemistry, but also the development of psychological, social and cultural phenomena, including various forms of scientific knowledge (Smith 2010).

Causal capacities are emergent properties that enable humans to transform material, mental or social phenomena and conditions. Smith (2010) shows that many causal capacities are distinctively human in scope, intensity and quality and thus distinguish humans from (other) animals. He gives some examples of what makes a human a human, such as understanding quantities, time and space, mental representations, abstraction, volition, tacit knowledge, emotions, empathy, memory, intersubjectivity, creativity, technology, symbolisation, identity formation and language.

These are aspects of subjectivity and humanity that in different ways apply to all humans, while at the same time each individual has his or her unique composition, form of expression and meaning-making. With subjectivity as our lens, we take this paradox as our starting point when we select qualitative methods as relevant and robust tools for developing new and valuable insights about people's lives, health and illness.

The instrumentalist error

Based on pedagogy and teaching practice, philosopher Hans Skjervheim (1926–1999) discusses research on human interaction. Inspired by Habermas, he emphasises the human being as a scientific subject and describes the researcher as a participant and observer at the same time (Skjervheim 1959, 2002). Skjervheim argues that the subjective is fundamental in social reality and in research about it—therefore, the social sciences must necessarily be subjective in their interpretation of meaning. Such views are just as relevant for medical and health research today.

Skjervheim also demonstrates how *objectification* takes place when I stop engaging with the other, distancing myself and turning the other into a category or a case. Skjervheim emphasises that people can be participants and observers at the same time, with the observer role providing a different technical relationship and insight than the engagement and understanding of the participant role. He warns against *the instrumentalist error*—an attitude in which technical rationality dominates the view of people in practice and research (Skjervheim 2002). Skjervheim points out that instrumental reason has a reasonable place in many contexts but also has its limits. He characterises the instrumentalist mistake as a transgression of boundaries—not a moral error, but as an intellectual and epistemological problem.

Knowledge-seeking activities—sensing, understanding and evaluating

In order to contribute to new understanding, the researcher will develop and read their data and look for patterns in the light of relevant theoretical perspectives (more on this in Chapter 5). Interpretation is a central act in the qualitative research process. When using qualitative research methods, I should not try to eliminate myself or my subjectivity, but, on the contrary, work actively to familiarise myself with my own role and position, consider and account for my influence, and consider the impact of this for my interpretations and conclusions (Braun & Clarke 2024b).

A well-known parallel from clinical practice is diagnostic work, where interpretation and subjectivity are central. This applies to both the mission (to understand what is wrong with the patient) and the data sources (symptom descriptions, bodily signs), which in various ways place the human factor at the centre. The theologian Bernard J. F. Lonergan (1904–1984) presents a theory of knowledge that we can use to understand clinical knowledge and diagnostics as an interpretive, subjective activity in three stages of perception, understanding and judgement (Lonergan 1992, Malterud, Reventlow, et al. 2019):

1. In meeting the patient, we first open ourselves to subjective sensations such as perception, preconceptions, experiences and ideas.
2. These form the basis for questions we can ask and concepts we can use to understand this information and move forward.
3. Finally, we evaluate our questions and possible answers.

This model differs from principles of biomedical research in that it recognises the subjective aspects of the doctor's interpretation as a relevant basis for sorting out impressions and information, and in that relevant questions can be more important than unclear answers. Lonergan emphasises that the knowledge-seeking activity—*knowing*—is at least as central as the result—knowledge (Lonergan 1992).

As researchers, we should proceed through all stages of the research process with an open mind, curious and alert to surprises and fresh connections that can transcend preconceptions and experiences and contribute to new understanding. To benefit from the subjective, both as empirical raw material and as an interpretive strategy, we must be open to creativity and utilise our human potential. At the same time, reflexivity and intersubjectivity oblige us to recognise, assess and communicate the conditions—what guides our gaze and interpretations.

Empirical data—the link to everyday life

Theoretical knowledge, often communicated in the form of models that provide new perspectives on clinical challenges, can be developed on the basis of key existing theories. In an article on how healthcare professionals can understand and prevent situations where we unconsciously humiliate our patients, for example, we used prevailing theories of objectification, distancing and indifference to examine the foundations of degrading behaviour and identify some concepts that can be used to understand such behaviour in the cultural context of medicine (Malterud & Hollnagel 2007).

But for most of the medical knowledge base that we call evidence, regardless of the research method, interpretation, analysis and synthesis are based on *empirical data*.

This is data from relevant sources developed with different methods, for example, from experiment, interview, register or observation. Qualitative research methods support the development of knowledge through the analysis of empirical, qualitative data. In this book, I use the terms *data development* or *data interaction* to highlight the fact that qualitative data is created in dialogue between researcher, participants and context. The term *data collection* is still widely used, but this implicitly states that data are ready and waiting to be harvested and further processed by us. Such an understanding is better suited to a register study. For research on people's subjective experiences and unique experiences, our sample—our empirical data—is something we should recognise that we are personally involved to create, so that we sharpen our reflexivity and assess the significance of this.

But empirical data are neither fact nor truth. In qualitative studies, the researcher's interpretation of the data is the path towards new knowledge. It is therefore a case of misguided loyalty to the material when the researcher tries to avoid leaving his or her own mark on the process, rather than taking responsibility for perspectives and interpretations (Kidder & Fine 1987). In such cases, the result can be qualitative studies characterised by obviousness and a lack of analysis, which the psychologist Steinar Kvale (1938–2008) describes as "boring to read" (Kvale 1996).

On the other hand, we can also see articles from qualitative studies where theoretical perspectives gain the upper hand, so that the empirical material only appears as quotes that embellish the theoretical considerations. Last but not least, unresolved attitudes to empirical data can lead to the researcher's voice and preconceptions taking precedence in interpretations and conclusions. Methodological knowledge can help to balance such challenges.

(Co-)humanity as added value in medical practice and knowledge

In clinical practice, the doctor has the role of both participant and observer, often at the same time (Skjervheim 2002). Diagnostic activities involve both analytical objectification and sensitive interpretation of multiple, quite indistinct clues (Sebeok & Sebeok 1981, Gatens-Robinson 1986, Malterud & Kamps 2021), often under a high degree of uncertainty (Malterud, Guassora, et al. 2017). Clinical knowledge grows from putting together the pieces of this puzzle from different sources of knowledge, so that we can better understand what they mean together (Malterud 2001a).

The interaction between healthcare professionals and patients on issues related to life and death, illness and health encompasses trust, security, fairness, dignity and openness. Responding to people's symptoms, grief, pain and fatigue requires knowledge of the uniquely human (Malterud 2001b, Malterud, Guassora, et al. 2015, Braun & Clarke 2019). Humanity and compassion are central aspects of the ontological landscape that we explore (Eriksson & Martinsen 2012). Seeing the other's face clearly in front of you is as important in medical and health research as it is in clinical practice (Lévinas & Hand 1989).

We develop knowledge at the intersection of perception, interpretation and action. The human factor is of great importance in data collation and analysis, and also later in the project when insights are to be shared with others (Latour & Woolgar 1986). This is particularly true for the exploration of people's experiences and perceptions from their own lives. Together we create the reality we live in, and together we develop words and concepts that convey our understanding of what we want to investigate. As a researcher, I am a participant in the field and influence my empirical data in different ways, whether data are developed from conversations that become transcripts, or from activities that become field notes.

Without a view of knowledge that explicitly embraces the (co-)human and subjective, medicine and health sciences will support the instrumentalist error (Malterud 2001b, Skjervheim 2002). Medical knowledge is supposed to contribute to both meeting patients and their illnesses in the best possible way, and to advance new ways of understanding illness and health (Malterud & Kamps 2021). Therefore, the research knowledge or evidence on which the health service is based must encompass more than biomedical and technical rationality. The practice of medicine and healthcare requires knowledge where metrics are not the only thing that counts. The ultimate question is what role subjectivity and humanity should play in the development of medical knowledge, and how humanism can have a more prominent place in medical research and practice. Qualitative research methods are well suited for this purpose.

CHAPTER 2

Unpacking assumptions underpinning qualitative methods

You do not need extensive in-depth philosophy studies to use qualitative research methods. Nor does anyone using statistical methods need to master the mathematical foundations, provided that the methodological assumptions are sufficiently clear. However, researchers with a biomedical background who want to use qualitative methods need to familiarise themselves with elementary knowledge of the philosophical foundations and preconditions for the how-to-do procedures. Without such a backdrop, it is difficult to grasp the meaning and implications of subjectivity and interpretation, as well as the crucial differences between qualitative and quantitative methods. Here, I present some key assumptions and concepts, along with a brief overview of the philosophical roots of qualitative research methods.

A gap between two cultures?

Chemist Charles P. Snow (1905–1980) coined the term *the two cultures*, referring to the gap between the natural sciences and the humanities in academia (1959). Despite the differences between the academic subject areas, medical knowing has substantial scientific roots in humanism, for example with medical symptom experiences and problem-solving (Gatens-Robinson 1986, Leder 1990).

The interdisciplinary field of medical humanities encompasses medical ethics and philosophy, the doctor–patient relationship, narrative medicine and the use of art and literature in medical education and practice, in some cases with ambitions to challenge and expand understandings of the medical profession (Viney, Callard, et al. 2015). In this book, I will present qualitative research methods as a contribution to humanistic medicine through influencing and expanding medical knowledge and practice.

Scientific paradigms

The philosopher of science Thomas S. Kuhn (1922–1996) writes about how scientific understanding proceeds in leaps and bounds when an unspoken agreement on basic

DOI: 10.4324/9781003786016-3

assumptions—*paradigms*—is challenged or proves inadequate (1962). Academic general practitioner Ian McWhinney (1926–2012) presents examples from medical theory and practice in which the premises of biomedicine fall short in understanding key issues such as medically unexplained symptoms, the mind-body relationship and the placebo effect (1984). Such disturbing elements, which Kuhn calls *anomalies*, contribute to the development of new paradigms that replace or supplement the prevailing "truths".

In everyday speech, opinions, attitudes and ideologies are sometimes referred to as paradigms and paradigm shifts, for example in connection with user participation or shared decision-making. In such contexts, the meaning differs from that of *scientific paradigms*, which refer to fundamental assumptions about the world and knowledge of it that are largely taken for granted. In medicine and health sciences, *the positivist paradigm* has had (and still has) a profound impact. Positivism represents a fundamental understanding that the world consists of phenomena that can be observed, measured and summarised as objective facts with realism as the yardstick, as assumed and approached by quantitative research methods (Crotty 2003). Research within this paradigm applies deductive logic, where conclusions are drawn from the general to the unique. Many researchers in medicine and healthcare are trained to believe that this is the only valid path to scientific knowledge (Loder, Groves, et al. 2016).

The *interpretive paradigm* (interpretivism) draws on a different set of assumptions than positivism. Here, subjectivity is placed at the centre in a binding manner. Interpretivism is nothing new—such a way of thinking has long traditions as a basis for knowledge in Western science, especially in the humanities (Crotty 2003, Braun & Clarke 2022, Thorne 2025). Skjervheim (see Chapter 1) was a key thinker when the critique of positivism was formulated in Norway in the 1960s. In the interpretive paradigm, subjectivity is recognised, practised and investigated with the researcher as a central and contributing tool, based on an understanding that the world can be perceived in different versions depending on one's point of view. The interpretive paradigm represents an *inductive* logic, where conclusions are drawn from the individual to the general (Pope & Mays 2020). Qualitative research methods belong in this paradigm.

As Snow declared, these paradigms give rise to significant contradictions in how knowledge, truth and scientific thinking are understood. Ontology and epistemology are central premises for the scientific paradigms, not least when it comes to subjectivity and objectivity (see Chapter 1) (Pope & Mays 2020). Within the positivist paradigm, the world is understood as unambiguous facts—a *stable ontology* with structural objects that can be standardised and categorised. This makes objectivity and generalisability relevant and key concepts in biomedical research. Seen from an interpretive perspective, a *fluid ontology* frames the world as taking form through shifting human, social and cultural processes, where values, meanings and experiences remain open rather than fixed. Thus, subjectivity, interpretation and diversity become central concepts for qualitative research methods.

As a result, there are substantial differences in how the research methods are operationalised, for example when it comes to the analysis of numbers or text, respectively, when it comes to sampling and transferability, and not least regarding the researcher's role in the research process (see Chapter 5). Both paradigms are useful and necessary platforms for knowledge development in medicine and health sciences. But neither of them is the best—it depends on what is to be investigated and what perspective we apply to what we want to investigate. Therefore, we need a sufficient understanding of the philosophy of science to understand, select, implement and justify our methodological choices (Chamberlain 2000, Carter & Little 2007)

Kvale illustrates this by describing two diametrically different *researcher roles*, where the researcher is either a gold miner or a tourist (Kvale 1996). The gold miner represents the positivist paradigm and views knowledge as valuable metal that is buried and can be discovered and uncovered by the researcher, untouched by human hands. Quantitative methods are the gold miner's tools for uncovering facts. The tourist, on the other hand, represents the interpretive paradigm and views knowledge as narratives developed while travelling through interaction and reflection that can provide new understanding when shared upon return. Qualitative methods are the tourist's indispensable strategies for interpreting and understanding different versions of reality, while quantitative research methods have several methodological measures to minimise human impact in the field of study.

Philosophical and ideological roots

In the *hermeneutic* tradition, understanding is grounded in the interpretation of meaning in human expressions. Texts from the Greek philosophers Aristotle and Plato formed the basis for what later became the methodical reading of biblical texts—exegesis. Over the years, hermeneutical understanding has formed the basis for research and practice in theology, law and history. Since the 18th century, this has been formalised by philosophers such as Friedrich Schleiermacher (1768–1834), Wilhelm Dilthey (1833–1911), Hans-Georg Gadamer (1859–1938) and Paul Ricoeur (1913–2005) (Gadamer 2004, Alvesson & Sköldberg 2018). In the interpretation of texts, hermeneutics emphasises the relationship between parts and the whole (*the hermeneutic circle*) and the importance of context and self-reflection. The hermeneutic understanding is an older tradition of understanding than the natural sciences on which contemporary biomedical science is based. Hence, we should not forget that Hippocratic medicine was originally a hermeneutic discipline (Gatens-Robinson 1986).

Phenomenology concerns understanding and knowing people's subjective experiences and consciousness. From the 19th century, this field was developed by philosophers such as Edmund Husserl (1859–1938), Martin Heidegger (1889–1976), Alfred Schütz (1899–1959) and Maurice Merleau-Ponty (1908–1961) (Merleau-Ponty 1962, Kohak 1978, Alvesson & Sköldberg 2018). A phenomenological prerequisite for understanding is to *bracket* previous knowledge to direct critical attention to the current subjective experience with a first-person perspective on the individual's *life world*. The *essence* of a phenomenon is described as accurately and carefully as possible, including relationships to other phenomena. Perception and bodily experiences have a particular place in phenomenology, which has become especially topical in physiotherapy science. Given nursing's longstanding orientation toward practice at the level of individual, lived experience, phenomenological approaches—marked by close engagement between researcher and participant—have appeared consistent with the discipline's moral commitment to recognising each patient as a unique and worthy person (Thorne 2025).

Social constructionism emerged in the 20th century and became a precursor to postmodernism (Lock & Strong 2010). From a social constructionist perspective, social phenomena are constituted through human interaction, privileging the relative and contextual rather than the absolute and universal. Text and dialogue create meaning, concepts and understanding, and diversity in subjectivities takes on greater impact than objective facts (Berger & Luckmann 1967, Lock & Strong 2010). Culture, society, narratives and symbols for understanding and knowledge are emphasised (Smith 2010, Alvesson & Sköldberg 2018).

For applied practice-based disciplines where professionals encounter individuals in different life situations with varying meaning content, these philosophical directions from other disciplines can offer access to new and valuable knowledge. In this book, social constructionism is my point of departure for several methodological considerations and recommendations and is therefore given a separate (still brief) section below.

The philosophical and ideological perspectives discussed here have matured as extensions of each other. There are many important differences between them, but together they have provided substantial theoretical assumptions for the interpretive paradigm and the qualitative research methods for exploring and knowing human subjectivity. All the qualitative methods contain elements of textual interpretation, movement between part and whole, and understanding human experience in light of their life conditions (see Chapter 1). Hence, none of these philosophical approaches "owns" such characteristics more than the others. It is also important to remember that research methodology is not the same as philosophy, although there are definitely links between them.

It is therefore misleading to refer to qualitative research methods as hermeneutics, phenomenology or hermeneutic-phenomenological without this being clearly and explicitly philosophically rooted. If you use these terms, your reader will expect a more specific explanation than that you want to use qualitative research methods. If this is not the case, it is better not to use the terms. However, some authors provide justification for such anchoring, while at the same time explaining the methodological approach that follows from this (Ricoeur 1976, Giorgi 1985, van Manen 2023). If you refer to these, you must also familiarise yourself with and respect the assumptions and procedures specified by the authors.

Social constructionism as a basis for cognition

Inspired by the phenomenologist Alfred Schütz (1899–1859), Berger and Luckmann coined the concept of *the social construction of reality* (Berger & Luckmann 1967). The authors question cognition based on rationality and objectivity, pointing instead to processes of knowing that embrace ideology, interests, institutions and power.

There are many variants of social constructionism. A common feature is to regard reality as socially created, contextual and changing over time. This means that research into this world must also take account of social, cultural and historical influences challenging realism, facts, truth or essences. The *hypothetical-deductive model* is challenged, not least since many different versions of the same reality may be valid at the same time, depending on people's experiences, consciousness and perspectives. *Social constructivism* is a related concept often used within mathematics and developmental psychology (Alvesson & Sköldberg 2018).

Social constructionism has been criticised for *relativism*—an understanding that everything is fluid and that there are no underlying structures (Smith 2010, Alvesson & Sandberg 2024). This version, known as *extreme* or *strong social constructionism*, may seem alien to healthcare workers who are familiar with biological and anatomical matters that most people will agree on. A version that is better suited to qualitative methods in medical and health research is therefore *moderate* or *weak social constructionism* (Smith 2010, Elder-Vass 2012). Here, knowledge is perceived as concrete, situated and rooted in human practice, while at the same time with room for realism, recognising and incorporating conditions that do not always need to be renegotiated or redefined (Alvesson & Sandberg 2024). Smith believes that strong social constructionism is more extreme than Berger & Luckmann's original conceptualisation (Smith 2010). He argues in favour of the moderate variant as the normal variant, better suited to social science and humanities research. As a basis for new and valuable knowledge developed with relevant and robust methods, this also makes sense for medicine and health sciences.

CHAPTER 3

Scientific rigour with a human face

Qualitative research methods are one of several routes to scientific knowing and evidence. Despite the growing recognition of methodological diversity in medical and health research, there remains a reluctance to acknowledge subjectivity as a foundation for knowledge meeting scientific standards. Many believe that only experimental designs, randomised controlled trials and registry-based studies with sophisticated statistical calculations can lead to scientific knowledge for healthcare. This book begins with the idea that no research method inherently ensures or rules out scientific rigour. It is the way knowledge is understood, developed and shared that determines whether it meets scientific standards. We will take a closer look at conditions for scientific rigour that apply to all kinds of medical and health research, not just qualitative studies.

Scientific knowledge and other kinds of knowing

There are many forms of knowing and knowledge. *Scientific knowledge (evidence)* is just one of these. Everyday knowledge that makes it possible to find your way from home to work every day, to obtain and prepare food and to live together with other people is more important to most people than scientific knowledge. Scientific knowledge is not a particularly precious form of knowledge, or something that is more genuine than anything else. It can be at least as true and important if I say that I have turned off the hob as if I say that the p-value for the difference between a and b is less than 0.05. As researchers, we therefore need to understand what delimits and characterises scientific knowledge or evidence.

When I buy jam, I assume that the manufacturer guarantees that the contents correspond to the product declaration on the label. Similarly, when knowledge claims to originate from a scientific study, we should be able to assume that its content corresponds to what is declared as constitutive of scientific knowledge. If, as a researcher, I make statements about how general practitioners relate to patients with subjective health problems asking for sick leave, I need more than my own experiential knowledge

DOI: 10.4324/97810037860´6-4

(Nilsen, Malterud, et al. 2015). If, as a researcher, I claim that gynaecological examinations are perceived as difficult by many women, the basis for this should be different from discussions with my closest friends (Larsen, Oldeide, et al. 1997). My reader should be able to rely on the fact that this is knowledge developed in accordance with certain basic requirements that scientific culture recognises and acknowledges. This is what distinguishes research knowledge from free imagination or random opinions and accounts.

There is nothing wrong with random opinions or accounts—that is how most people talk to each other on a daily basis. When I share my clinical experiences with a colleague, I must also be allowed to say what comes to my mind or emphasise what I myself am most concerned about. But when the researcher presents their results, we have specific anticipations of how these have been developed. Nevertheless, the criteria for this declaration of contents often come implicit in the form of inarticulated principles and rules rooted in paradigms (see Chapter 2) (Kuhn 1962), where we take for granted that everyone agrees on what is meant by scientific knowledge. This is particularly true within the biomedical culture, which has paid little attention to epistemological and philosophical issues.

Standards of scientific rigour are not universal constants, but implicit norms moulded within specific social and cultural contexts and their historical conditions. Science is understood differently today than people did 300 years ago. In many ways, medical and health researchers think otherwise about scientific rigour than humanists or social scientists (Thorne 2025). Social constructionist and postmodern perspectives raise fundamental challenges to our understanding of knowing and knowledge in general (Berger & Luckmann 1967, Foucault 1970, Lock & Strong 2010). Nevertheless, there is a substantial agreement of common metaunderstanding across paradigms and academic cultures about what is required from knowledge-seeking processes for the result to be acknowledged as scientific knowledge and evidence.

Research is the practice of developing, systematising and abstracting scientific knowledge. The results must stand up to scrutiny based on observations, reasoning and arguments. Scientific knowledge is somehow accountable and open to scrutiny. However, procedures for assessing transparency vary according to the aim and type of the research methods. For example, while a purposive sample (see Chapter 7) may be relevant in a qualitative study, a representative sample is usually necessary in an epidemiological study.

A brief definition of research, likely acceptable across different methodological strategies, entails a systematic and reflexive process in which the development of knowledge is open for scrutiny and can be shared, with the ambition of transferability of the results beyond the context in which the individual study was conducted (Malterud 2001b).

Systematic critical reflection

Scientific knowledge should be the result of systematic, critical reflection, as opposed to random impressions and self-affirming assertions. If I, as a researcher, am to investigate a phenomenon, the data, interpretations, results and conclusions need to be part of a larger context that I have related to and taken a position on.

Knowledge is power and should be shared with others. Scientific knowledge is currency that can be compared to deposits into a shared pool of professional expertise—not just a private experience that I have made in my practice. Abstraction and transferability (see Chapters 7 and 20) are therefore important ambitions for the researcher, so that the results can in some way be original, shared and utilised as an understanding that others can benefit from in contexts beyond the one in which I conducted my project. When knowledge is shared, others can also interject with critical reflection, preferably from angles different from the researcher's (Malterud 1993, 2001b).

In this way, we can learn more about the scope and limits of knowing and realise that the process and the questions may be just as important as the answers. Different ways of understanding can create opportunities for knowing in different colours and shades that together provide a broad picture of what we want to explore. We can also use scientific methods to highlight the contradictions, paradoxes and complexities that characterise human life and health. Knowledge about knowledge—philosophy of science, history of ideas and epistemology—encourages humility, reflection and new questions and can inoculate against the notion that evidence is the same as eternal truth. Incidentally, it is rare for medical research to generate knowledge of unlimited validity.

With qualitative methods, scientific rigour cannot be checked with simple procedures or calculations (see Chapter 24). Rather, it involves an attitude of systematic, reflexive processing leading to knowledge (Hamberg, Johansson, et al. 1994, Pope & Mays 2020). Therefore, the researcher's most important tool in the service of accountability and trustworthiness is to make the reader an informed companion, given insight into the conditions under which the knowing takes place (Malterud 1993, 2001b, Stige, Malterud, et al. 2009). This is called *intersubjectivity* or *transparency.*

In this book, I summarise my version of the basic conditions for scientific knowledge in three points, namely reflexivity, relevance and validity, with the former as an overall heading. Reflexivity entails the researcher's assumptions and interpretive framework. Relevance is about the utility of the knowledge. Validity concerns the soundness of what the researcher has come to understand, and the scope within which that understanding holds.

Similar *meta-criteria* appear in all scientific paradigms and activities, regardless of qualitative or quantitative method (Malterud 2001b). But how these premises are put into practice in the form of procedures and practices is determined by epistemological assumptions, such as data consisting of text or numbers, or exploring people or things. This is why validity takes on different forms in different research traditions. Nevertheless, overarching meta-criteria can help us ask questions about the scope, limitation and meaning of knowledge and provide us with tools to assess whether and in what sense it is scientific knowledge. In the sections that follow, I will elaborate on and concretise these concepts.

Reflexivity

In the process and outcome, the researcher must demonstrate *reflexivity* as a willingness and capacity to question their own procedures and conclusions as doubt and questions (Stige, Malterud, et al. 2009, Alvesson & Sköldberg 2018, Braun & Clarke 2019, 2022, 2024b). If I think I know in advance that the GP always gives sick leave to patients who want it, there is no point in wasting time on research—I can just say that this is the case. Call into the forest and the echo will answer in kind. The researcher is a human being with motives, inner images and perceptions. For the research process to produce something else than I know in advance, believe or have taken for granted, I need an open mind with room for doubt, considerations and surprises.

The significance of *the researcher's role* is an important part of this (see Chapter 5) (Haraway 1991, Alvesson & Sköldberg 2018). Therefore, the researcher needs to clarify his or her preconceptions and hypotheses and share access to these with the reader (Malterud 1993). It is equally important to consider the social and cultural context of the study aim and the project and consider the consequences of this. This permits the reader to understand how the researcher arrived at a particular result, even though the reader might have chosen a different interpretation based on his or her starting point that would have led to a somewhat different result.

Reflexivity is an active attitude—a position that the researcher must learn, seek out, practice and maintain. The researcher cannot take the state of affairs for granted or wait for surprises to arrive but must seek out confrontations with their own ideas and positions. The proficient researcher creates positions that challenge field knowledge, preconceptions and stereotypes previously held. As a researcher, I must be prepared for the possibility of having to reject results and conclusions that I thought were in place.

The philosopher of science Karl Popper (1902–1994) claimed that a hypothesis can never be verified; it can only be disproved or *falsified*. A classic example (*The Black Swan*) concerns the question of how many swans we need to see to conclude that all swans are white. No matter how many white swans we see, we cannot say that all swans are white. But once we have seen a black swan, we can reject the hypothesis that all swans are white with a high level of certainty. In the same way, our research results must be able to survive systematic attempts at falsification, by us and others asking fundamentally critical questions about what we see and about our methods.

Most of us have blind spots where we do not always realise that we are following tracks we have laid out ourselves. The *confirmation trap*, where we forget to consider alternative interpretations when we get a good idea, is a serious pitfall for the researcher. That's why it is indispensable to include active questioning in all phases along the way, as a systematic part of the work we do. This approach is supported by *metapositions*—points of view in the research process that enable us to look at what we are doing from the side with a fresh perspective (Stensland 2003, Guassora, Reventlow, et al. 2022) (more on this in Chapter 16). Reflexivity cannot be claimed. The article that will ultimately describe what we have done and arrived at can demonstrate reflexivity in that the researcher recognises their tracks and examines the specific significance of these in the process of knowing.

At the same time, there are reasonable limits to scepticism. A falsificationist attitude does not mean that we should simply try to disprove what we have arrived at. Ultimately, we must be encouraged to argue that the results are sufficiently appropriate answers to the questions we have asked. Because a case always has several sides, where an observation usually has multiple valid interpretations, I must decide why I consider my own conclusion to be the strongest and most relevant alternative. The researcher should be able to show the reader which competing versions have been considered.

Inflated proximity to the material may obstruct reflexivity. As researchers, we sometimes identify so strongly with a particular interpretation that we are unable to see alternatives. When researchers who are themselves clinicians study GPs' strategies in challenging situations, this can, on the one hand, make the interviews targeted and relevant, but also, on the other hand, lead to a lack of a critical view of the data (Aase, Nordrehaug, et al. 2008, Nilsen, Malterud, et al. 2015, Thaulow, Eide, et al. 2023). This applies regardless of whether a qualitative or quantitative method.

Therefore, I must always ask myself what establishes my seeing and knowing—what is my vantage point for observations and interpretations, what glasses am I wearing when I read my data, what is the impact of my cultural and theoretical tradition on the questions I have asked? Do I have any strong opinions in this field? Only when we have asked such questions and acknowledged our positions can we assess more specifically how this has influenced the development of knowledge, and reflect on alternative paths to knowledge that, from this standpoint, we did not choose to follow.

Some call this *bias*. In certain forms of experimental design, it may be necessary, realistic and relevant to work to eliminate bias. In most other forms of medical research, bias is impossible to eliminate and may even represent a resource in the research process if the researcher's point of view and field knowledge offer special conditions for insight and understanding. In qualitative research, aiming to eliminate bias is epistemologically inconsistent (the small q, see Chapter 4) since it excludes the researcher from active participation in the process (Varpio, O'Brien, et al. 2021).

At the same time, it can still be a goal to reduce unintentional or undesirable tilts and declinations in the development of knowledge, such as allowing preconceptions to dominate at the expense of empirical data. Reflexivity then becomes a key tool, by highlighting the researcher's position and reminding us that multiple interpretive perspectives are available (Haraway 1991). It is only when we believe that we have eliminated our own influence on the development of knowledge that bias really threatens the opportunities for critical reflection.

The demands for doubt, reflection, falsification and recognition of one's point of view are part of what is often called *objectivity*. However, as the term is used today within biomedical research culture, it has acquired a much more restricted meaning. Impersonal distance and technical logic emerge as an ideal, in a manner comparable to Skjervheim's understanding of objectification. (see Chapter 1) (Skjervheim 2002). Technical rationality will then reject the positive impact of the researcher's involvement in the development of knowledge.

The norm of objectivity from the positivist paradigm has also contributed to a devaluation of subjectivity as relevant to the development of knowledge. As a result, objectivity is an inadequate basic criterion for scientific knowledge in general, and for qualitative studies in medicine and health sciences in particular. In this book, reflexivity is an overarching prerequisite for scientific knowledge. Systematic considerations of relevance and validity are tools for managing reflexivity (Malterud 2001b). *Robust and relevant* strategies for knowing are methodological ideals we recurrently will return to throughout this book.

Relevance

Even if the research process has followed all applicable rules, it is not a foregone conclusion that the outcome will constitute scientific knowledge. In addition to technically correct methodological conduct, scientific knowledge must have relevance as knowledge with some form of utility. As researchers, we want others to learn from what we have done and for it to lead to development and change. This also relates to the transferability of knowledge. The relevance requirement is particularly relevant for research in applied practice-oriented disciplines such as medicine and health sciences (Patton 2015, Thorne 2025). I must consider what role this particular contribution can play in the large pool of shared scientific knowledge—where and how it can make a difference. Then we will see if others can use our insights for something *new and valuable*—another utility ideal for qualitative studies that you will encounter in various places throughout this book.

When the police officer reads the figures on the radar meter, the requirements for accuracy and validity must be satisfactorily met. They assume that the radar meter provides an accurate measurement of the speed of the car that has just passed but also knows that figures measured in a bend may have greater uncertainty than measurements from a straight stretch of road. The police officer does not accept the first number that comes along on the screen—they know that it is easy to confuse 5s and 6s and therefore have a reasonable doubt built into their professional attitude. If the radar meter is known to have good stability from several tests, and the police officer has new glasses, the measurements become highly reliable.

These numbers belong in a context where it is clear-cut what they mean and what they can be used for. Nevertheless, we do not consider the collection of this type of data to be research. Nor would we give a high relevance score to qualitative studies that merely answer questions that have previously been satisfactorily answered countless times. Knowledge about how GPs talk to patients about possible alcohol problems carries more weight when it can inspire change than if it is about something everyone already knows (Lid & Malterud 2012).

What is then the difference between scientific evidence and knowing derived from *routine data* collection? Medical and healthcare research is rarely truly original, in the sense that the questions, methods and answers have never been put on the agenda before. Truly groundbreaking breakthroughs are few and far between. Nevertheless, we expect scientific knowledge to add something new to what is already known. We may disagree about the impact of this novelty, or how strict the requirements for *originality* should be in scientific endeavours. For qualitative studies, the aim is not to repeat or confirm previous research, but on the contrary to see something new and fresh—to utilise subjectivity to focus on the unique for the benefit of emergence and abstraction (see Chapter 1), thereby unfolding something we did not know before.

The criterion of relevance can equally be applied to the project's study aim as its results. A new question can give rise to original knowledge development. Originality and relevance may also include methodological strategy. Developing a new way of knowing about a well-known topic can provide nuances and facets that change our understanding of an old problem (Malterud 1990). Relevant theoretical perspectives can also help to unwrap fresh insights, both in research and practice (Malterud 2016, Guassora, Reventlow, et al. 2022, Malterud, Reventlow, et al. 2024).

When a scientific article is rejected, it is usually because the text does not convincingly present knowledge considered new and valuable. Therefore, a thorough literature search, critical reading and careful assessment and prioritisation of what this study adds are important tools. Remember that common search terms do not always cover what you are looking for. A simple search on PubMed or in the Cochrane databases is rarely sufficient to provide a comprehensive overview, especially when it comes to qualitative studies.

Validity

No knowledge is universally valid in the sense that it applies in all circumstances for every purpose. Therefore, *generalisability* is a problematic concept, regardless of the ideals of transferability (Sandelowski 1996, Malterud 2001b, Varpio, O'Brien, et al. 2021). The researcher must assess the validity of what the interpretations indicate, as well as their transferability. (Kvale 1996). We can rarely answer yes or no to the question of whether what we have found is true. Such an ideal belongs in research within the positivist paradigm, with matters within a stable ontology (see Chapter 2). It is more important to consider what the interpretations and conclusions are "true" about—what the method and material allow us to say, and what scope and transferability the results have—to assess the soundness of what we have come to understand and the scope of that understanding.

The domain and context in which the knowing is conducted will always determine the reach of the knowledge in time, space and culture (Haraway 1991). Even though we are mapping the typical symptoms of heart attacks in men, these are not necessarily the most typical symptoms of heart attacks in women. GPs in Spain may have different strategies for negotiating sick leave than those found in a study of Norwegian doctors (Nilsen, Malterud, et al. 2015).

The first question about validity is therefore what it is "true" about (*internal validity*) (Kvale 1996). Is there consistency between the study aim, method and conclusions? Were appropriate concepts, theory, design or sample to study the actual phenomenon in question applied? It may seem obvious that there is no point in measuring litres by the metre. It is perhaps less obvious to the medical researcher that symptoms are subjective phenomena that are experienced, interpreted and communicated in unique ways (Gatens-Robinson 1986, McWhinney 1989, Malterud et al. 2015). We often run the risk of people answering "true" about something other than what we mean to ask them, and sometimes we do not even understand this. Such are the core challenges of subjectivity in empirical research with people.

The risk of weak internal validity is particularly current for research on topics or people from another culture or with a language other than our own. In such cases, we need to look carefully at the tools we use to develop knowledge and ask ourselves to what extent the methodology and theoretical perspectives are robust, relevant and likely to strengthen the validity of our conclusions. No matter how accurate data our methods can facilitate, internal validity is weak if the study is not conducted according to its purpose—with epistemological congruence (see Chapter 4). Asking questions about validity may be helpful to prevent systematic errors in the research process. This means, for example, assessing whether we have pointed our investigative tools in the right direction in relation to what we wanted to look at, or whether we have made the fundamental mistake of setting up our camera facing east to photograph the sunset.

The second question of validity concerns transferability (*external validity*)—the scope within which the researcher's interpretation holds. A useful keyword for this is *context*. To which contexts can our results provide new insights beyond the context in which we have mapped them (Malterud 2001b)? If we conduct a statistical survey on a representative sample of the Norwegian population, it is not a given that the answers apply to a different ethnic, social or cultural context, such as the Japanese population. If we talk to Norwegian patients about their experiences from long-term sick leave, this may be completely different to countries with different sick leave rules (Aamland,

Werner, et al. 2013). The question of transferability and context can also apply to gender. If we interview men about their living habits, it may well be that the answers do not cover women's everyday lives.

External validity is weak if we only relate to the local context without abstracting and synthesising our interpretations and thereby consider the conditions for transferability. We cannot limit our ambitions by dismissing questions of transferability, for example by stating humbly that we (only) investigate experiences of dance as a physical activity in six people with Parkinson's disease in a Copenhagen suburb. Finally, transferability also relates to *abstraction*—the process of interpretation, analysis and transformation from the unique to the more general (though not generalisation).

The transferability of results from qualitative studies is always linked to sampling and Information Power (see Chapter 7), but it also raises the question of relevance and utility—how can these results be relevant to a comparable issue in another context? Can the experiences of lesbians and gays who conceal their sexual orientation teach us something about other situations where people, for various reasons, conceal an important aspect of themselves (Malterud & Bjørkman 2016)? Can concepts developed from conversations in general practice about alcohol use provide insights that are useful in conversations about relationship problems (Lid & Malterud 2012)?

Repeatability—achieving identical results through repeated data development—is often used in biomedical research as a measure of reliability, verifiability and validity. This idea originates in laboratory research, which seeks to control most aspects of human behaviour. But even in the laboratory, observation, analysis, interpretation and presentation are all influenced by the researcher in some way (Latour & Woolgar 1986), not only in interviews about people's health perceptions, but also in the interpretation of mammography images (Elmore, Wells, et al. 1994).

The strength of qualitative research methods is to draw on diversity, acknowledging several valid versions of knowledge and evidence. A GP is perhaps more likely to get colleagues to talk about different nuances of sick leave strategies than an interviewer who is a sociologist (Nilsen et, Malterud, et al. 2015). We recognise that different researchers may adhere to different nuances even when reading the same material, without us thereby considering all versions to be equally interesting. Therefore, repeatability and consensus are misconceived criteria for validity in a qualitative study (Malterud 2001b, Braun & Clarke 2024b). When researchers examine a process involving the introduction of a health measure in a municipality, repeating the study a year later to test for identical results serves little purpose. You cannot turn back the clock and pretend that nothing else has happened. Also in qualitative health services research, trustworthiness and utility are better ensured with strategies other than repeatability. Validity assessments require a different logic in the interpretive paradigm than in the positivist paradigm.

Questions of validity lead to an overall obligation towards *consistency*—a visible common thread—which should be a clearly coherent line between the project's study aim and the theories, methods and data that feed into interpretations, analyses and new knowledge. We can call this *epistemological congruence* (see next chapter). It is therefore crucial that the method is determined by the study aim, and not the other way round.

In qualitative studies, people's experiences and perceptions (what was it like for you?) are best investigated using interview designs, while observation designs are better suited to studying people's behaviour (what happened?). Validity considerations should be made at all stages of the research process. You can read more about validity in Chapter 21.

Compromises
It is naïve to believe or expect that the meta-criteria I have presented here can be completely fulfilled in a research project. Our tools are inadequate, our data will always reflect only a limited part of the reality we want to explore, and the unique person of the researcher will always have an impact on interpretations and conclusions (Haraway 1991). Therefore, the goal is not to eliminate challenges and subjectivity, but to make it visible and to actively engage with its impact and meaning (Stige, Malterud, et al. 2009).

In all projects, we make compromises that, in one way or another, conflict with some of the criteria we request of scientific knowledge. However, for the outcome to qualify as scientific knowledge that is both new and valuable and developed through a relevant and robust strategy, we must ensure that the choices entailed by such compromises are recognised, made visible and discussed (Malterud 1993). When we are obliged to consider the consequences of our choices as researchers, we will also learn more about the foundations for knowing.

CHAPTER 4

What makes research qualitative, and why it matters

Qualitative research methods are strategies for scientifically knowing, describing, interpreting and analysing the meaning, traits and properties of the subject of inquiry. Most often, the empirical data consist of text from conversations or observations. Qualitative methods can be relevant and robust tools for systematic reflection in developing nuanced and complex knowledge about people's lives, health and illness. Grounded in the interpretive paradigm, subjectivity offers added creative value for knowing with the researcher in the proactive role of interpreter. While one and the same reality can be described and interpreted from different perspectives, not all perspectives are equally relevant to our study aim.

What kind of issues can we explore?

Biomedical or epidemiological research methods with statistical processing of numerical data collected under standardised conditions provide only limited access to the inquiry of people's experiences, values and interactions. Considering health and disease as dynamic processes in living people, we need more than generalisable knowledge (Varpio, O'Brien, et al. 2021). The same applies to studies of the health service systems in social and cultural contexts and in encounters with different user groups. We need scientific approaches that acknowledge such processes as specific to the unique individual in a sociocultural context. At the same time, however, phenomena experienced by the individual may hold the potential for abstraction, leading to transferability that provides insight into how others feel and understand (Gatens-Robinson 1986, McWhinney 1989). *Qualitative research methods* enable scientific exploration of questions of the following type:

- What do women with chronic muscle pain think about their ailments (Johansson, Hamberg, et al. 1999)?

DOI: 10.4324/9781003786016-5

- What strategies do general practitioners (GPs) use when patients with subjective health problems request sick leave (Nilsen, Malterud, et al. 2015)? When is advice on smoking cessation relevant (Guassora & Baarts 2010)?
- What experiences do lesbian women have in their encounters with the health service (Bjørkman & Malterud 2009)?
- What explanations do people with obesity have for their weight problems (Smith & Holm 2011)?
- What is the significance for the GP of having an immigrant background (Diaz & Hjorleifsson 2011)?
- How can the health service safeguard public health in the face of climate challenges (Brubaker, Bell, et al. 2011)?
- What are patients' experiences of home-based rehabilitation after shoulder surgery (Eriksson, Lindström, et al. 2011)?
- What issues do surgical nurses emphasise in their communication with patients and relatives (Jangland, Larsson, et al. 2010)?
- What does it mean for people to live with different forms of medical risk status (Reventlow, Hvas, et al. 2001, Bach Nielsen, Dyhr, et al. 2005, Frich, Ose, et al. 2006, Malterud & Ulriksen 2010b)?
- How do teenage girls experience sexual harassment from boys at school (Slåtten & Malterud 2024)?
- What do medical staff on the emergency number (113) experience with video support in contact with callers (Idland, Iversen, et al. 2022)?

These are just a few examples of different questions where qualitative research methods contribute to fresh knowing.

These methods give access to understand people's experiences, perceptions, thoughts, expectations, motives and attitudes. We can ask about the meaning, significance, conditions and nuances of events and behaviours, and we can strengthen our awareness of why people do what they do. By involving ourselves in such research contexts, we can develop living knowledge in its natural contexts. These potentials characterise the terminology used in the field, where qualitative methods are also referred to as "human science" after their field of activity (Riessman 2008), "naturalistic inquiry" after the context (Lincoln & Guba 1985), or "ethnographic approach" after ways of conducting fieldwork (Maanen 2011).

Qualitative studies are well suited to explore dynamic processes such as interaction, development, movement and complexity, for example:

- What kind of efforts do women with chronic muscle pain make to appear credible in their encounters with the doctor (Werner & Malterud 2003)?
- How do the physiotherapist and the patient negotiate the course of a long-term treatment process (Øien, Steihaug, et al. 2011)?
- When does it make a difference for lesbian women that the doctor recognises their sexual orientation (Bjørkman & Malterud 2007)?
- What experiences do patients have of discussing relationship problems with their GP (Berge, Brekke, et al. 2024)?
- How do GPs utilise linguistic modes to organise and edit consultations with multiple issues (Guassora, Johansen, et al. 2021)?

- What is everyday life like for children who grow up with parents with alcohol problems (Werner & Malterud 2016a)?
- What is the impact of early abuse on the development of symptoms and health problems in adulthood (Kirkengen 2001)?
- What happens to the balance in families where a family member has a serious, hereditary disease (Røthing, Malterud, et al. 2014)?
- What does the doctor learn when the patient brings written home notes about their ailments to the consultation (Stensland & Malterud 1999)?
- How are the activity patterns of patients with osteoporosis affected by cultural perceptions of this condition (Reventlow 2007)?

Qualitative methods can make a broad range of medical issues accessible for exploration and understanding. Notice, however, that it is not only the humanistic, social and cultural elements of the subject that are relevant topics for qualitative methods (Malterud 2001b). Tacit practical knowing in clinical procedures such as abdominal palpation, perception of heart sounds, deviations from guidelines, or terminology for breath sounds are phenomena that are only to a limited extent available as systematic descriptions and analyses in medical literature (see Chapter 19) (Maragh-Bass, Appelson, et al., Nelson 2016, Thaulow, Eide, et al. 2023). The same applies to issues as diverse as surgical techniques, experiences of rehabilitation and training, and the implementation of administrative reforms in the health service.

We should avoid the term "qualitative researcher"—it is the research methods we use and the studies we conduct (qualitative inquiry) that are qualitative. Remember that concepts like qualitative methods are also used in "hard" natural science such as geology and chemistry. There, the task of these methods also includes exploration of properties and characteristics, as opposed to measurements, quantities and distributions, but still within academic rigour and standards. Qualitative methods are useful for describing, analysing and interpreting phenomena, and are especially valuable in medicine and health sciences for studying human interaction and experience.

In medicine and healthcare, ontology and epistemology (O&E) (see Chapter 1) and thus also our methodological strategies are often different from the use of these methods for knowing within the social sciences or the humanities (Smith 2010, Guassora, Reventlow, et al. 2022). With the intention of developing medical and healthcare knowledge, often to investigate applied practice-based questions, the qualitative methods must be tailored for the purpose. Working from this context, Thorne (2025) presents *Interpretive Description* as an approach in which a coherent disciplinary logic provides the rationale for drawing on a wide range of analytic techniques and procedures beyond their customary methodological settings. This strategy intends to offer an organising logic for the development of evidence in ways where application and knowledge translation are embedded from the outset, responding directly to the particular knowledge needs of applied fields.

Understanding content and meaning

With qualitative methods, we can shed light on questions such as "What is...?", "What does... mean?", "What are the conditions for..." or "How does... take place?". The goal is insight and understanding rather than explanation and prediction. We are aspiring to make sense of what something consists of, how it is experienced, how it can be defined, what it can be called, and how it relates to something else (Kvale 1996, Malterud 2001b, Patton 2015, Miles, Huberman, et al. 2018, Pope & Mays 2020, Denzin & Lincoln 2023). These questions are particularly helpful in unfamiliar terrain, where little is known about what is there or what is happening, and where the central phenomena have not yet been extensively described or defined. If we are uncertain of how our hypotheses and study aim can be formulated as relevantly and precisely as possible, or if the terminology in the field is vague or poorly developed, qualitative studies can lay the foundation for progress and fresh insights.

Qualitative methods enable research on topics when the knowledge base initially is thin, with complex and multifaceted issues, provided that we are open to a variety of possible answers. Such methods are suitable for research that wants to place new questions on the agenda, or for matters where we do not have a prior overview of relevant answer alternatives. To develop new and valuable knowledge, we must pursue new questions rather than old answers.

The study aim determines the choice of design, sample and analysis method—What types of questions does this project seek to clarify or answer? We should not decide in advance which method to use but choose the one that is most relevant and robust for the purpose. The researcher therefore needs appropriate breadth in their methodological expertise to make the best possible choice, choosing between different qualitative methods and designs. If we want to develop a hypothesis, it may make sense to use qualitative methods. If, on the other hand, we want to test a hypothesis, we might rather go for a quantitative method.

Qualitative studies can be conducted sequentially with quantitative studies on the same topic, i.e. before or after them, see below. It is also possible to conduct qualitative studies in parallel with quantitative studies in a mixed methods design (see Chapter 22) (Mengshoel 2012). Qualitative studies most often function as self-contained contributions to scientific knowledge.

Before the numbers speak

If the purpose is to map the extent, scope, distribution or effect, or conclude about difference or correlation, qualitative strategies are not suitable. Qualitative methods should not be chosen if the questions such as "How much...?", "How often...?", "... more effective than...?", "What is the cause". Qualitative methods are not the right strategy if we want to know how often GPs meet patients who request sick leave for subjective health problems, or how common it is for such requests to be granted. In such cases, we need data that can be processed statistically.

But for quantitative methods to work, several conditions must be met. We must be sufficiently familiar with the phenomenon we are investigating to provide a meaningful, unambiguous definition and operationalisation of the variables we want to study. We cannot count medically unexplained symptoms among GPs' patients and calculate what proportion of consultations this accounts for without defining "medically unexplained physical symptoms" (Aamland, Malterud, et al. 2014). But even when the concepts are well known and that categories and variables have been clarified in advance, we must also understand the problem well enough to present a well-formulated hypothesis that can be tested using numbers and statistics.

Research that maps extent, scope, distributions, effects or differences logically starts with a qualitative phase in which concepts and categories are established, and hypotheses are formulated. In medical and health systems research, this phase is often implicit, taking place as the researcher invents a questionnaire or formulates definitions based on existing theory and empirical data. We may conduct a preliminary pilot study to check if the programme works. It also happens that the researcher creates a home-made survey questionnaire, without considering possible ambiguities in translation, data or coding, or hidden guidelines that later affect processing and statistical analysis.

Scientific rigour is weakened, especially for validity, when such parts of the research process are not identified and made visible, no matter how solid the subsequent procedure is. In such situations, it may be better to map conditions and context thoroughly in advance, for example, as was done with focus groups and ethnographic field studies in a large intervention study from India when the effect of skin contact with premature babies ("kangaroo mother care") was to be investigated (Kumar, Mohanty, et al. 2008). Mixed methods strategies (see Chapter 22) aim to integrate results from different methodological perspectives into a coherent synthesis (Creswell 2022).

In other projects, the basic understanding may already be appropriately established, for example with standardised and validated questionnaires, or with results from previous studies allowing for relevant hypotheses and alternative outcomes. Where an appropriate conceptual framework and well-founded hypotheses already exist, we will pick up where others left off. It is not necessary to reinvent the wheel every time a research project is carried out, unless traditional methods or results have demonstrated their inadequacy for what we want to understand. Therefore, a systematic review or a qualitative metasynthesis can be a useful starting point for a research project, surfacing and synthesising the available evidence in the field (see Chapter 18) (Fosse, Schaufel, et al. 2014, Gough, Oliver, et al. 2017b, Malterud 2019b).

If I want to investigate the relationship between workload and health in women and men, I can use established categories for categorising occupations, which in this context should represent the independent variable. However, I may sense reservations about relying on categories that include only paid work, as this risks obscuring a significant part of women's workload, namely unpaid work. In that case, it might be appropriate to return to the starting point, put the categories aside for the time being, and start by asking: "What is work for women, and how can it be categorised in a meaningful way?" (Forssen & Carlstedt 2001). This is an example of a qualitative study that can lay the groundwork for later quantitative mapping and enumeration of the result categories from the qualitative study. Similar questions can be asked in the opposite direction: What is work for men, and how can this be categorised in a meaningful way?

Even when well-tested instruments are available, we should not take it for granted that previous researchers in the field have asked questions from the perspective we ourselves want to investigate. In that case, we may risk that the conceptual framework in question provides answers to questions other than those raised by our study aim. It is also possible that previous research has been carried out in a significantly different context to our own, so that the validity of the study may be questionable. It may be worthwhile to do thorough qualitative preparatory work, even when planning a main study where quantitative methods are to be used (Beich et, Gannik, et al. 2002).

A qualitative study with empirical data can also be used to develop models that form the basis for further qualitative or quantitative studies, for example with an interview study on how significant weight reduction can be maintained by people with severe obesity (Natvik et, Råheim, et al. 2019). The model may indicate new directions for research, such as shifting the focus from behaviour to intentions. Asking open-ended questions without predefined response categories is one of the important strengths of qualitative research methods. Only then we can get answers to questions we did not realise we could ask. Such answers can serve as a basis for precise and well-defined questions in a later questionnaire. Perhaps the answers to the open-ended questions will also help to resolve which hypothesis is most relevant to our study aim. In this way, qualitative methods promote a systematic approach to the foundation on which quantitative studies are built.

After the numbers have spoken

Qualitative research methods can also be used to expand and elaborate on questions following a quantitative study where the field of knowledge turns up as unclear, deserving further development and exploration. Imagine that, in an epidemiological survey on smoking habits, we ask participants to tick our boxes about why they do not quit smoking. We can imagine that the researcher has set up six possible answers, and the last answer option is "other". If a lot of people tick this box, we will know that our imagination regarding the other categories was inadequate and that there is potential to find out more about what we are wondering about.

Then we plan a qualitative study to explore this residual category more systematically. The aim would then be to provide a presentation of the various reasons people have for not quitting smoking that were not covered by the alternatives we had initially presented (Graham 1987). Such a study can help to answer the question of why people do not quit smoking but should not attempt to answer how many people this applies to.

Although I have emphasised above the strength of qualitative methods for preparing or elaborating on traditional medical research methods, I would like to emphasise again that a qualitative method is most often accomplished as a self-containing research strategy. Qualitative studies are well suited to explore the unique characteristics of various phenomena and are not required to precede or follow quantitative research (see also Chapter 22).

Methods and methodology

Qualitative research methods (in the plural!) represent a diversity of approaches that together constitute a common strategy for knowledge development, rooted in the interpretive paradigm with vital sources from hermeneutics, phenomenology and social constructionism (see Chapter 2). Qualitative methods offer a wide range of practices for the systematic development, organisation and interpretation of empirical textual material from conversations, observations or written data sources.

The common denominator is the exploration of the subjective meaning of social and cultural phenomena, as experienced by those involved within their natural context, and turning this into scientific knowledge with systematic interpretation using relevant

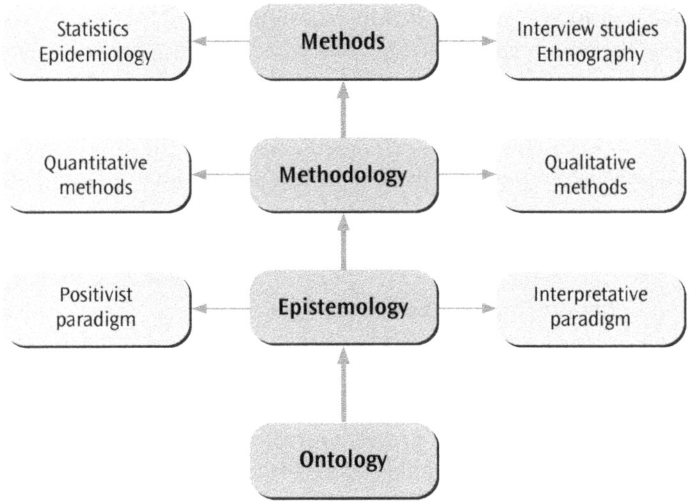

Figure 4.1 Ontological and epistemological assumptions underlying different research methodologies (after Malterud (2016))

and robust methods. Jointly, we call this *methodology*—a family of methods that have some differences between them, but also some strong commonalities. A *method* is a family member—a concrete, specific formulation of the methodological principles. If you are going to use a qualitative research method, you need to know where in the methodological family tree it belongs and why you have chosen it.

Figure 4.1 illustrates connections between ontology, epistemology, methodology and methods in different paradigms.

Qualitative research traditions—a rich diversity of methods

Inspiration from various academic disciplines has contributed to the development of different qualitative methods, each with their own distinctive characteristics. Some of these have a specific theoretical basis, such as *Grounded Theory (GT)*, developed by sociologists based on symbolic interactionism (Glaser & Strauss 1967, Blumer 1969). Participant observation became the tool of social anthropologists' *ethnographic method* based on theories of culture, society and symbols (Malinowski 1944, Garfinkel 1967, Atkinson & Hammersley 1994). Psychologists and literary scholars developed *discourse analysis* from pragmatic linguistics and semiotics (Austin 1962, Skagestad 1981, Potter & Wetherell 1987), and sociologists presented *narrative analysis* with roots in literary studies and sociolinguistics (Labov 1972, Riessman 2008, Eagleton 2011). *Phenomenology* was used by psychologists and anthropologists for analyses of the lifeworld and first-person perspectives based on individual interviews or participant observation (Giorgi 1985, van Manen 2023).

In addition to their distinct theoretical starting points, the various qualitative methods represent diverse designs with varying approaches to data development and analytical strategies. These are some examples of the rich diversity, partly discipline-specific, in the qualitative methodological traditions, demonstrating the importance of choosing a methodological approach that best matches what we want to investigate.

At the same time, we must admit that there are partial overlaps between these methodological categories. It is, however, difficult to present an overview or classification tree that simplifies similarities and differences. Some of the qualitative methodological traditions have clear common ground (even if this is expressed differently); for example, both ethnomethodology (Garfinkel 1967) and GT (Strauss & Corbin 1990) are inspired by phenomenology (Alvesson & Sköldberg 2018). Other traditions are far apart and may only have the interpretive paradigm in common, such as queer theory (Butler 1990) and phenomenology (Giorgi 1985).

Creswell discusses different classification systems for different qualitative designs, suggesting a "Big Fives" group of method categories that often appears as an overarching taxonomy (Creswell & Poth 2024). However, this selection only covers a part of the landscape available, and there is no general agreement on how to draw the map of the various methodological family members. Therefore, please stay awake, although you may be temporarily confused.

Furthermore, we may notice in the research literature that there is not always a correspondence between a declared affiliation with a particular tradition and a correspondingly clear theoretical approach (Malterud 2016). For example, if the researcher presents his or her study as a narrative analysis, we expect something more specific than the narratives from the participants that make up the empirical material. The focus of a narrative analysis may also be sharpened with a substantive theory (Guassora, Reventlow, et al. 2022) (see Chapter 20), for example on identity in a study of cancer patients in palliative care (Ricoeur 1992, Synnes 2015). Claiming to belong to a particular methodological tradition does not exempt the researcher from theoretical reflection.

We also find a significant proportion of qualitative studies from medicine and health sciences without a specific *philosophical affiliation*, even though the interpretive paradigm is a clear prerequisite. Such studies are often referred to as *pragmatic*, generic or eclectic. In this context, the term "pragmatic" refers more to everyday speech and practical considerations than to pragmatic philosophy, which emphasises usability, practice and consequences (Skagestad 1981). In pragmatic studies, empirical data from semistructured interviews or focus groups are often used for thematic analysis. The degree of theoretical immersion can vary from relatively modest (Malterud & Ulriksen 2010b) to more committed (Werner & Malterud 2016a).

Applied, practice-based qualitative studies in medicine and the health sciences are often pragmatic, which can make it somewhat problematic—though not necessarily impossible—to situate the project within a traditional philosophical category (Bradbury-Jones, Breckenridge, et al. 2017). Perhaps a more suitable contribution to intersubjectivity is to present key assumptions for the research question, data development, interpretation and analysis method in a relevant and transparent manner, and to ensure consistency between the study aim, design and procedures, as recommended by Thorne (2025).

For the purposes of this book, moderate social constructionism is chosen as the philosophical platform for qualitative methods within the interpretive paradigm (see Chapter 2) (Berger & Luckmann 1967, Lock & Strong 2010, Smith 2010). We will review different types of design, empirical data and analysis, with an emphasis on qualitative methods that are widely used in qualitative studies in medicine and health sciences today. I will prioritise discussion of methods for data development (interviews and observations) and analysis (thematic analysis) which, in my experience, have a low threshold for beginners in medicine and health sciences—an important target group for this book. At the same time, I would like to present the diversity that is also available and well established in this family of methods, so that we can develop our strategies as our experience grows.

Epistemological congruence—the Big Q

Across paradigms and methods, some basic principles apply to the development of scientific knowledge and evidence. Intersubjectivity should make the process (relevant and robust method?) available for scrutiny and challenge. The results (new and valuable knowledge?) should be shareable and understandable to others, emphasising intersubjectivity and transferability beyond the local context (Malterud 1993, 2001b). We must therefore be able to ask and respond to critical questions about reflexivity, relevance and validity in all kinds of research projects (see Chapter 3).

With qualitative research methods rooted in the interpretive paradigm, the researcher has an interpretive mission and mandate as an active participant in the development of knowledge that can never be complete and comprehensive, and which is more about new questions than about universal truths or old answers (Kvale 1996). Understanding the researcher's role and the relationship between subjectivity and objectivity is essentially different in qualitative methods compared to biomedical and epidemiological research methods rooted in the positivist paradigm.

Some important differences between qualitative and quantitative research methods are related to purpose and study aim, where qualitative methods are used to understand, not explain or predict as with quantitative methods. We should not use a hammer if the task is better solved with a screwdriver. *Epistemological congruence* presupposes correspondence not only between study aim and paradigm (O&E) (see Chapter 1), but also between paradigm and methodology (Pope & Mays 2020). A related idea is that qualitative research should demonstrate *epistemological integrity*, understood as a defensible line of reasoning that connects assumptions about knowledge to the methodological principles used to justify decisions throughout the research process (Thorne 2025).

Within the interpretive paradigm, textual data are handled very differently from numerical data. Appropriate strategies for establishing a relevant sample of empirical data are also closely linked to these assumptions. Therefore, for example, a purposive sample is a better choice for a qualitative study than a representative sample (see Chapter 7). Similarly, transferability at the conceptual level requires a fundamentally different understanding than transferability at the population level.

No research method can deliver proof of truth—at best, we can make something probable. The researcher using qualitative methods knows that there are many scientifically sound alternatives for substantiation and consideration of transferability. To conduct a qualitative study, the researcher therefore needs basic insight into relevant philosophical issues such as paradigms, as well as specific methodological expertise suitable for the actual study aim.

The concepts of *the small q* and *the Big Q* were first introduced by Kidder and Fine (1987). Based on reflections on triangulation, they showed how ideals from the positivist paradigm are alive and thriving, even deep into studies presented as qualitative. Such ideals can manifest themselves as ambitions for realism, precision, measurement, hypothesis testing, consensus or facts. In such studies, where the research process is fixed and stable from the outset, the results are more about descriptive confirmation of previous knowledge than about interpretation leading towards new questions. This propensity was labelled *the small q* as an expression of the fact that the basic conditions for qualitative research methods were met only to a limited extent.

Its opposite, *the Big Q*, on the other hand, reflects the interpretive paradigm in a committed way, where inductive, organic and flexible strategies give access to investigation of diversity and movement (Kidder & Fine 1987). Braun and Clarke (2019) show how the researcher's mission of interpretation and subjectivity is augmented with the Big Q, for example in describing the analysis process where themes or result categories are developed, not discovered. They also refer to the small q as a *post-positivist* position, here implying that the positivist paradigm has a strong (and erroneous) impact (Braun & Clarke 2024a).

This is a matter of pervasive differences between qualitative and quantitative methods. The small q is a variant that, despite weak epistemological congruence, has had (and continues to have) a considerable visibility in qualitative studies from medicine and health sciences. This reflects the two cultures (Snow 1959), where the positivist paradigm seems to function as an autopilot with preferential rights and legitimacy.

There are many opinions about where the boundaries lie for what can be called qualitative research methods. The methodological position represented by the Big Q is the starting point for this book. The consequence of this is that we no longer talk about qualitative methods when analyses based on subjectivity and interpretation are absent or justified with positivist concepts and arguments. Thus, for example, I will not use the term qualitative methods to describe strategies for quantifying qualitative data. We can also discuss whether purely descriptive studies that neither mediate subjectivity and interpretation nor present new and valuable knowledge can be called qualitative studies, even with text data as the empirical material. You may find this harsh, but epistemological congruence is a mandatory assumption underpinning robust and relevant research methods.

CHAPTER 5

You are the interpreter—your most powerful research instrument

The idea of the researcher in an objective and neutral role, with no influence on the development of knowledge, is poorly suited to methodologies rooted in the interpretive paradigm. Instead, qualitative research methods make the researcher responsible for the proper conduct of subjectivity—both their own and that of the matters being interpreted. The researcher's point of view, professional interests, motives and personal experiences establish the study aim, perspectives, design, sample and methods. This determines which of the interpreted patterns most appropriately address the questions posed, and how the conclusions are emphasised and communicated. The question is therefore not whether the researcher influences the process, but how, and then so what. A relevant and robust research method leading towards scientific knowledge and evidence requires that we recognise and understand the importance of our own role.

About using yourself as a research instrument

In all kinds of research, regardless of methodology, interpretation is the basis for analysis and conclusions. The actors in the research processes are people, not just dead objects or numbers. Thus, the interpersonal game in its social and cultural context is also an organic part of knowing and knowledge development (Latour & Woolgar 1986, Kvale 1996).

With qualitative research methods, reflexivity is a crucial means for subjectivity to be transformed to scientific knowledge (see Chapter 3). The same value could also help to make quantitative research methods more relevant and robust. However, in the medical research tradition, this question has not been problematised to any great extent, even though clinical knowledge and decision-making primarily rest on subjectivity and interpretation (Gatens-Robinson 1986, Malterud 1995b, 2001a). The social anthropologists Latour and Wollgar demonstrated in their study of the renowned Salk laboratory (Latour & Woolgar 1986) that the human factor is intimately woven into

DOI: 10.4324/9781003786016-6

the research process, even in a classical experimental laboratory context that traditionally symbolises the positivist paradigm.

The term "the interpretive paradigm" can therefore function as a false contradiction, since this paradigm does not have an exclusive right to interpretation or to exempt the positivist paradigm from interpretation as a scientific mission. However, since the interpretive paradigm is a well-established concept within the philosophy of science, I will continue to use this term as discussed in Chapter 2, that is, with subjectivity and interpretation understood as substantial sources of valid knowledge about human life, health, and disease.

With this framework, the researcher's mission, role and tools for developing valid scientific knowledge are notably different when using qualitative and quantitative research methods. The assumptions and approaches for interpreting empirical data in the form of text or images are different than when objectivity and numbers provide the framework for quantitative studies. Subjectivity provides an indispensable platform for the researcher to use human resources such as emotion, empathy, language, creativity, identity, abstraction and symbolisation for the development of scientific knowledge in a creative, though systematic way, anchored by reflexivity (Smith 2010).

In qualitative studies, we expect the empirical data to embody the experiences and meaning of the participants. We are not interested in reading summaries from conversations guided by leading questions or answers suggesting that the participant primarily wants to convince the interviewer that they are a decent human being. Interview questions that begin with "You also believe that..." or "Don't you agree that..." indicate that the researcher's voice may have drowned out the participant's voice. We need to consider who the statements really refer to. That is why researchers somehow need to keep themselves in the background, although we should never imagine or try to become invisible in our material. A rule of thumb is that you can reflect upon what you yourself need to put aside to be able to faithfully forward the participants' story and take responsibility for interpretation, abstraction and synthesis. To be a competent interpreter using relevant and robust methods, you need to know yourself well enough to handle your own participation with honest and humble reflexivity.

If I have a strong commitment to the field I want to explore, it may be necessary to seek advice from others so that I can develop and correct my interview technique and thus prevent my data from serving as a disguise for asserting or confirming my own opinions (see Chapter 14). If the researcher's personality is too clearly present in the material, the validity and trustworthiness of the conclusions are weak. Working in a research group together with others can serve as a helpful inoculation against blind self-absorption, which can otherwise unconsciously colour what I interpret from my data. Reviewing the data with others early in the research process can serve as a strategy for establishing metapositions and identifying one's own blind spots, making it possible to take them into account along the way (see Chapter 16). The goal is neither objectivity, facts nor consensus, but the qualified accomplishment of the researcher's role as an interpreter guided by reflexivity (Braun & Clarke 2024b).

It is therefore naïve to deny one's own role and to imagine that, in the name of objectivity, the researcher will become an invisible and inactive pawn in the game where the data are developed. That is a small q attitude (see Chapter 4). The researcher must always ask themselves, their colleagues and their advisors about how (not whether) the process, interpretations and conclusions are affected by the researcher's specific points of view. If I, as a female general practitioner (GP), am conducting a study on female patients' experience of the consultation, my gender will certainly have an impact on the questions I ask and the responses I receive (Malterud 1990, Larsen, Oldeide, et al. 1997). If I am interviewing male patients about impotence, it is probable that, due to my gender, I miss out on important knowledge that the participant would have shared with a male interviewer. In this way, the knowing and the knowledge that we develop in the project are situated (Haraway 1991).

Situated knowledge

When a researcher encounters the participants and reviews their contributions, the patterns they see will depend on what kind of patterns they have learned to recognise. The historian of science Donna Haraway (1944-) writes about *situated knowledge* (Haraway 1991). She claims that knowledge is always developed from a specific context that is determined by the researcher's gaze and perspectives.

This is an important assumption underlying all qualitative research methods. Drawing on mammalian biology, Haraway argues that all eyes are actively sensing systems, where sensory impressions are translated and filtered through interpretation, reflection and refinement. Therefore, meaning is shaped from the given perspectives. These biology metaphors can be transferred directly to the research process, where there are many simultaneous and sometimes contradictory versions of the same "reality", as we also know from social constructionism (Berger & Luckmann 1967) (see Chapter 2).

Haraway dismisses the notion that the researcher's neutral gaze forms the basis for universal and generalisable knowledge—she calls this *the "God trick"*, which means that the researcher does not recognise his or her status as a human being. She argues that the researcher is situated and therefore speaks from a discernible place of origin that should be open to intersubjective scrutiny. Situatedness thereby constitutes a more appropriate criterion for scientific rigour than the traditional understanding of objectivity, as a key aspect of reflexivity and intersubjectivity (see Chapter 3). Only when we acknowledge and consider the positions that situate our knowledge, others can understand the assumptions underpinning our interpretations and conclusions.

It is therefore legitimate for different researchers to adhere to different main features of the material and thus report on different aspects of a phenomenon. In a qualitative study, such a diversity will enrich the interpretations and contribute to negotiations and nuances. As readers, we expect to be acquainted with the researchers' point of view—about how the knowing is situated—to be able to understand why the prioritised and presented interpretation appears to be the most relevant, given the study aim and the empirical material in question.

In the qualitative research process, the researcher must concentrate especially on the significance of their own *preconceptions* and the *theoretical perspectives* chosen, see Figure 5.1 (Haraway 1991, Malterud 1993, Kvale 1996). In the interaction between these elements, the progress of knowing can grow. These concepts, which I elaborate on below, are useful resources for the researcher's conduct of their role as interpreter.

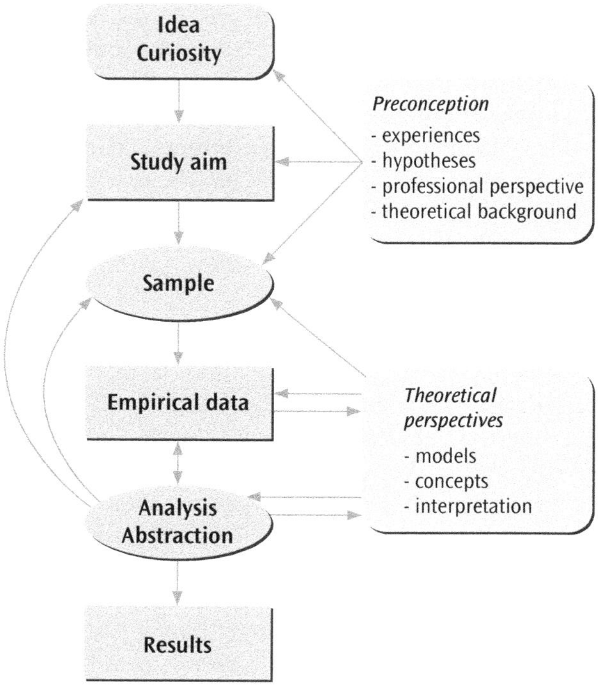

Figure 5.1 The researcher's role shaped by preconceptions and theoretical perspectives (after Malterud (1993))

Preconceptions

Gadamer was an important contributor to hermeneutic philosophy—the theory of the interpretation of texts as a basis for understanding (see Chapter 2). Among other things, he emphasised the impact of historical and individual assumptions and experiences that people bring with them as conscious or unconscious parts of their basis for interpretation (Gadamer 2004). Such prior awareness may be referred to as *preconceptions*.

Our preconceptions are the backpack that we bring with us into the project, before the research has started. The contents of this backpack inform knowing—the way we articulate our study aim and then develop, read and interpret our data. This luggage can, at best, nourish and strengthen the project and act as a packed lunch, but which, at worst, can become a heavy burden that causes us to interrupt the journey because it is all about what we are carrying and not about what we see along the way. Our luggage contains experiences, hypotheses, professional perspectives and the theoretical perspectives (see below) as they are implicit or stand out at the start of the project.

For medical and health researchers, preconceptions are often an important and adequate aspect of the motivation for embarking on a qualitative study. The general practitioner (GP) who wants to learn more about patients with medically unexplained symptoms may have encountered so many such patients without being able to provide beneficial help (Malterud 1990). The public municipal medical officer who wants to improve the services for people with major mental health problems may have the experience that multidisciplinary cooperation is necessary to make interventions work (Thesen

& Kuzel 1999). The nurse who would like to learn more about patients' experience of being on a ventilator brings a caring perspective for seeking this knowledge (Gjengedal 1994). The gender researcher who is going to study women's experience of undergoing a gynaecological examination aspires to have an impact on the gender power relations of this procedure (Larsen, Oldeide, et al. 1997). The GP who is critical of notions of the menopause as a negative phase of life would possibly ask for women's positive experiences of this part of life (Hvas 2001). The sociologist who explores the experiences of children growing up with parents with alcohol problems may be keen to shift the focus from mental health pathology to social interaction (Werner & Malterud 2016a).

All these aspects of preconceptions are legitimate motivations that may be helpful to the research process. However, preconceptions can also lead us to enter the project with blinders and limited horizons. The most common pitfall is that our preconceptions drown out the message from the participants and our empirical data. This is often the case in projects where it is difficult to distinguish the project's presentation of results from the project outline. In qualitative studies of limited quality, descriptions of what is at issue tend to remain largely unchanged before and after data collection and analysis. At worst, this may mean that the researcher neglected the knowledge resources from the empirical data—in which case these are flaws approaching the threshold of scientific misconduct. The reader has the right to expect the results to be derived from the empirical material.

On the other hand, such a situation may occur when the researcher has had extensive prior field knowledge and experienced that the process did not add anything new and valuable along the way. In that case, it is worth considering whether the project was a waste of resources and ethically problematic to carry out, or whether the empirical data were used exclusively to strengthen and confirm the researcher's own hypotheses (see Chapter 25). Perhaps the originality of the project is ultimately not up to scratch. If the researcher has established a reflective relationship with their preconceptions, such difficulties can be prevented. Here is some specific advice on how this can be conducted.

Before you start developing and organising your data, it is a proper investment to set aside time to identify the factors that guide your knowing, write them down in the decision trail (see Chapter 6) and check them out regularly throughout the research process. Of course, my gaze is automatically guided towards what I already know or believe. What is my experience of the topic I'm about to investigate? How does this make my position as a researcher different from researchers with a different experience base? What are my expectations of what I might find? Why is this exactly what I expect to find? How can I best mobilise my curiosity? What is my professional standpoint when I seek knowing about this topic? What would have been different for a researcher with a different professional background than me? What are my theoretical perspectives before the project, starts—which models, which conceptual framework and which research traditions are guiding my way of thinking about this? And what would have been different if I had read different literature or relied on a different methodological framework at the start of the project? How can I contribute to this project delivering scientific evidence that is new and valuable, developed by means of relevant and robust methods? In the project outline, your preconceptions and such considerations should be visible, though without dominating.

To benefit from your *creative subjectivity*, you need to sharpen your ears and eyes to sense the knowledge from your data. For this purpose, you can make a note to yourself, ending with a list of the results you, at this early stage, expect to make later, preferably as concrete as possible. This note contains an expression of your knowledge at the starting line, which along the way should be challenged, confronted and supplemented with the living knowledge from the empirical field. Think of this as a *positional statement*, where you anticipate the results to avoid by just following your own tracks. You write down what you expect to find, well before you have had a chance to find anything in the research project.

Feel free to use the same format as the abstract of the article you will eventually write, and write your preliminary version of the results section of the abstract based on your preconceptions. Your text can function as a reflexive positional statement, capturing a concentrated version of what you think you knew beforehand. You can paste this into the decision trail (see Chapter 6) and use the text to challenge and further elaborate your perspective and interpretations later in the analysis and writing process. The positional statement is a working note and not supposed to be included in the article you are writing.

When the results are later synthesised and you are writing your article, you can retrieve the bonus and place your positional statement next to what you think you developed in the analysis. If these are completely or almost identical, it is necessary to re-examine the data and analysis strategies. If, on the other hand, it is very different, it is also useful to look for possible explanations. A rule of thumb is that the more surprises the empirical material brings you, the better you have succeeded in generating new and valuable knowledge from the data.

Theoretical perspectives

A *theory* is a consistent and well-founded set of assumptions that can be used to predict or explain a phenomenon or relationships between phenomena, while a *model* is a simplified representation or image of the theory (Malterud 2016). Let us imagine that the *theoretical perspectives* are the glasses we wear when we encounter the participants, develop and interpret our data and elaborate the patterns of knowing. In this way, theory is an integral part of our research methodology that helps us understand results and conclusions in a larger context (Malterud 2016, Guassora, Reventlow, et al. 2022). To some extent, we take these glasses from our backpack—we build our project on preliminary reading from a particular theoretical position, for example when gender perspectives form the starting point for understanding depression experiences (Danielsson & Johansson 2005). But we are not always aware of how and where we are theoretically situated.

In qualitative studies from medicine and health sciences, we rarely use theories as elements of a deductive logic and analysis strategy with predetermined result categories (see Chapters 6 and 11). Instead, theoretical perspectives and result categories should be inductively established along the way, in close interaction with data development, analysis, reading and conversations with others (Morse 2002). Applied health disciplines do theorise—frequently with great insight—but their theoretical work is usually directed toward improving application rather than abstraction for its own sake (Thorne 2025). Theoretical perspectives may change as fresh data reveal better ways to align theory with study aim and empirical data.

This is a common and legitimate indication of ripened understanding and realisation during the process. It is necessary to identify and explain the theoretical perspectives and their significance for both the researcher and the reader to understand why the presented versions and interpretations appear to be the most relevant.

The theoretical perspectives include the theories, models, concepts, definitions, and research traditions I use to understand meaning, structure my interpretations, and situate the project in context. Theory is most important for the analysis part of the research process, but it contributes—often implicitly—to the whole process. When it comes to the sampling, development and processing of data, and not least the summary and discussion of the results, the researcher's theoretical perspectives will also determine which version of patterns is prioritised and how this is communicated (Guassora, Reventlow, et al. 2022). It is therefore necessary to account for this, without the theory floating around as an unconscious phenomenon.

Intersubjectivity means, among other things, that the researcher gives the reader insight into the theoretical perspectives that have had an impact on the research question and analysis and contributed to situating the knowledge (Malterud 1993). For example, the interpretation of interview data about lesbian women's understanding of their identity will be completely different if I use theoretical perspectives from psychoanalysis (Lingiardi & Capozzi 2004) or from queer theory (Ohnstad 2011). In the first case, I will probably concentrate on unconscious processes, established through childhood and adolescence, that govern self-understanding and sexuality, while in the second case, I will emphasise how social categories are defined and understood in our culture.

The importance and utility of theory in qualitative studies can vary widely from discipline to discipline. In medicine and health sciences, theoretical perspectives function more to situate the project and support interpretation than as an independent goal (Thorne 2011, 2025, Guassora, Reventlow, et al. 2022). *Grand theories*, developed by theorists such as Freud, Bateson or Heidegger, tend to miss the mark when it comes to situate and focus a qualitative study. While educational models such as the patient-centred clinical method or the biopsychosocial model may offer a starting point, they are too broad to inform the researcher's specific interpretive choices.

In a qualitative study, it may therefore be more relevant to talk about theoretical perspectives as tools for situating and understanding than about theory as a fixed platform and means of control. Practice-orientated substantive theories addressing specific conditions, experiences or activities can contribute apt and relevant concepts. These kinds of theories are helpful vantage points to situate your study and set your gaze in a direction that gives access to new and valuable knowledge (Guassora, Reventlow, et al. 2022). Theoretical perspectives from substantive theories can, for example, deal with recognition (Schibbye 1993), speech acts (Austin 1962) or metaphors (Lakoff & Johnson 1980). You can read more about substantive theories (Guassora, Reventlow, et al. 2022) and theoretical perspectives in Chapter 20.

Beyond a descriptive study

A qualitative study necessarily consists of descriptions as well as interpretations. It is not possible to develop one without developing the other—every description is coloured by interpretations, and every interpretation is based on descriptions. But even if we recognise that description and interpretation go hand in hand, the researcher may choose to emphasise one of these dimensions more than the other when developing and analysing qualitative data.

At one extreme of the scale, we find the researcher adopting a distinctly *interpretive standpoint*. Data are used to explore underlying meaning, perhaps at a level that for the participant represents an unconscious understanding, or with an excessive respect for theory. For example, a psychoanalytic frame of reference could be relevant in this position. Is the patient's discomfort during the gynaecological examination due to unconscious traumatic childhood experiences? Here, the researcher is confronted with many challenges, both of an ethical nature and in terms of analysis and communication. Do we have the right to claim on behalf of someone else that their expression means something other than what they said? Is the researcher's interpretive standpoint more valid than the participant's own? How do we account for such an interpretive process in a trustworthy and transparent way that demonstrates for the reader the path from data to conclusions?

Some of these problems can be avoided if we choose the opposite position and try to adopt a markedly *descriptive standpoint*, conceptualising our project as a descriptive or exploratory study. Our intention is then to represent the participant's voices as faithfully and accurately as possible, with the least possible disturbance caused by preconceptions and theory. With this approach, we accept data and statements without asking whether they are true or correct but consider this to be the knowledge that the participant in the given situation shares with the researcher. However, if the researcher compiles the knowledge in a way that is completely loyal to the individual participant's expressions and experiences, without making an independent interpretation, we end up as a microphone stand for the participants. In this way, the researcher abdicates their role as interpreter and neglects the task of knowing and abstraction towards new and valuable knowledge. Treating the data as "objective truth", such a project is demonstrating positivist ideals from the small q position (see Chapter 4).

However, we do not usually find the researcher in one of these extreme positions, but in more intermediate positions. Descriptions that are not constrained by preconceptions enable interpretation that can generate new knowledge—by contrast, description without interpretation signals that the analysis remains incomplete. This book is based on an understanding that the development of new and valuable knowledge requires active and creative interpretation of data—in other words, something distinct from and beyond a descriptive study that provides nothing more than a well-organised reiteration of the participants' stories (see Chapter 12) (Braun & Clarke 2024b). For knowledge development in applied practice-based disciplines, we also assign empirical data a strong impact for interpretation, analysis and synthesis, not to be overruled by theory. Still, relevant theoretical perspectives will build a creative bridge between description and interpretation, so that both aspects are connected and raised to a new level (Malterud 2016, Guassora, Reventlow, et al. 2022).

PART 2

Traversing the research process

CHAPTER 6

Planning, flexibility and field notes along the path

A research project deserves good planning. A thorough literature search is a necessary foundation for formulating a precise study aim. Only then can you develop a project outline presenting an interesting study aim with relevant design and theoretical perspectives informing your positions and interpretations. At the same time, flexibility and reflection are key words in a qualitative study, because you need to learn from experience during the process and adjust your course accordingly. With quantitative methods, the premises are the opposite, with a stable structure and standardised experimental conditions. To manage and benefit from the dynamic elements of a qualitative study in an accountable and trustworthy manner, the researcher must make them available to themselves and others. We are constantly creating process data that requires attention and reflection. It is helpful to establish a decision trail to leave traces wherever we go that we can return to.

From research ideas to project outline

A project idea must be digested and structured before it becomes a researchable and conceptualised study aim in a feasible scientific study. There is no point in setting up a video camera in the doctor's surgery and seeing what comes out of it, other than possibly as a basis for brainstorming that can contribute to a more distinct focus and questions. It is often said that you should go into a qualitative study with an open mind. This is correct, but it does not mean that the researcher should be blank on the starting line without appropriate preparations.

What do I really want to find out about? What has already been thoroughly studied? What are my personal and unique prerequisites for creating insights that can be transformed to relevant and robust evidence that can be shared with others? Who can help me structure my ideas so that my questions are converted to a researchable format? How can I establish sound framework conditions for a large or small research project? What are my motives for embarking upon this in the form of research?

DOI: 10.4324/9781003786016-8

These are all questions that require time, consideration, resources and relationships. The first thing you should do is establish a connection with a research institution in your own field—initially preferably in a non-binding way, so that you do not commit to carrying out something that turns out to be bigger or different than you thought. You should not decide in advance that you want to do a qualitative study, that a focus group design is your priority, or that you want to do a PhD. An experienced researcher, preferably with expertise in both qualitative and quantitative methods, can discuss your ideas with you so you can progress soundly.

Regardless of paradigms and research methods, you need to start by ascertaining what knowledge already exists about what you want to know more about. Perhaps a researcher in New Zealand has already done extensive and excellent studies about these matters? If your idea has been comprehensively explored by others, there is no need to conduct a new qualitative study on exactly the same question. It is always useful to build on the work of those who came before you. If you are embarking on a research project, it is also important to be or become familiar with the context—where in this substance area will my study fit, and how can it contribute to expanding or challenging existing knowledge? An experienced researcher who can act as your supervisor can help you initiate a relevant literature search so that you can get an adequate overview of existing research knowledge.

Only then can you begin to formulate an overall *study aim*—about what do you want to develop more knowledge? Then, with the support of your supervisor, you can draft a more specific study aim to delineate more focused what you choose to explore to feed your study aim. My recommendation is to put a lot of effort into this phase, because a well-developed and precise study aim is crucial for the project to be feasible and develop new and valuable knowledge (Alvesson & Sandberg 2024). In this step, you should also articulate an adequate and precise project title. Still, throughout the project you must challenge, develop and adjust the study aim as intimate contact with empirical data and theoretical perspectives strengthens your understanding of what you actually want to know more about. A challenging combination of flexibility and clear direction is therefore necessary.

Your *project outline* will serve several purposes. Initially, this is a text that may help you to compile your thoughts in a committed and organised way. You will probably need funding for the project so that you can set aside enough time to do this properly. Your supervisor will know the possibilities and procedures for applying for project funding, with the project outline as a crucial document for this purpose. There are often strict formal requirements for such applications—this is therefore not something you should wrestle with on your own. A thoughtful description of the study aim, design and method is required for someone to grant funding for this—not least when it comes to a qualitative study. In other words, it is not enough to write that you might want to carry out a focus group study when you see how the rest of the project develops.

Along the way, you should make many adjustments to your plans and focus, preferably by elaborating and updating the study aim and project title. You can write a new version of the project outline and save it with a new date, but this is primarily a process document for your own use. You should not feel constrained by your very first project outline or by the application that gave you the research funding. It is important to make the problem's focus clearer over time. This is very different from a project with a quantitative design. However, if the transformations along the way deviate significantly from what your funding source has approved, you must, in consultation with your supervisor, secure approval of the amended plans.

Decision trail—why and how?

In the past, the *decision trail* was mainly used mostly to prove methodological accuracy, i.e. that the process can be documented in detail, point by point (Koch 1994). Today, we would consider this to be positivist legitimisation and indications of the small q (see Chapter 4). Intersubjectivity is a strategy that better matches the flexibility of qualitative methods. However, the decision trail is still a useful tool for handling process data, in that you draw a map of where and when you go.

Your decision trail is continuously updated with selected *field notes* from the journey that together will make it easier for you to recapitulate decisions and choices from the research process. Such moments can be important when interpreting your data, by explaining your strategies and enabling you to take three steps forward and two steps back and make different choices than those you initially made. With the decision trail, you can leave tracks behind you in the forest, making it easier for you to navigate your way back to where you were and understand why you got lost. With the support of the decision trail, you can prevent yourself from just following a set track where you do not have the chance to discover what you did not know you could look for.

It is a waste of time and energy to put a lot of effort into structuring the editing of the decision trail. This is not a diary that someone imposes on you and demands you to present, but a bank account for depositing small and large resources that can grow and earn interest. Although the research process seems to follow intuitive tracks and leaps, there is usually a logic behind it. We do not always realise this in the moment, but it can become clearer with a little distance from the decision point or the fuzzy feeling. That is why you do not know in advance which notes will be useful later.

Create a continuous document in your word processing programme where you start at the top and write downwards. Trail notes are dated and recorded in chronological order. It does not matter what style you choose when writing—the addressee is yourself, your supervisor and selected collaborators. Only a minimum of what is stored in the decision trail will later be reported in the article or thesis. This text is a working memo and primarily serves as reflective capital. Feel free to use the same file name for the document all the time, so you do not have to keep track of which version of the text you are updating.

The decision trail is where you store text, dialogue and reflections. Relevant email correspondence between you and your partners can be cut, dated and pasted into the notes. But with extensive dialogue, it is too much to include anything other than what you think is most important. If you have comments or questions that you choose to keep to yourself, feel free to include these in too. Eventually, the decision trail will become a long and confusing document. That is not a bad thing, because the most recent and relevant entries are always at the end of the document. However, you should bear in mind that this is not your complete document repository, but an account specifically designed to safeguard process tracks of possible future importance.

Therefore, you do not need to enter voluminous texts from the project outline in many versions with small corrections—instead, briefly and immediately enter your reactions to what once again requires a new review in the planning phase of the project. Do not use the decision trail to summarise all articles you have read. However, if you find something that seems to have a significant impact on how you think about the problem or approach, you can make a small note of this. Do not use the log to store raw data—such texts must be handled with special procedures regarding privacy and research ethics (see Chapter 24).

We must always make compromises in a research project. Do not let the perfect be the enemy of the good. On the other hand, we should try to develop an awareness of the limitations and opportunities for compromise, for example when it proves more difficult than we thought to recruit participants for a purposive sample with a particular composition. When everyday life confronts us with something that leads to deviations from the original plan, the decision trail comes in handy. Here we can enter what we do and why, especially when we have not followed our own plans and procedures.

Learning from experience

When we prepare for the development of empirical data, for example by creating an interview guide for individual interviews or focus groups, we do not know in advance how our questions will work. Often, the researcher thinks about his or her problem in a more theoretical language than is suitable for dialogue with the participants who are going to share their experiences. Therefore, the interviews should always be adjusted in line with methods of questioning and follow-up that turn out to lead to data with the best possible Information Power (see next chapter) (Schaufel, Nordrehaug, et al. 2011, Malterud, Siersma, et al. 2021).

This does not mean that we should enter the field unprepared, but that we must remain prepared to refine our focus on where new and valuable knowledge can best be developed. For this reason, we should for example not classify the first interviews as a *pilot study* that is excluded from the analysis—it is often precisely at the beginning that the researcher's enthusiasm takes the sting out of awkward interview questions and points the way to dialogues that provide insight and surprises. Recording afterthoughts in the decision trail when encountering the field will provide useful material for reflexivity.

The same applies to projects where we have underestimated practical or ethical challenges, which is not so rare. It is better to change the strategy before we have developed large amounts of data with limited Information Power regarding our study aim, or before we have contributed to discomfort or negative reactions of those who will share their experiences. If you make a brief note in the decision trail of what happened and the practical consequences of this, it will be easier to put aside the idea of following the original plan. What the researcher understands along the way is empirical process data that are also included in the development of knowledge, although not reported in detail later.

Three steps forward and two steps back

Analysing qualitative data is not a linear process where the researcher goes from A to B and then reaches the finish line. In Chapters 10 and 11, you will read about analysis as a dynamic process, where we steadily move forward, repeatedly focusing on our empirical data and assessing which of the alternative patterns of interpretation best illuminates the problem. We will organise the material in different contexts in a systematic way until the result categories can be conceptualised and communicated as clearly as possible, with interpretations and messages voicing something fresh about what we are wondering about. Therefore, in this process, the researcher must never choose the first and best alternative but consider different possible interpretations against each other.

It is not always easy to take a few steps back when you realise that the path is not leading clearly enough. The decision trail can be priceless for self-awareness and intersubjectivity, especially in the analysis process. The trail notes help you get back on track when you realise that you have made choices that are not working so well. Therefore, make a note of substantial interpretive steps, such as how you and your colleagues negotiate the coding strategy and how you agree upon differences between the various codes. In a qualitative study, the writing is an extension of the analysis. Making notes on your reasons for organising interpretations makes it easier to later adjust categories that are not working.

CHAPTER 7

Sampling guided by Information Power—advancing transferability

Empirical data from our sample offer several possible answers to the questions that the study aim presents. The content and size of the sample determine what we can make claims about—what is this, what is it valid for and in what context? There are fundamental differences in sampling strategy with qualitative research methods compared to quantitative methods due to the different philosophical assumptions. You need to understand why this is so and how to choose the most appropriate approach. In qualitative studies, we often use purposive sampling. Reflexivity related to the scope of the sample is necessary for assessing internal and external validity. Information Power is a more compelling concept than saturation for planning, organising and assessing a qualitative sample.

Transferability rather than generalisability

Sampling strategy is key to determining the transferability of a study, regardless of whether the research is quantitative or qualitative. But in this regard, the conditions are divergent for numbers and text. In intervention studies and epidemiological research, *generalisability* is a scientific ideal. In such designs, the selection criteria are determined by statistical conventions to calculate statistical significance and complex relationships between standardised variables.

Furthermore, epidemiological studies require representative samples to support transferability to the target population, whereas intervention studies require arbitrary or randomised samples compared with a control group to estimate effects. In the end, evidence derived from group-level data is here translated to the individual level, for example for screening programmes or blood pressure medication. What is more, generalisability is a concept that invites unrealistic and positivistic assumptions about universal applicability. Only in exceptional cases can research deliver generalisable results—conclusions that apply to all people in all kinds of societies under any historical condition (Haraway 1991).

DOI: 10.4324/9781003786016-9

Sample selection based on this logic will jeopardise internal as well as external validity in qualitative studies. Here, *transferability* is a more appropriate concept, referring to opportunities and limitations of the capacity of interpretations to make sense for contexts beyond the one where the study was carried out (Malterud 2001b). Intersubjectivity and relevance indicate that knowledge is both communicable and applicable. This applies not only to the research process and methodology, but also to interpretations, conclusions and results. Thus, transferability becomes a central ambition in a qualitative study, but with different goals and means than in a quantitative study (Sandelowski 1996).

Research presenting completely local or private results is rarely of scientific interest to others. An interpretation from a very specific context may nevertheless represent a breakthrough in understanding, suited for a case study (Haas 2001) (see Chapter 15), and descriptions, concepts or models developed under specific conditions may be used for purposes of a more general nature. The same applies to an anomalous interpretation that can put the ordinary into relief in a particularly clear way. If I study a phenomenon that affects doctor-seeking behaviour in a small rural community (such as ferry timetables or roads at risk of collapse), the results may be of considerable local interest without having strong external validity. If I develop a clinical method in my own practice that no one else can use, the transferability is very limited.

However, if I put forward research evidence that specifies what the clinical method consists of, how it can be used and what can come of it, transferability may be strong (Malterud 1990, Stensland & Malterud 1997). Transferability depends on whether the results make sense beyond themselves, abstracted in the form of interpretation and concepts, or in a larger theoretical context.

In this way, progressing towards transferability from the *unique* via abstraction to the *general*, we are not seeking generalisability (Sandelowski 1996, Varpio, O'Brien, et al. 2021). For example, Rudebeck shows how "body empathy"—the ability to empathise with another person's bodily experiences—constitutes a fundamental aspect of the general practitioner's (GP's) clinical knowledge. With his meticulous elaboration of this concept, we do not need significance values to agree that this is also valid for other GPs (Rudebeck 1992). Pragmatic case-finding, a strategy developed from qualitative studies of how GPs talk to patients about possible alcohol problems, can also provide ideas about alternatives to screening for other lifestyle conditions in general practice (Lid & Malterud 2012). *The 'aha' effect*—the fact that someone else understands something more about the problems they face based on what I have handed over—is an important indication of transferability in qualitative studies from applied practice-based disciplines.

In other words, we are talking about epistemological assumptions that are neither suitable nor available for statistical calculations, and therefore, other concepts and strategies are required. In the planning and implementation of the research project, the researcher's skilled interpretations and knowledge of the field will strengthen the transferability of the results. Our selection of empirical data as a point of departure is key here. Principles and procedures for establishing samples should ensure relevant and robust data about what we want to explore, with appropriate validity also outside the study context. In the article, we will present and discuss conditions, opportunities and limitations for the scope of knowledge— how and where our results have validity.

A section in the article reflecting on the scope and conditions for appropriate transferability is an important sign of quality, indicating that the researcher is aware of the strengths and limitations of their interpretations. Ultimately, however, the responses from colleagues in research and practice will recognise and determine the external validity of the knowledge we developed.

For a researcher with a biomedical background, the sampling strategy in qualitative studies may seem alien, contributing to undue scepticism towards qualitative research methods (Loder, Groves, et al. 2016). The novice will soon realise the benefit of understanding and communicating the (methodo)logical arguments underpinning transferability and sampling in a qualitative study. This is better than trying to adapt to ideas of transferability that violate basic principles of subjectivity as the starting point and core of knowledge development, as with *the small q* (see Chapter 4) (Varpio, O'Brien, et al. 2021). We will therefore first look at some concepts that are almost regarded as natural laws for sampling strategies in traditional medical research, which are still not very suitable as qualitative selection criteria.

Why representativity is a misplaced concept in a qualitative study

Epidemiological research provides knowledge about health and disease in different population groups. For logistic and resource-related reasons, such studies are conducted on a limited part of the whole group we want to say something about. In epidemiological designs, the logic for transferability rests on specific sampling procedures with the *representative sample* as a key tool.

In biomedical or public health intervention studies, *Randomisation* is a common means of drawing a probabilistic sample, and *a control group* is established to provide a standardised basis for comparison with the study group receiving the intervention. We can then use statistical methods to calculate associations, differences and margins of error.

When the sample or study group in these ways convincingly represents the target group, and the margins of error fare acceptable, the results can be *extrapolated* to the target group (see Figure 7.1). These procedures are based on a logic where randomness ensures representativeness, and conventions on how given p-values or confidence intervals provide relevant measures of margins of error for comparison.

It is, however, essential not to confuse means and ends in this matter. In the biomedical knowledge tradition, representativeness, randomisation, control group and significance are appropriate scientific concepts signifying ideals that determine the transferability of a particular form of scientific knowledge. In quantitative studies, this provides a logical and legitimate operationalisation of deductive procedures as the basis for transferability and validity. Belonging to medicine and health sciences, we must take into account that these are design-specific tools from the positivist paradigm (see Chapter 2), but neither universal criteria for scientific rigour nor relevant sampling criteria for a qualitative study.

We see this more clearly, for example, when we explore marginalised phenomena. If we want to know more about lesbians and gays whose sexual orientation remains disclosed, we cannot—even in a quantitative study—expect to obtain data of appropriate validity on this issue from a random population-based sample (Malterud, Bjørkman, et al. 2009, Anderssen & Malterud 2017). Firstly, the proportion of the *population*

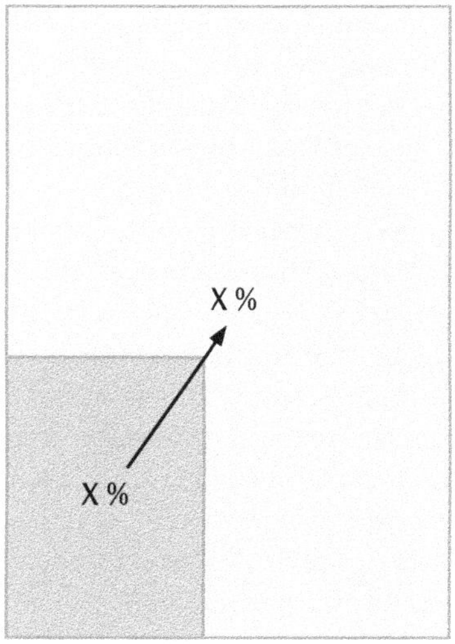

Figure 7.1 Extrapolation from study group to well-defined target group

that is queer is relatively low, and secondly, there are still many who will not respond honestly to questions about sexual orientation. The transferability of qualitative results developed from a random or representative sample will have major limitations with such a problem, because diversity and breadth of variation will be inadequate (Malterud & Bjørkman 2016). There will also be substantial challenges associated with making sense of the relationship (see Figure 7.2).

Hence, neither representative samples nor control groups are universal criteria for scientific validity and rigour, independent of research design and methods. The question is what kind of knowledge we are after, from where our sources of knowledge are drawn, and what kind of validity and transferability is relevant to the issue at hand. Only when these questions have been considered is it time to assess which sampling strategies are best suited to contribute to validity and transferability.

Researchers conducting qualitative studies continuously face flawed demands for generalisability, representativity and control groups from colleagues working with traditional biomedical or epidemiological designs (Loder, Groves, et al. 2016, Clarke, Braun, et al. 2024). When confronted with such peers, it can be useful to ask for their justification for such requirements—then it may be possible to discuss specifically what opportunities and limitations this could add to the research project in relation to the study aim and design. Basic knowledge about subjectivity and the relationship between the interpretive and positivist paradigms provides good arguments for such discussions (you may want to repeat Chapters 1 and 2).

But also in qualitative studies, the researcher must establish a sharp focus on the content and size of the sample and assess the impact of this regarding the internal and external validity of the knowledge being developed. The sample must be carefully composed so that it contains sufficiently relevant and robust material. Lean or skewed material offers limited access to the field that the researcher wants to investigate. Here we will look at some common principles for establishing appropriate samples of qualitative data.

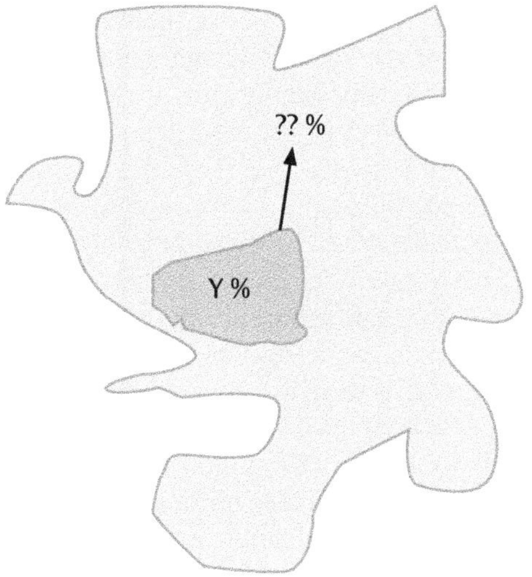

Figure 7.2 Extrapolation from study group to target group with fluid boundaries

Purposive, convenience and snowball sampling

Most often in qualitative studies, interpretations and analyses are based on data from a *purposive sample*. This is the opposite of a random or representative sample. Preparing a qualitative study, you need to make active choices, based on experience, theory and knowledge of the specific field in order to recruit appropriate participants so that your empirical data can best shed light on the problem (Kuzel 1999, Patton 2015).

This is about more than transferability and external validity. Your sample must also be established with the best possible internal validity in mind. What kind of empirical data can provide a relevant and robust basis for interpretations and conclusions that demonstrate something new and valuable about the matters we are puzzled by? Relevance and utility are therefore also important keywords when deciding what kind of data sources you want to establish and organise. Preconceptions, previous research, study aim, design and theoretical perspectives provide a scaffold for what you should emphasise in order to develop data containing the phenomenon in question in sufficient depth and breadth.

To establish a purposive sample, we first consider the direction of focus, ensuring that data collection does not drift away from the study aim. We want to avoid systematic errors that arise if our sample has the wrong focus. Perhaps we know or assume that there may be differences in the way younger and older GPs talk to their patients about possible alcohol problems. Our data may then become more robust if the sample does not only originate from consultations with doctors with long practice experience. In an interview study on doctor-seeking behaviour in families with children, Ertmann put together a purposive sample of parents from a cohort where she had information on the range of variation from questionnaires, symptom diaries and telephone contact (Ertmann, Söderström, et al. 2005).

Field knowledge and everyday logic are also helpful qualifications for choosing relevant and varied data sources. We do not go to the local nursing home to conduct interviews about young people's smoking habits. We need to know where such knowledge can be found, for example during break times at the school gates. However, we do not always know in advance where the most informative data live. We often get to learn about different relevant sources of knowledge during data development. With a flexible design, we can take the consequences of this and expand our purposive selection along the way. Experience-based field knowledge is therefore an important asset for planning and establishing a relevant and robust purposive sample.

If data is highly homogeneous, it can be difficult to bring out sufficient variations of nuances that invite new questions. A purposive sample with strong variation can provide effective challenges to conclusions that initially seemed obvious. A breadth of variation also makes it possible to describe several sides of the same issue. However, the researcher must also decide which dimensions of the matter are particularly valuable to enhance variability for. For example, we cannot automatically assume that gender and age are everlasting key dimensions for a purposive sample, and we cannot include all kinds of variations. We need to prioritise strategically, purposefully and focused.

The study aim determines our emphasis, considering prior empirical studies and theory (Sandelowski 1995). In a study on experiences of physical activity in patients with chronic fatigue syndrome, the sample comprised participants with experienced different movement activities, and with varying degrees of illness (Larun & Malterud 2011a). Here, exercise variability together with level of symptom burden were key dimensions for a purposive selection. In another study on resource-orientated consultations, the sample actually comprised a series of consecutive patients (Malterud & Hollnagel 1997). We can also exceptionally call this a random purposive sample, because the sample was composed to ensure data from many different types of consultations. More usually, the researcher chooses a few, well-considered issues of variation with rough, but relevant categories (level of experience, gender or type of symptoms).

However, such strategies can mislead us into thinking that we are dealing with *stratification* and randomisation in a statistical sense, which is certainly not the case (Sandelowski 1995). It is therefore necessary to make the premises for the purposive selection explicit, so that it is clear to the researcher and the reader what thought was behind it. The researcher must make this clear in the description of the methodology so that the reader can consider whether this was a relevant choice.

We often make pragmatic choices based on the art of the possible. Sometimes it can be hard to recruit an optimal purposive selection. We should not make the best the enemy of the good. On the other hand, we must be prepared to account for any limitations that result from this sampling strategy.

Sometimes, it is a more appropriate alternative to establish a *convenience sample*. We include participants who are easy to reach, such as relatives of patients with a rare disease (Røthing, Malterud, et al. 2015), or lesbian women who want to talk about their experiences with the health service via a web-based form (Bjørkman & Malterud 2009). Another option is *snowball sampling*, where we take advantage of the network of someone who has already opted in, to get hold of further, relevant participants. Especially in studies based on convenience or snowball sampling or other forms of self-recruitment, we expect careful arguments in the method discussion about the strengths and limitations of this particular sample.

Data from a relevant and robust purposive sample strengthens the opportunities for doubt and reflection and allows for reflexivity about the validity and transferability of the interpretations. Taking a small time-out for reflection during data development, we can use our experiences and reflections to adjust the sampling strategy. The material can then be optimised with complementary nuances that lead to competing or compelling results and conclusions. A sample that allows for multiple interpretations and different outcome options demands of the researcher to consider which answers offer the most relevant responses to the questions asked, rather than accepting the first and best answer.

Information Power—the content and size of the sample

Even when we have decided to establish a purposive sample, several important questions remain to be clarified before we can get started. To fulfil the assumptions of reflexivity and intersubjectivity, we need concepts and models that can be used to assess and communicate the assumptions and criteria underlying our sampling strategy. Numbers are rarely of great importance in a qualitative study. Still, for sound project planning, it is legitimate and necessary to consider numbers in terms of resources to develop relevant and robust data with the best possible potential for developing new and valuable knowledge.

While often debated, the use of limited samples in qualitative studies reflects a deliberate and well-founded methodological position. Validity and transferability do not increase in proportion to the size of the sample—in fact, the situation is often the opposite, because an extensive sample can make the data confusing and the analysis superficial— "*the 1000 page problem*" (Kvale 1996). Nevertheless, the arguments are often rotating around *the N-question*—how many participants or interviews do we need?

Researchers with extensive experience from qualitative studies tend to have their own rules of thumb for how many are needed (Mason 2010). The methodology literature states quite casually that N must be sufficient to shed light on the study aim (Marshall 1996, Kuzel 1999, Patton 2015). *Saturation* is often referred to as a criterion for the adequacy of the sample (Glaser & Strauss 1967, Charmaz 2024) (see critique of this concept below). Similarly to quantitative studies, methods for statistical power calculation of sample size have also been proposed (DePaulo 2000, Guest, Bunce, et al. 2006), which appear inconsistent, demonstrating simplistic, small q ideas (see Chapter 4).

But in these matters, it is about more than N. We need to think beyond the numbers. The content of the sample interacts with other elements of the study's design and process, contributing at least as much as N to the conditions for internal and external validity. Together with research colleagues Siersma and Guassora (2016), I have developed the concept of *Information Power* (IP), which is intended to give a qualitative study the best possible conditions for development of rigorous and creative knowledge.

IP is a term we recommend for specifying requirements for the content and size of the sample in relation to the design and process of the study. With strong IP, we need fewer interviews, while a study with weaker IP requires a larger sample size. An overall assessment of IP provides indications of what kind of sample will best serve the purpose.

We developed a model with criteria for systematically assessing IP illustrated by examples from a fictional qualitative interview study. The model was developed in two stages, and the final version of the model is the most appropriate for the message we

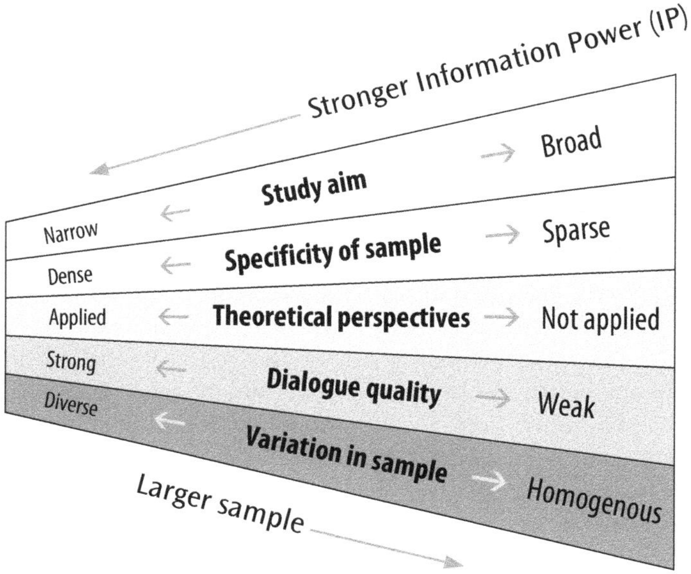

Figure 7.3 Dimensions for assessment of sample Information Power (IP) (after Malterud, Siersma and et al. 2021)

want to convey. If you want to understand this concept and use it, you need to read more than what you will find in this chapter, preferably the latest version (Malterud, Siersma, et al. 2021).

The model demonstrates how IP can be assessed by systematically reviewing the following dimensions of the study in question (see Figure 7.3): narrow vs broad study aim, dense vs sparse specificity of the sample congruent with the problem, applied vs no level of theoretical grounding, strong vs weak quality of the dialogues, and diverse vs homogenous variation in the sample (Malterud, Siersma, et al. 2021).

By reviewing these five dimensions, first individually and then collectively, we gain indications of the sample size considered necessary. We systematically consider the impact on IP from each dimension, and then as a whole. This is not a checklist of points or percentages—in the review, we use our best judgement in dialogue with a research colleague.

With a narrow and focused study aim, a group of participants who are tailored to the study aim, entailing robust and relevant application of an appropriate theoretical perspective, dialogues with lively exchanges, as well as diversity in the sample, we need the fewest participants. But each of these dimensions contributes in different ways and often in opposite directions when it comes to IP. It is the combination of the different dimensions that affects IP. This is by far more helpful than starting by asking for the N number (Malterud, Siersma, et al. 2021).

Because IP is dynamic, we can compensate for certain weak dimensions, both initially in the project and along the way. With strong IP, data from a small number of participants (4–7) can be sufficient to provide rich material for an interview study. For example, in the project on everyday life for children growing up with parents with alcohol problems, nine interviews were the empirical source for three different articles (Werner & Malterud 2016a), and in the study on physical activity in chronic fatigue syndrome, we conducted two focus groups with a total of ten participants (Larun & Malterud 2011a).

Qualitative studies are often based on individual interviews with 10–25 participants. However, the substance, nature and scope of the data can vary greatly, depending on more than how long and how many conversations are included in the data development. For example, if we are planning an interview study that requires the use of a language interpreter because participants speak a foreign language, there is a risk of weak dialogue. Then, it may be helpful to sharpen the approach with a relevant theoretical perspective. Emphasising interview technique and constant revision of the interview guide can also strengthen IP. But the analysis becomes prohibitive if we try to compensate for low IP by significantly increasing the number. Even with computerised tools for handling qualitative data, the requirement for an overview is still absolutely necessary. A large number of participants may suggest a superficial analysis.

If you have used IP as a tool to present and discuss the composition and size of the sample in your article, you must write more than simply that you found satisfactory IP. For this term to make methodological sense, you must rather systematically (preferably briefly) comment on each of the five dimensions of IP for the project in question and say something about how this together characterises the content of the sample and the subsequent issues of size. Remember also that IP represents a sampling logic that is fundamentally different from saturation (see below). These terms should therefore not be confused or applied side by side.

A qualitative study with data that contributes to strong IP can enhance unusual patterns and interpretations. But we should neither believe nor claim that our results have the same kind of extrapolation and transferability to a population that we will achieve with an epidemiological design. We should stay far away from quantified claims and issues relating to measures of effect and causality. Moreover, we need to be cautious about saying that something is larger or better or truer than something else. This does not, however, exempt us from thoughtful reviews of transferability. The researcher may aim to enhance the transferability of knowledge and clarify its scope: transferable in what respects, to whom and under which conditions?

The trouble with saturation

In the qualitative methodology literature, saturation has been used almost as a universal criterion for deciding that the sample size is sufficient (Braun & Clarke 2024a). The term comes from Grounded Theory (GT), which entails the analysis strategy Constant Comparative Method (Glaser & Strauss 1967). In GT, the Constant Comparative Method prescribes that every new observation be compared with prior data in order to identify similarities and differences in the categories developed. Saturation is reached when additional data does not add new knowledge to the development of a theory. However, close studies of qualitative articles reveal that the defined procedure is not always followed and that the concept of saturation is often poorly specified (Carlsen & Glenton 2011).

There can be many different explanations why the researcher does not find anything new in subsequent data. The interview technique may be poor, the focus blurred, or perhaps the end of the funding period is approaching, and the researcher does not have the opportunity to immerse themselves sufficiently. It could also be that you do not know the field or the methods well enough to notice a few small pearls between several large grey stones of empirical data.

In addition, saturation refers to having a limited, manageable set of facts needed to describe the entire field. Such a notion contradicts important assumptions for qualitative research methods, where knowing and knowledge are inherently partial, temporary and dependent on the researcher's situation (see Chapter 5) (Haraway 1991, Kvale 1996, Varpio, Ajjawi, et al. 2017). Therefore, aiming for completeness is not only illusory, but also an (epistemo)logical fallacy. Qualitative methods are first and foremost a strategy for developing knowledge about the particular and unique in the whole, although this type of knowledge should also be abstracted and provide transferability (Sandelowski 1996).

Moreover, it is not obvious that the GT concept of saturation can be transferred to any other qualitative method, where the analysis may unfold in a distinctly different way than with constant comparison in the GT.

In principle, an adequate material based on a purposive sample with $N = 1$ can be conceived of, such as in traditional medical case studies (Sandelowski 1996). Then it is the unique story containing knowledge with a potential for new insights about conditions outside itself. From Nordic general practice research, we have several examples based on experiences and data from a single doctor's practice (Malterud 1990, Rudebeck 2000). Such designs raise particular methodological challenges that are discussed in more detail in Chapters 15 and 19.

Real-life sampling

The IP of the project and the sample will determine our capacity to respond to the study aim through interpretation and analysis. The less we know prior to data development about what we want to look at, the greater the likelihood that our sample will provide lean and arbitrary data with weak IP. Skilled theoretical groundwork and step-by-step analyses are therefore important tools for strengthening the internal validity of a qualitative study.

A flexible research process allows the researcher to sharpen their focus as data interaction, interpretation and analysis supply more nuanced insight into the phenomenon we want to study. The likelihood of establishing a rich sample of manageable size for an interview study increases if we conduct a preliminary analysis as soon as data from the first few units are available, without committing ourselves to any specific number of participants, see Chapter 11 (Malterud 2012b). This will allow us to consider alternative or complementary sources of knowing that can strengthen IP and provide at least equally relevant data.

It is a good rule not to decide on the size of the sample in advance, but along the way, ensure a sample that contributes to appropriate IP through step-by-step recruitment and analysis. In other words, you need to resist the pressure from the positivist research tradition (the small q, see Chapter 4) that N should preferably be a large and predetermined number. A vivid results section with credible stories that can make a difference (Stige, Malterud, et al. 2009) gives good indications that you have conducted the analysis with a sample of strong IP, regardless of N or "saturation".

Selection bias is a calculated risk when establishing a purposive sample. Of course, knowledge is affected by where we have collected our material, and field knowledge comes with both positive and negative aspects. If we collect material only from our own closest peers, we should not expect data that challenges our preconceptions. Nevertheless, the goal is not to eliminate bias, but to reduce or highlight conditions that contribute to disturbing the development as hidden assumptions (see Chapter 5) (Varpio, O'Brien, et al. 2021). We can reduce undesirable selection bias if, well in advance of developing and organising data, we familiarise ourselves with aspects of our preconceptions that could otherwise contribute to narrow, skewed or self-affirming knowledge development. Then it will be easier to seek out sources or metapositions supporting a broader perspective that can challenge our own hypotheses.

CHAPTER 8

Data creation interacting with various sources of knowledge

In qualitative research, data consist of selected information relevant for the study aim drawn from experiences, attitudes, perceptions or observations and transformed into empirical material, commonly from audio or visual formats into text. In this step, you establish and organise the sample that you will further elaborate through systematisation, interpretation, analysis and synthesis. The text is a co-creative product in which the researcher becomes part of the data by virtue of personal participation. For development of new and valuable scientific evidence, you need data with strong Information Power. Informal advances to analysis begin with sample development and continue well into the writing process. You should not try to eliminate or objectify yourself in this part of the process, but on the contrary exercise reflexivity by recognising your impact and exploring its significance.

Different designs and sources of knowledge

The qualitative research tradition offers various paths to knowledge, each distinguished by specific qualities—that is why we talk about qualitative research methods in plural. To choose paths that lead to data with strong Information Power (IP), you need to familiarise yourself with the distinctive features, assumptions, rules, potentials and pitfalls of the various methods. Here I will present a brief overview of commonly occurring strategies for developing and organising qualitative data. In Chapters 14–19, you will find more detailed presentations of some types of designs or data sources that are well established in qualitative studies in medicine and health sciences.

By talking with people, we gain first-hand knowledge of their experiences (see Chapter 14). If we want to explore how experiences from childhood and adolescence shape experiences of illness in adulthood, we can, for example, co-create data from *semistructured individual interviews* (Kvale 1996, Kirkengen 2001, Seidman 2019, Berge, Brekke, et al. 2024). The familiarity and tranquillity of the interview situation may offer a safe framework for stories about memories and connections (Mjølstad,

DOI: 10.4324/9781003786016-10

Kirkengen, et al. 2013). In the project on children growing up with parents with alcohol problems, data were developed from retrospective individual interviews with participants in adulthood (Werner & Malterud 2016a).

Necessary for the development of strong empirical data is that the participants feel secure and cared for, and that the interaction takes place without the interviewer having the answers ready in advance. Listening with an open mind, so that we as researchers can be aware of the new or unexpected, is a methodological interviewing skill that can be learnt and developed. As healthcare professionals, we often ask questions where we believe we know the answer, seeking confirmation of a hypothesis. But talking with people in a sufficiently open mode as data interaction, aiming for concrete and down-to-earth interview data about something more than what we already knew, is a distinct and different research.

The novice interviewer is often left with data replete with general and abstract statements, such as "you should…", "most people think that…" or "I always tend to…". In this kind of material, it can be difficult to tell what stems from the participant's own experience and what they said to perform with a positive social role, interacting with the interviewer. The most evocative material is cocreated when you get participants to tell very specific stories, preferably from last week or the last time something happened (Flanagan 1954).

Focus groups can produce rich data for exploration of phenomena related to shared experiences (Morgan 1993, Malterud 2012a). Group interviews facilitate associations and imagination, and the group dynamics will prompt different narratives than those we get one-to-one. This may be relevant, for example, if we want to learn about symptom experiences from a patient perspective (Søderlund, Skoge, et al. 2000, Undeland & Malterud 2007, Larun & Malterud 2011a). We can use focus groups to study the experiences and views of healthcare professionals (Malterud, Fredriksen, et al. 2009, Modin, Törnkvist, et al. 2010, Hana & Rudebeck 2011, Lid & Malterud 2012, Nilsen, Malterud, et al. 2015, Idland, Iversen, et al. 2022). Focus groups are also well suited to share and compile the experiences of different groups of patients encountering the health services (Bjørkman & Malterud 2007, Malterud & Ulriksen 2010b, Aamland, Werner, et al. 2013, Ree, Harris, et al. 2014, Idland, Iversen, et al. 2022).

Focus group interviews will create a lot of data, considering the resources required, especially if the alternative is individual interviews. However, we must remember that the group dynamics in a focus group may preclude dissenting views or prevent information about sensitive issues from being disclosed. Data from focus groups can also be superficial or one-sided, because the conduct of a group discussion requires structured and skilled guidance from the moderator. This can to some extent be mitigated by developing data from several different groups. The moderator should take an active role and must therefore be well-trained to prevent and recognise situations where the participants' voices are drowned out by questions and guidance or where the conversation devolves into trivial platitudes.

Narratives provide indirect access to actions and events, with subjective experiences as a filter. On the other hand, *observational studies* with varying degrees of participation can offer a different, more direct insight into what is going on (see Chapter 16). We can study interaction and dialogue between doctors and patients without being part of the event, for example by using prospective audio or video recordings from real-life events as empirical data (Nessa & Malterud 1998a, Schaufel, Nordrehaug, et al. 2009, Guassora, Reventlow, et al. 2014). Video recording is particularly relevant when non-verbal issues are highlighted. It is worth noting that observational data from audio or video recordings provide limited insight into participants' opinions and experiences. Instead, we can study behaviour, engagement and the surrounding context.

Participant observation gives access to the interaction between professionals in the health services and stakeholders in society, for example when introducing a new programme (Thesen & Kuzel 1999, Lykkeslet, Gjengedal, et al. 2016). A prerequisite for this is that the researcher is able to enter the relevant context without unduly disrupting the natural course of events. The better we know the field in advance, the easier it is to slip unnoticed into everyday life. But experience can also be blinding, so that the researcher with extensive field knowledge may fail to recognise the most important events.

Medicocentrism—perceiving the world from a medical point of view—represents an important challenge if we intend to carry out participant observation on professional home ground. The naïve questions asked by an observer without the medical taken-for-granted—such as a social anthropologist—may open access to kinds of knowing beyond the view of researchers in medicine and health sciences. Our knowledge horizons can be expanded by inviting other disciplines into the project. But we must also be prepared for multidisciplinary collaboration to raise uncomfortable questions or discoveries that challenge what we consider obvious. This is a risk we must be willing to take when we want to develop new knowledge.

Document analysis is a tool for studying written data, for example if we plan to look into the meaning of life stories written by patients starting cognitive therapy with their general practitioner (GP) (Ehrenreich, Hilden, et al. 2007). Document analysis can be prospective, where the material is produced for the purpose (Bjørkman & Malterud 2009), or retrospective, based on existing data produced for a purpose other than research (Aarseth, Natvig, et al. 2017). In retrospective document analysis, we must rely on what is at hand, while carefully considering whether the sample offers sufficient IP, containing data that can inform the study aim. For example, data drawn from medical patient records are often insufficiently detailed to serve as robust research material, being incomplete and heavily dependent on abbreviations and codes that may be opaque to those without insider knowledge or taken for granted by professionals. Questions about internal validity appear—what is being conveyed in this text? It is crucial that the researcher is sufficiently familiar with the context of the written material to decode the meaning and whether it is usable for the purpose.

The same applies to *open-ended responses from self-completed questionnaires*, which can create scope for understanding aspects of a phenomenon other than frequency distributions of predetermined response categories (see Chapter 22). The anonymity of a questionnaire provides the participant with a safer opportunity to answer sensitive questions or give negatively charged answers than with face-to-face data interaction (Bjørkman & Malterud 2012). For example, we might choose such a strategy if we want to know more about what words patients with lower urinary infections use to describe their symptoms (Malterud & Bærheim 1999) or why GPs do not want to participate in a randomised controlled trial on sick leave (Mæland, Magnussen, et al. 2011). This type of qualitative data is less robust than interview data, and the interaction factor is limited. Such answers easily become superficial, stereotypical or ambiguous, and must therefore be interpreted with considerable caution. Critical assessment of the IP of the material is also crucial for appropriate analysis.

Metasynthesis—identifying, summarising and synthesising results from published qualitative primary studies—may also be a relevant strategy for knowledge development with qualitative research methods (Noblit & Hare 1988, Bondas & Hall 2007b, Sandelowski 2012, Malterud 2019b). For example, it may be advantageous to familiarise yourself with existing qualitative evidence about the experiences of patients, relatives and doctors about chronic fatigue syndrome, and what the various studies convey as a whole (Larun & Malterud 2007). At the start of a major project, metasynthesis can be a strategy to establish an overview of the field, allowing new sub-studies to add to the knowledge base that already exists (Fosse, Schaufel, et al. 2014). There are also detailed methodological rules for metasynthesis to ensure transparency and systematic reflection (Gough, Oliver, et al. 2017a, Malterud 2019b). You can read more about qualitative metasynthesis in Chapter 18.

From experience, interaction and observation to raw data

Empirical data originate from many different sources, referring to different research designs. In the analysis, data are compiled and organised into a larger puzzle in which solid media such as field notes, documents, audio tape recordings, and video recordings together substantiate and complement memories and insights. Loose pieces of paper need to be assembled, speech must be turned into text, and the text has to be organised before coherence and meaning become accessible. When data are organised and prepared for analysis, the metacriteria of reflexivity, relevance and validity (see Chapter 3) are put to the test.

In the field notes, the researcher accumulates their observations and reflections along the way. Notes along the path constitute an important element of the decision trail (see Chapter 6). In a project with data from participant observation, field notes are a key source of data. However, in projects based on interview data or video recordings, the field notes and the decision trail can also be helpful to capture impressions and reflections that would otherwise not end up in the footage. The analysis cannot rely solely on the researcher's recollection of the events. A research project that aims for scientific knowledge, with subjectivity as a starting point, requires trustworthy documentation, leaving visible traces in the final text. Data are the binding agent and the link between experience and analysis. Our empirical data are also the solid basis for conducting reflexivity when analysing, interpreting and synthesising what we have seen and heard.

The most helpful field notes compile brief descriptions, comments and mixtures of these. Accounts of actual events are framed by the researcher's point of view. Therefore, they also represent comments, where elements of descriptions also occur. Your decision trail can also be your treasure trove where points from theoretical, empirical or methodological literature can lie dormant and then progressively become crucial for your understanding of meaning.

It is easier to treat field notes as data reflexively if we can later distinguish, to some extent, between descriptions, comments, and literature-based elements. It is essential to handle excerpts from others' texts responsibly to avoid plagiarism and textual similarity. Personally, I use a yellow marker to indicate verbatim records from other authors, as a reminder during writing that these are not my own formulations.

We must be able to account for the sources of our results and conclusions. The reader is entitled to know which parts of the results originate from the field, from our own preconceptions and experience, from articles and theory we have read, or from the meeting points between these sources of knowledge. On the other hand, we must not believe that such a distinction can be made consistently. Empirical data always provides an indirect, filtered view of reality that necessarily incorporates us in some way. But this should not prevent the conscientious researcher from considering the different sources of knowledge and their impact.

Audio recordings are appropriate raw data for analysis of talk and interaction, although they capture only the linguistic and near-linguistic elements of the conversation (pauses, hesitation, laughter) (Malterud 1990). Nonverbal communication is not recorded. The project's study aim determines what kind of data the audio recording should include. You will probably use digital audio recorder, and there is no need for expensive and technically advanced equipment. Transcribing audio recordings with AI speech recognition requires additional reflections (see Chapter 9). In any case, it is always necessary to ensure that your recording proceeds as planned. Find out how the equipment is best positioned for optimal sound reproduction and consider whether an external microphone is needed. Do not forget extra batteries or a fresh charge.

Informed consent is a prerequisite for all research involving human subjects (see Chapter 24). Audio recordings from real-life situations with patients, such as medical consultations, require prior written consent from every participant, who must also have the right to delete the recording without further explanation or negotiation. Notes from the interview can provide useful additional information that later supplements the audio recording. Keep in mind, however, that the conversation may be disturbed if the interviewer's attention is focused on the notes at the expense of contact with the participant.

Video recording can compile data on many different phenomena complementary to talk, especially non-verbal phenomena such as movement and interaction (Steihaug & Malterud 2002, Øien, Steihaug, et al. 2011). Video recording may also enhance the interpretation of linguistic conversation data (Nessa & Malterud 1998b). These strategies entail data co-creation of a more sensitive nature than audio recordings, but the intervention effect is still lower than with a live observer present, for example in a consultation. If we prefer data where other observers (with the participants' consents) subsequently can access what happened, video recordings may be appropriate. However, data in the form of video recordings provide large amounts of information, and the researcher needs a well-focused study aim for the analysis to be manageable.

But field notes, audio recordings and video recordings are only media for raw data. The project outline presenting design and method must therefore contain more detailed information about what kind of phenomena the researcher aims to explore in this way, how this material will be handled and stored and what analytical approach will be adopted.

Step-by-step process

Flexibility is typical for all stages of the qualitative research process. As researchers, we have the right and responsibility to learn from our experiences, and it is appropriate to fine-tune the course of the project in accordance with what we realise and learn along the way. Engagement with the field and proximity to the data may contribute to a more clearly specified and focused research problem than was possible at the stage of the initial project outline. Quite often, the researcher realises along the way that the study aim can be better illuminated from a different angle than the one that the preconceptions originally pointed towards.

Therefore, the *data interaction* must establish material that is appropriate for the purpose, also when the study aim changes character or is refined. Such processes are more difficult if the project outline locks data development and analysis as sharply separated parts of the research process. If we manage to implement a flexible process where data development and analysis go hand in hand in a stepwise process, we will have come a long way with the analysis when the last interview is completed. Assumptions and approaches for analysis can be read in Chapters 10–12.

Filtering and further development of data

Empirical data must encompass the most relevant aspects of what we want to study. In qualitative studies, human activities that do not originally appear in a written form are translated into representations in the form of text. The text has the power to create its own reality, where different accounts of the same phenomenon can be available and become data that we must choose among.

Reality consists of living events in time and space that can never be fully preserved for posterity. All data only partly represent actual events or statements, shaped by the decisions made during data co-creation (Kvale 1996). New versions of subjective reality are developed through texts designed to articulate and consolidate a particular new version of that reality.

Social constructionism recognises the researcher's involvement in all stages of the knowing (Berger & Luckmann 1967, Haraway 1991, Lock & Strong, 2010, Smith 2010) (see Chapter 2). In the interpretive processes of data co-creation and analysis, we employ systematic procedures to read human meaning from our material. The researcher's journey through this terrain is not trackless. We must be able to identify our own progress—only then can we advance further. We strive to ensure that our personal inner voices and subjectivity are played without drowning out the voices from others' experiences.

The researcher's motives, characteristics, interests and positions leave their mark on the material in the form of questions asked (or not asked) and responses given (or not given). Already in the interview, interaction takes place that shapes the participant's narrative and the subsequent data that follows from this. At best, we can hope to gain access to a particular historical version of this narrative—the one that the participant chooses to tell us under given circumstances. As researchers, we should endeavour to find out which version we apply for further analysis.

A note of caution: Audio recordings and transcripts, while valuable, are not absolute Facts or Truth. Our empirical data provide filtered representations of our research focus, shaped at each stage of interaction and organisation. Raw data are usually converted into text before being analysed, and the transcription process also shapes the material. No transcription procedure allows us to escape this.

Therefore, we should not believe that we are holding "authentic facts" in our hands but demonstrate humility and reservations due to the handling we have subjected the material to. Knowing what happens to the text as it is narrated and further developed is an important prerequisite to assess the material during analysis. This is one of many good reasons why the researcher should be personally responsible for transcribing, and why such assessments should be made regularly during the data development process (more on this in the next chapter).

CHAPTER 9

Transcription—capturing voices, not just words

All research involves interpreting some or other representations of what we want to study. Several possible versions will always be available to provide insight into different aspects of the problem, and some representations provide more relevant insight than others. In the qualitative research process, we transform experiences and events from conversations or observation into text and meaning. After the first turn of data interaction with the participants, for example interviews, the material must be organised, developed further and prepared for analysis. Qualitative analysis commonly depends on transcribing material into a form that is accessible and manageable. This invites a closer look at the transcript as an analytical tool and how it can be prepared and used effectively.

A depiction twice removed from its source

People's subjective experiences and understanding in the context of time and space of what has happened constitute the raw data for a qualitative study. In the interaction between researcher and participants, a limited version of this is established for a specific purpose, adapted to elucidate or respond to the researcher's study aim. Even a technically appropriate video recording that is abundant with information will only provide an indirect representation of selected aspects of what took place. The transcript based on the recording becomes an indirect representation of an indirect rendition that lacks many of the crucial meaning-making properties of what happened or was said. The researcher's interpretation of this text is, regardless of analysis method, a key element in any qualitative study. This is so obvious and unelaborated that it does not make sense to conceptualise this as "text analysis".

The transcription must as faithfully as possibly signify the original material, as the participants' experiences and opinions were communicated and perceived by the researcher during the data interaction. The text should also to some extent make it possible to read between the lines, in the sense that we can recall the situation and

DOI: 10.4324/9781003786016-11

context in which the stories were told, in addition to the words that were spoken. At the same time, we must admit that we may not perceive or understand everything that was said, for example when several participants talk simultaneously in a focus group, or when participants tell a story where important background knowledge about the preconditions for what was said is missing. We will still transcribe to the best of our ability but be careful with interpretations where the meaning of the text or recording seems blurry.

Beyond doubt, you should not mistake the text in the transcript for "reality". Even the most accurate transcription can never provide more than a limited and situated access to our study aim, rigged for the purpose (Haraway 1991, Lock & Strong 2010). In addition, translation links from spoken to written language will always involve filtering, where meaning is lost or distorted along the way. This is particularly relevant when the researcher was not present during the event and may therefore misunderstand the meaning of what was said and done. As a researcher, I must therefore decide which procedures best safeguard the content and meaning of the subsequent transcript (Lapadat & Lindsay 1999).

Technical devices

Digital methods and devices are the obvious choices to record qualitative data. You rarely need top technical quality to get satisfactory sound to transcribe recordings from individual interviews or focus groups, but you should check in advance whether you need an external microphone. Often this is not necessary.

If possible, select equipment and software for recording that allows you to connect a foot pedal to the computer for transcription. The foot pedal software makes it easy to fast-forward and rewind, and you can also choose the playback speed that best matches your own keyboard capacity. There is also playback software that can be set up with customised speed and automatic rewind. For most people, this provides better ergonomic conditions than when we manually fast-forward and rewind all the time to catch everything.

Audio and video files should be stored securely and encrypted immediately after recording. Easy-to-use encryption software is available (see Chapter 24). Find out what rules and procedures for safe storage of the encrypted files your research organisation requires and offers.

From speech to text

People normally do not speak in a manner where a strictly verbatim transcription of the conversation presents a valid and meaningful representation of what was said and heard. Natural spoken language is much more fragmented and informal than written language. When a spoken conversation is transformed into written text, there is always a distortion of the event, even in the case of a meticulous transcription. The natural context of the conversation supports the structure of oral expressions that may seem incomplete in written form. Non-verbal aspects of the communication and the actors' common background of experience can represent a shared knowledge capital that greatly shapes the meaning of the conversation, but which nevertheless cannot be traced in the audio recording. Remember that the purpose of writing is to capture the conversation in a form that best conveys what we believe the participant wanted to communicate, considering the study aim. When transcribing recordings from focus groups, it may be handy to assign pseudonyms to the participants already in the transition from audio to speech as a contribution to privacy.

Here we may experience a confrontation between validity and reliability. Validity is weakened when we are (mis)guided by positivist ideals conveying a mechanical understanding of trustworthiness. If we write down exactly what was said, we do not necessarily get an adequate reproduction of what was meant or heard. Verbatim transcription of oral communication may provide the reader with a different idea of the conversation than what the interlocutors heard in the situation, especially if one or both actors use a dialect or a mode of oral expression with fill-in characteristics: "And then you could say I—well, I do not really know how—but in any case, I went and talked to her then, so." Such a sentence can sound precise and coherent when spoken, even if it does not preserve coherence in written form. You should be particularly aware of the risk of ridiculing the participants' expressions by striving for the most exact verbatim transcription of a conversation. To prevent this, rather try to carefully edit the text during transcription ("slightly modified verbatim mode"). It is not uncommon for transcribed material to undergo a further stage of translation when a researcher whose first language is not English writes an article in English. Hence, there are many challenges when we try to preserve the meaning in the best possible way.

In some projects, we may want to investigate linguistic and near-linguistic elements, such as interruptions and other subtleties, for example in dialogues between doctor and patient. In such projects, it may be appropriate to use specific and detailed transcription methods, developed from different linguistic research traditions (discourse analysis, conversation analysis), which are capable to capture such phenomena (Potter & Wetherell 1987, Nessa & Malterud 1990). It is, however, possible that what we find most interesting is so language- and culture-specific that it simply disappears, even when the translation is of a very high quality. Therefore, there are limits to which linguistic nuances in a foreign language can be researched if the result is to be presented as an English-language article.

Nor is it a given that a verbatim and complete written reproduction will lead to the best presentation of the conversation in the article. A 15–20-minute transcript of a general practice consultation extends the format requirements of an article in a medical journal, and it can be difficult to get an overview of the communicative process. If the researcher's intention is to show what takes place during the consultation, it may be appropriate to use or develop transcription methods created to compile the linguistic interaction (Nessa 1995a, 1995b, Nessa & Malterud 1998a, Undeland & Malterud 2002, Schaufel, Nordrehaug, et al. 2009).

To obtain epistemological congruence, we must choose a method that is fit for eliciting what we are going to study, and we must be prepared to justify and explain our choice of method. If you want to study the conversation in linguistic detail, you must therefore first learn enough about the available transcription methods to be able to choose the one that is most appropriate, considering your study aim. Using a standardised transcription method will make it easier to make comparisons with other researchers' results and conclusions. A fixed procedure can also strengthen intersubjectivity, because the path we follow is thoroughly described. However, rigid procedures, perhaps developed in other disciplines for other epistemological purposes, can also weaken precision and relevance. In qualitative studies in medicine and the health sciences, attention is often directed more towards the content of the conversation than to how it unfolded.

Complete the transcription yourself rather than delegating it

Transcribing from audio or video recordings is time-consuming and quickly leads to extensive written material. It takes time to listen to the raw material. Often there are also uncertain points in the flow of speech where it is difficult to know for sure what was said. Even though it takes time, there are many good methodological reasons why the researcher should do this job themselves. Those who were present in the conversation will remember perceptions that can clarify ambiguities or that are important for understanding the meaning of the text. This can play a major role in validity and Information Power, even with minor editing, when the oral conversation is to be translated into text.

However, the benefit of carrying out the transcription yourself is chiefly linked to the early access to the material that such a detailed review provides. By acting as an intermediary between speech and text, you get to relive the experiences of the data interaction and familiarise yourself with the material from a new perspective. Transcribing allows for a new encounter with the text that leads to more thoughts and interpretations than when the recording was made. Such reflections provide fertile ideas for questions that we ask more explicitly in the analysis phase. When we have difficulty understanding what was said, we may still identify key knowledge relevant to our purpose.

At the same time, such assessments may reveal, sometimes disappointingly, that a particular interview did not provide sufficient access to the matter in question. Through the transcription work, it also becomes clear how much "dead" material an interview can contain. This may reflect a limited capacity to create dialogue on the participant's terms, or an unresolved relationship between the researcher and the research question. Furthermore, not all participants are equally articulate.

Transcription is more than producing a transcript. Material that attracts little attention during the interview may acquire significance only in retrospect, particularly in the case of *grey participants*, whose voices were less evident at the time. Early engagement with such material can temper a later analytical bias toward participants whose accounts are especially articulate. Sometimes, during the transcription process, the researcher needs to admit that the proportion of inert material is more extensive than anticipated. It is crucial to take such discoveries seriously. Excessively voluminous material may also push the researcher towards superficial analysis. When the researcher personally does the transcription work, the possibility of revealing weaknesses in the material is strengthened, and the risk of collecting countless unnecessary pages can still be reduced by adjusting the recruitment or interview strategy.

We should be respectful of the transcription phase of the research process. Although it is only a text, it is also a filtering and interpretation stage (Lapadat & Lindsay 1999). Any close contact with the material means that the traces from the researcher in the material constitute data interaction with that will have an impact on the meaning of the text. This is not something to be avoided, but since the act of transcribing is not a passive act of reproduction, it becomes embedded in and may be an asset in the interpretive–analytical process. Some transcription methods involve more explicit and extensive interpretation, such as Nessa's method for summarising a consultation text into a synopsis (Nessa 1995a). Reflexivity is particularly challenged by such strategies, because the researcher must account for how their own position has coloured the creation of the text that is subsequently made the subject of more detailed analysis (Lapadat & Lindsay 1999). But the transcript is not a sacred "fact".

External resources for transcription

In large projects with extensive funding and data material, it is not unusual for transcription to be carried out by someone other than the researcher who will analyse the material in the subsequent stage. For example, this could be a secretary or a student assistant. This saves time and effort for the researcher, but in my experience, it leaves many important gaps for the analysis step. The researcher misses out on early close contact with the text and may be less likely to adjust the interview guide or dialogue style along the way. The transcript can be misleading at some points without the researcher realising this. It may also turn out that the problem requires a specific method of transcription that it is too late to implement once the text is completed and closed.

Similar challenges apply when using digital speech recognition programmes based on artificial intelligence (AI). Such software can be useful for streamlining certain aspects of clinical practice, but when handling qualitative data for research purposes, the assumptions are different. This applies to the privacy of the participants, the protection of the researcher's data material and the safeguarding of and respect for the subjective aspects of the analysis (see Chapters 14 and 23). Dialect variations are also easily lost in AI translation and may contribute to a lack of coherence.

Audio data

Since transcription is time-consuming, it can be tempting to skip the transcription phase and conduct the analysis directly from audio data (sound recordings) (Beich, Gannik, et al. 2002, Halcomb & Davidson 2006). However, a written text provides substantially better opportunities for thorough and methodical investigation, which is an important prerequisite for a committed, systematic qualitative analysis of scientific standard. In conversations where the researcher was present, either as an interviewer or a participant observer, taken-for-grantedness and blind spots can be reinforced by re-listening to audio data. Beginners should therefore not skip the step of transcription for convenience, but rather use it to strengthen the proximity to the data and invest in the systematic nature of the research process. The more experienced researcher can also benefit from the committed reflexivity that written text invites (Lapadat & Lindsay 1999, Halcomb & Davidson 2006).

CHAPTER 10

Analysis—the creative art of rigorous reflection

Analysis bridges the gap between empirical data and the interpretations from a scientific study, guided by the study aim and the analysis method. The researcher's role as interpreter is an instrumental resource for developing new and valuable knowledge through close, yet rigorous, engagement with data, providing the highest possible Information Power. Qualitative analysis is inductive and interpretive, in that the unique provides access to understanding more general phenomena through abstraction and transferability. Strategies for abstraction may be primarily theoretically based or empirically based. Subjectivity entails a distinctive analytical creativity drawing on empirical data, particularly suited to the exploration of complex human and social phenomena familiar from clinical practice, such as unpredictability, nonlinearity and interaction. In such contexts, theoretical perspectives will usually inform abstraction, even when the strategy is primarily empirically based.

What is analysis?

Many methods are available for the analysis of qualitative data. If you are a novice, do not start analysing with the idea that you will find your way on your own or craft your own method. The *analysis method* serves as a compass, providing direction and structure along the way. That is why you should put time and effort into choosing, learning and using a method that best matches the problem and the material. The analysis starts informally already during the data interaction, when we form thoughts and hypotheses that we bring with us to the analysis phase, and continues right up until the article is finished. In this chapter, analysis is treated as a distinct phase of the process, through which scientific knowledge is developed from subjectivity and through subjectivity.

We start with the end: The outcome of qualitative analysis is the analytical text in the results section (see Chapter 12), complemented by your reflection in the discussion section. The analysis involves asking questions from the study aim of the empirical

DOI: 10.4324/9781003786016-12

material (what can this tell us about x?). With this type of question, you can systematically read, organise, interpret and develop data and synthesise the answers in a comprehensible way, expressed as concepts and analytical text. The answers you develop and synthesise depend on the questions you ask. Along the way, you will mutually maintain and reshape the subjectivity of your empirical data. Reflexivity towards your assignment and your position is essential for the scientific rigour and quality of your analytical interpretations (Malterud 1993, 2001b). Your preconceptions and theoretical perspectives determine your position, influence your gaze and situate the knowledge you develop (see Chapter 5) (Haraway 1991). Therefore, you need to know where you stand.

You ought to approach the analysis with an open mind. Still, you need to be clear about what you seek to explore and the strategy you intend to follow. Initially, we decide which analytical questions and which theoretical perspectives can best form the basis for relevant and robust interpretations (Malterud 2016, Guassora, Reventlow, et al. 2022). The question expressed through your *study aim* should be consistent and logical and is usually more clearly reformulated and specified during the analysis. The broader the problem statement, the lower the Information Power (IP) (see Chapter 7), and the more ambiguous your interpretations and results will be. At the same time, be receptive to the progress of new questions and possible changes in direction. Your empirical data will show you which aspects of your original question are most meaningful and possible to answer.

Do not hesitate to draw on new insights and adjust your study aim as the work progresses. Flexibility is useful and necessary in qualitative analysis (see Chapter 6). When data development proceeds stepwise, well integrated with the analysis process, we will notice that the questions we ask of the material gradually change according to what leads to the most relevant answers. In other words, it is not a goal to stick to the original conceptualisation of your study aim—on the contrary, it is important to draw on experience and insight to develop the project through analysis conducted at the points of intersection between data, theory, and interpretation. Alvesson & al emphasise "the quest for interesting phenomena", i.e. elaborating a focused study aim that leads to something truly new and valuable (Alvesson & Sandberg 2024). The sampling strategy also helps to determine which questions we can work out. If the material cannot answer questions that we perceive to be central to our project, we must revise the study aim and the sample in accordance with the knowledge we are seeking to develop (see Chapter 7).

The same material can yield different answers depending on the analytical position adopted. The sharper the question, the clearer the answers we will get, provided a sample of appropriate IP concerning the project's study aim and design (Malterud, Siersma, et al. 2021). In the project on general practitioners (GPs) and challenging sick notes, for example, the problem was refined in the analysis phase to include negotiation strategies in a conflict-filled position, while the empirical material contained a lot of further interaction information that, with a different focus, could otherwise have been interesting (Nilsen, Malterud, et al. 2015).

For a quantitative study, it may be an appropriate strategy to repeat other people's questions and answers to standardise and strengthen the knowledge base. In a qualitative study, on the other hand, we aim for new knowledge, not the reproduction of what is already known. The task is not to confirm previous research but to contribute something that expands or challenges the actual knowledge base (Alvesson & Sandberg 2024). It is therefore essential that we familiarise ourselves sufficiently with the empirical literature, so that we know what has already been done. Then we can credit our predecessors and proceed in new directions. In our own analysis, we must distinguish what is key and focus on the potential for the generation of new insights. Prioritising text that can facilitate new knowledge in the analysis, while setting aside old answers, is also an essential research skill.

Analytical reduction

Qualitative data contain large amounts of information. Taking the raw data as a starting point, we select text elements that can support the best possible IP. This process is an extension of the sampling strategy and involves *filtering*, implying that considerable parts of the original material are set aside. Quantitative research methods are often criticised for reductionism, in that reality is broken down into elements so small that the overall picture may be lost (see Chapter 1). However, all scientific analyses, including qualitative studies, require some form of *reduction* (see Chapter 5). That is why it is particularly important to maintain the context for different parts of the material throughout. If the empirical material becomes too extensive, this can be demanding or impossible. When you are a participant and an observer at the same time, you must combine analytical reduction with active proximity to the living knowing, involving plenty of challenges. For novice researchers, realising that not everything can be included and that appropriate delimitation is necessary is often a demanding but important attitude. Thinking in terms of relationships and interconnections involves loyalty to what we perceive as the meaning of the participants' statements, and a commitment to knowing in the subjective and unique context in which it belongs. The analysis involves more than repetition when the goal is new and valuable scientific evidence. Central to this process is interpretation, abstraction and synthesis that encourages the transferability of results and conclusions. The analysis method leads the way with principles and procedures, and theoretical perspectives contribute to critical reflection, meta-perspectives and fresh possibilities for interpretation.

Qualitative analysis always involves some form of decontextualisation and recontextualisation (Tesch 1990). Through *decontextualisation*, parts of the material can be temporarily lifted out of the whole and explored in relation to other elements that speak to the same phenomenon. Through *recontextualisation*, reductionism is avoided by assessing whether the answers derived from decontextualised material retain a justifiable reference to their original context. We validate the interpreted partial aspects against the whole and the context. Without such a perspective, results tend to become disjointed and fragmented, a tendency reflected in results sections dominated by lengthy quotations and sparse analysis.

Inductive and data-driven or deductive and theory-driven?

With *inductive* logic, we pursue transferability by abstracting and drawing conclusions from the unique to the general (bottom-up). With *deductive* logic, we conversely draw conclusions with transferability from the general to the unique (top-down) (see Chapter 2). Inductive logic is often based on experience, while deductive logic is often based on theoretical models. When it comes to research methods and analysis, inductive analysis starts openly, without predetermined response categories, while deductive analysis starts with the organisation of data, hypotheses and categories derived from existing knowledge (Pope & Mays 2020).

When planning design and research methods and assessing analysis strategies, we are committed to some basic assumptions from the scientific paradigms. We often talk about this as a polarised dichotomy, where we choose one or the other. It is perhaps more correct to imagine a continuum, with inductive and deductive as extremes, where many position themselves between these extremes. With *Interpretive Description*, Thorne (2025) for example does not set out a fixed procedural template. Instead, she frames it as a guiding logic with very few explicitly prescriptive guidelines within which rigorous qualitative studies in applied, practice-based disciplines can be designed and carried out in ways that yield meaningful results.

Put simply, the interpretive paradigm—with subjectivity and uniqueness at its core—can be positioned toward the inductive end of the scale, whereas the positivist paradigm, typically associated with quantitative research methods, aligns more closely with the deductive end. At the same time, the ideals of reflexivity and metapositions remind us that we never enter knowing with a clean slate, untouched by deductive cognition logic (see Chapter 16). Relevant theoretical perspectives can thus function as metapositions and strengthen reflexivity in a qualitative study, without the analysis being governed by deductive logic with predetermined result categories. These are key premises for situating the knowledge that we develop (Haraway 1991).

Miller and Crabtree (1999) present concepts for different qualitative analysis strategies according to how strongly the theoretical perspectives influence the analysis process, particularly for the organisation of the result categories. The *editing analysis style* is an analysis strategy that is mainly data-driven, but the researcher uses the theoretical perspectives as support and backdrop to interpret relevant patterns in the empirical material. This hybrid analysis strategy, which is widely used in qualitative studies from medicine and health sciences, involves an active dialogue between theory and empirical data. Theoretical perspectives and concepts help to focus the analytical gaze without predetermining the result categories. With the editing analysis style, the researcher must clearly demonstrate how empirical data constitute the substance of an inductive analysis, while at the same time clearly situating the study, otherwise this becomes a non-committal concept (see Chapter 20).

Template analysis style is a deductive analysis strategy where theoretical concepts from are used as an overarching, predetermined organising principle for the result categories (Miller & Crabtree 1999), for example the communication theory of Habermas (Walseth, Abildsnes, et al. 2011). Yet, with a theory-driven analysis strategy, rich and contextual interpretations and results can help balance and counteract a deductive logic. For example, in a study of interactions between healthcare professionals and women with chronic muscle pain, the dimensions of listening, understanding, acceptance, tolerance and affirmation from a psychological theory (Schibbye 1993) were used to show how these could play out in practice as recognition in this specific context (Steihaug, Ahlsen, et al. 2002). But theory-driven analysis, also known as *framework analysis*, can easily become static, without sufficiently creative approaches to knowledge development.

A sharp polarisation does not necessarily provide the best picture of the methodological terrain. Nevertheless, an inductive and data-driven analysis strategy, supported by relevant substantive theories, generally affords the best conditions for knowing as conceptualised as the Big Q (see Chapter 4). In this way, theory contributes to better immersion in empirical data and thus supports an inductive strategy, while a deductive, theory-driven analysis strategy runs the risk of stumbling into positivist ideals of stability and objectivity, modelled by the small q.

A *theoretical model* expresses an understanding of relationships that may be the outcome of our interpretations and analyses. But most often, qualitative studies in medicine and health sciences aim to develop empirical knowledge that can contribute to improvement and change cognition and practice—only rarely is *theory development* (Natvik, Råheim, et al. 2019) specifically on the agenda. A precise figure can summarise our inner images in a pedagogical way that gives new meaning, but boxes and arrows alone do not provide a theoretical model (Wilson & Hutchinson 1996, Morse 2006). A figure that illustrates a model should be immediately understandable, while at the same time conveying relevant and new insights. If you modify a model developed by another researcher, you must consider what, why and how you are changing it, and you must credit the originator.

Analyses aimed at the development of theoretical models require thorough knowledge of existing theories in the field, so that we know and show sufficiently clearly what new insights we can contribute. Within medicine and the health sciences, researchers sometimes present extensive and complex, home-made figures to illustrate how they believe the elements are connected. But perhaps someone else (probably researchers from other disciplines) has already presented more elaborate theoretical models and figures, representing thinking and interpretation rooted in data and theory.

This is not made any easier by the fact that some qualitative research traditions (particularly those rooted in Grounded Theory) use the concept of theory to denote any result that is properly anchored in data. Such terminology contributes to an unclear understanding of what theory entails and may also invite unrealistic ambitions to develop theory in studies that do not provide sufficient scope for results at that level.

Systematic reflection

Structured analysis using relevant and robust methods for interpretation and abstraction of results—methods that enable the development of new and valuable knowledge—is what fundamentally distinguishes research from superficial opinion. The analysis implies closeness and distance at the same time. We therefore need to employ orderly procedures alongside creative logic. Bear in mind that the analysis is not an impressionistic stroll, but a targeted and well-organised journey from study aim via interpretations to results.

The novice may benefit from a travel guide that outlines underlying assumptions as well as tangible procedures, with a supervisor serving as a knowledgeable travelling companion. Following an established and well-described analysis method makes it more straightforward to stay on course through unfamiliar terrain, while also remaining attentive to subtle traces and impressions along the way. Regardless of the analytical method chosen, it is important to be familiar with what characterises the method, as well as the strengths and weaknesses of this choice.

The key to a good outcome is that you follow a set route where you have a clear foothold and know where you are going. A few specific methodological steps can help ensure that the road goes forward and not just backwards or sideways. The novice researcher must become skilled at a well-described analysis method, rather than inventing or modifying something themselves. If, as a researcher, I claim that the results I present are the outcome of qualitative analysis, it is not sufficient to claim "thematic emergence" (Varpio, Ajjawi, et al. 2017). As we sort and organise the material, we will, during the analysis, clarify the hidden systematics of the patterns we come up with and share this with the reader. This is considerably easier when we follow a method that shows the way than when we try to do it blindly.

In the analysis, the researcher stops, thinks, examines relevant patterns that can elucidate the study aim and compares alternative interpretations. The analysis method guides your course so you can do this systematically, with appropriate intersubjectivity. Citing a clearly explained analysis method allows readers to trace the process from data to results, provided the procedure was truly followed. But there is no point in adding a reference that just fits, without committing to what it says. Such shallow practices are unfortunately more common than you might think, even in articles published in good journals (Bondas & Hall 2007b, Glenton & Carlsen 2019, Braun & Clarke 2024d).

Hence, you have a lot to gain by following one of the methods that has been thoroughly described and extensively used. Examples of this are Giorgi's psychological phenomenological analysis (Giorgi 1985, 2009), Grounded Theory (Glaser & Strauss 1967, Charmaz 2024), Reflexive Thematic Analysis (Braun & Clarke 2022), Qualitative Content Analysis (Graneheim & Lundman 2004) or Systematic Text Condensation (presented in more detail in the next chapter) (Malterud 2012b). Some argue that such recipes turn the analysis into rigid and mechanical approaches. An opposite point of view is that it is then easier to focus on the content and meaning of data development and interpretation.

Do not sit alone the first time you do a qualitative analysis. If you are an experienced researcher with a quantitative background, you also need to properly familiarise yourself with the rules of the game and then follow them. Only when the researcher can account for the path followed is it possible to share this with others (Malterud 1993, 2001b, Stige, Malterud, et al. 2009). The analysis should be presented so that others can later follow the path we have taken, recognise our systematic approach along the way, and understand our interpretations and conclusions. Intersubjectivity in the analysis means that this process should not only be carried out but also communicated.

Analysing within or across cases?

Qualitative analysis methods can be classified in various ways (Creswell & Poth 2024). Some are based on specific philosophies (e.g. phenomenology or hermeneutics) (Ricoeur 1976, Giorgi 1985, van Manen 2023), others categorise according to different methodological traditions (e.g. Grounded Theory or ethnography) (Glaser & Strauss 1967,

Atkinson & Hammersley 1994). Different classification methods may reflect what the researcher prioritises and how the analysis is situated.

The prevailing analysis methods have many similarities and some differences. On an overall level, the distinction concerns whether analysis proceeds within cases or across them—akin to reading a grid vertically or horizontally. These two directions of analysis are used for different purposes and require different strategies. In analysis within cases, we explore a single or a few courses of events over time, while analysis across cases compiles and synthesises information as themes from several participants or units of analysis.

Analysis within cases is not better than cross-case analysis or vice versa—it depends on the purpose of the analysis. Therefore, you need to be fully aware of what kind of knowledge you are aiming for, what your data covers and what the strengths and weaknesses of the different analysis methods are. Thematic analysis carries the risk of fragmentation and a lack of focus on individuals' specific conditions if we are not sufficiently alert throughout the analysis and manage to stay in touch with the context of the data. Analysis within cases provides better opportunities to go into depth but often requires more expertise in theory and methodology. It can also be more challenging to explain conditions for transferability in an analysis within cases.

Most qualitative studies from medicine and health sciences are conducted with different variants of cross-case analysis (Glaser & Strauss 1967, Graneheim & Lundman 2004, Malterud 2012b, Patton 2015, Braun & Clarke 2022). Many of these methods are called *thematic analysis*. For novices, it can be less challenging to conduct thematic analysis than analysis within cases. I therefore emphasise these strategies the most in the following.

Methods for thematic analysis include guidelines for interpreting and synthesising similarities, differences and variations in experiences, feelings, experiences or attitudes from several participants. The aim of the study on sick leave for patients with subjective health problems, for example, was to investigate different negotiation strategies among Norwegian GPs (Nilsen, Malterud, et al. 2015). Another study explored GPs' experiences of how they could be of help to children of parents with substance abuse problems or serious chronic illness (Gullbrå, Smith-Sivertsen, et al. 2014). However, although experiences are compiled across studies, this does not allow conclusions to be drawn about the frequency or distribution of the phenomenon in question.

Discourse analysis, conversation analysis, narrative analysis, semiotic analysis or phenomenology can serve as relevant methods for *analysis within cases*, such as case reports, individual accounts or issues where the time dimension plays a role (Potter & Wetherell 1987, Nessa & Malterud 1990, Have 2007, Riessman 2008, Frank 2012, van Manen 2023). For example, microanalysis of two dialogues between doctor and patient was used to understand the impact of different consultation styles when the doctor perceives some health problems as medically unexplained (Undeland & Malterud 2008). In another study, narrative analysis was used to explore how seemingly trivial everyday stories can serve as identity carriers for patients in palliative care (Synnes 2015).

Giorgi's psychological phenomenological analysis aims to develop knowledge about the participant's life world within a specific domain (Giorgi 1985). Here, we focus on the essences or basic characteristics of the phenomena we are studying when we interpret the material. We endeavour to silence our preconceptions when encountering the data (bracketing) and recount as faithfully as possible the participants' experiences and the content of their meanings without using our own versions as a basis. In this analysis method, the meaning units and the analysis encompass the entire text, not a selection of the text as in most other methods. The content from the meaning-bearing units is abstracted without the material being organised through coding. This analysis method requires a certain degree of familiarity with phenomenological philosophy (Kohak 1978, Giorgi 2009).

van Manen's practice-oriented phenomenology is widely used in education, psychology and nursing science (van Manen 2023). The method is based on phenomenological philosophy, in which the researcher studies people's life worlds by means of attitudes characterised by reduction or bracketing (see above) and "epoche"—an attitude of wonder about what we do not know for sure. These guiding principles involve both research methods and writing practices that are closer to fiction than is usual in scientific texts. This method used to be called hermeneutic phenomenology, but the name was changed because it was used in so many ways.

Thematic analysis—different options

Within thematic analysis, several different methods are available. Most of them start with the researcher establishing an *overview* of the entire material with an open mind, with varying degrees of attention to the individual participant's story. Data are then usually *coded*, leading to decontextualisation. From this point, we organise relevant text to allow parts of the material to be studied and interpreted alongside other elements that speak to the same matter. Such chunks of text are often called *meaning units*. Groups of text with relevant common features are used as a starting point for *abstracting* and summarising what the joint reading of these text elements, considering the study aim, implies. Finally, the interpretations are recontextualised and designed as a *synthesis* and *presentation* of the new understanding we have arrived at. We then need to carefully consider whether our interpretations still appropriately refer to a context with the whole from which they initially belonged, both in terms of the individual participant, the conversations from which the texts originate and the conditions under which the questions were asked. These analytical advances often overlap in practice, and the selection of one method over another is rarely critical to the quality of the outcome.

Here are some examples of cross-case analysis methods that are widely used in medical and health research with brief comparative comments. The most important thing when deciding which method to use is your supervisor's expertise and support in the choices you make, and that together you choose a method congruent to your study aim. However, once you have chosen an analysis method, it is important that you thoroughly familiarise yourself with the rules of the game and follow them, as described in your reference. One of these methods—Systematic Text Condensation—is presented in more detail in the next chapter (Malterud 2012b). If you choose one of the other analysis methods, you will need to read more about the specific procedure than what you find below.

Grounded Theory (GT) accentuates the development of theories that are anchored in empirical data (Charmaz 2024). The researcher begins with an open stance and adopts an inductive approach, applying little or no prior theoretical framework. The analysis procedure is stepwise, with open, axial and selective coding (Glaser & Strauss 1967). Open coding involves dividing the data into incidents that are coded and grouped, and axial coding identifies the connections between preliminary categories developed through repeated comparison. Finally, with selective coding, you establish a consistent narrative and a core category as a basis for what in this context is called theory development. (It may be debatable whether these are results or theory, see above.)

Interpretative Phenomenological Analysis (IPA) is based on phenomenological philosophy and is used to investigate how a given person, in a specific context, experiences and understands a given phenomenon (Smith, Jarman, et al. 1999). With this method of analysis, data from the individual participant is first summarised as a phenomenological reading within each case, and then these are placed next to each other for further cross-case thematic interpretation. To maintain the overview, the sample should not consist of more than 10 participants.

Braun and Clarke present a detailed procedure for *Reflexive Thematic Analysis* (RTA) that does not assume guidelines from specific methodological traditions, theories or philosophies (Braun & Clarke 2019, 2022). This is a pragmatic and flexible method with reflexivity as a prerequisite for situating the analysis sufficiently clearly. The purpose is to develop, interpret and report patterns towards themes in the empirical material. The analysis may be descriptive and content-oriented or interpretive with an emphasis on meaning and understanding, often a cross between these positions. In the initial steps, the material is coded broadly and comprehensively (splitting) into groups that are later lumped together (lumping) and further developed. In recent years, the authors have significantly developed the analysis method with a much stronger focus on subjectivity and the epistemology of qualitative methods known as the Big Q (see Chapter 4) (Braun & Clarke 2019, 2024c), in the same sense as in this book you are now reading. If you choose Braun and Clarke's analysis method, you should apply the latest version of their method (Braun & Clarke 2022).

Qualitative Content Analysis is a pragmatic analysis method that has many similarities with thematic analysis as described above (Graneheim & Lundman 2004). Here, each individual meaning unit is condensed and assigned a code. The codes are compared and further organised into sub-themes, which together make up the results in the form of themes (again: first splitting, then lumping). The analysis is organised around the issues from the interview guide, which are also followed through to the result themes. The authors distinguish between analyses that focus on *manifest meaning*—the immediate—or *latent meaning* (the underlying). Note that "content analysis" is a term that is also used more informally for analysing content, i.e. with no specific approach. The same term is also used to describe strategies for quantifying qualitative data (see Chapter 22).

Systematic Text Condensation (STC) has many elements from several of the methods mentioned above (Malterud 2012b). This analysis starts with a few preliminary themes (lumping), which are later refined into code groups and subgroups (moderate splitting) as the data are organised. An inductive, flexible analysis process is accomplished to keep an open mind about interpretations that are not initially accepted. STC has a specific procedure, different from the other methods of thematic analysis for condensing and abstracting data in a feasible and rigorous way. You can read more about this in the next chapter.

If you compare different analysis methods, you will notice that the terminology is not consistent. This is particularly true of the terms "theme" and "category", which in different analysis methods refer to, respectively, the first and the last steps of the analysis. There is no consistent methodological consensus on what is right or wrong here. "Meaning units", however, mean essentially the same thing no matter which method you choose, but the different methods differ in whether you use a selection or all meaning units, and also in what analytic element you subject to abstraction or condensation. The same applies to "coding" as a description of a process in which related text elements are grouped together. However, the term "code" can have slightly different meanings from one method to another. Here too, you will make it easier for yourself and your readers if you carefully organise your use of concepts in accordance with the method description in the reference you have chosen.

CHAPTER 11

From complexity to knowing—Systematic Text Condensation

Systematic Text Condensation is a method for thematic analysis of qualitative data. The method is appropriate for qualitative studies of many different types, including data from semistructured individual interviews, focus groups, observational studies or written answers to open questions from questionnaires or social media. The method is based on inductive logic, where preliminary themes are systematically elaborated further via code groups, subgroups with condensation and result categories into analytical text. Through four stages of analysis, you follow a systematic procedure that will support your knowing by relevant and robust interaction with data towards new and valuable knowledge.

Background and development

Today, several established qualitative analysis methods are available. Your priorities must be congruent with your study aim and context. Qualitative analysis is best learned through concrete efforts with your own data, supported by a supervisor or partner who has methodological experience and expertise. For the novice, it is therefore crucial that the supervisor has experience with the chosen analysis method.

Systematic Text Condensation (STC)—a method I have developed over many years interacting with students and research fellows—is not necessarily your first choice. Still, I choose to present STC here in detail as a concrete example of how the method can function as a compass that leads the way and helps you navigate steadily through the analysis.

Initially, my purpose was to offer a simple roadmap for conducting qualitative analysis in a systematic and affordable way, without the requirement for comprehensive immersion in the philosophical roots or grand theories. I soon realised that the method could just as easily be used by experienced researchers to analyse many kinds of qualitative data, with varying degrees of theoretical depth. Over the years, I have become

DOI: 10.4324/9781003786016-13

increasingly aware of the importance of the researcher recognising and respecting the theoretical assumptions associated with subjectivity and interpretation (see Chapters 2 and 4). Only then can the strengths and idiosyncrasies of qualitative research methods lead to new and valuable knowledge.

Since the original version was published (Malterud 2012b), STC has been further developed, consistent with my own methodological maturation. Feedback from teaching and observations from my own peer reviews have revealed misunderstandings explained by unclear wording in the original version, which means that the method is not always used as intended. Revised versions have subsequently been published in book chapters (in Norwegian).

If you are familiar with STC from earlier, it may therefore be a worthwhile update to read this chapter extra thoroughly, especially the paragraphs on condensation in steps 3 and 4. Below is the latest version in 2026.

Theoretical and methodological platform

Within the interpretive paradigm, STC relies on moderate social constructionism (see Chapter 2), where knowledge is assumed to be constructed and reconstructed through people's interactions and narratives in a social context, while still maintaining a realist grounding (Berger & Luckmann 1967, Nagel 1986, Lock & Strong 2010, Smith 2010). The exploration of subjective phenomena is thus recognised as a valid starting point for scientific knowing. At the same time, empirical data has a strong value—not as facts and truth, but as foundations for interpretation and analysis and as a committed material link to the ontological level of health and social care.

A well-designed study aim and prolific empirical data are crucial for strong Information Power (IP) with analysis of appropriate quality. As health researchers, we are often close to practice with an expectation from ourselves and others to develop knowing that can support better understanding and services (Malterud 2001a, Thorne 2025). We may already draw on field knowledge that supports the meaning and IP of our empirical data. STC embodies an inductive logic in accordance with the Big Q (see Chapter 4), with theoretical perspectives nevertheless substantial to situate interpretation, sharpen focus and enable abstraction (Malterud 2016, Guassora, Reventlow, et al. 2022).

It is worthwhile to conduct the analysis together with another researcher—not for consensus, but to create an analytical space with more nuances. However, the more researchers who conduct the analysis together, the more extensive and time-consuming the process becomes. It is not a given that the more people we have, the better the result. Personally, I find two preferable to one, and three preferable to four. Ten is simply too many. A recipe-like presentation of how to proceed, step by step, as presented below, may give the impression that the analysis is carried out as a technical and linear procedure. However, interpretation and subjectivity can never be organised in a manual without losing their distinctive features and being digested by the instrumentalist error (see Chapter 1). The analysis must be conducted as a flexible process, where three steps forward and two steps back are the norm. In a project with appropriate IP, your creative interpretations of data determine whether the analysis leads to new and valuable scientific evidence. Nevertheless, follow the recommendations in the method description quite closely until you are sufficiently familiar with the terrain to leave the compass at home.

Table 11.1 shows an overview of the different steps in the analysis process in STC and presents the key terms with their site and meaning in STC

Analysis step	*Terminology—Systematic Text Condensation*
1	**Preliminary themes** (5–8?) are identified at the first reading
2	Preliminary themes provide the basis for negotiating **codes** for sorting meaning units into **code groups**. Codes are adjusted and defined in the coding process
3	Each code group is subdivided **into subgroups** (2–3) that each highlight different aspects of the content of the code group. Abstraction is carried out by developing a **condensate** from each subgroup
4	**Result categories** (3–5) are developed by synthesising the meaning content from each of the code groups based on the condensates from the subgroups. This forms the basis for the subsections in the results chapter.

Terminology

Methodology literature often demonstrates how the same term can have different meanings for different authors. In this book, I try to keep the terms as close as possible to their meaning in everyday speech (Table 11.1).

Symptoms of irritable bowel syndrome—an example

Below, I present the specific procedure for conducting a thematic analysis with STC. My presentation is illustrated by a fictional project where we explore symptom distress among patients with irritable bowel syndrome (a chronic and troublesome digestive disease) based on empirical data from ten semistructured individual interviews.

To give you an overview of the process, I describe the analysis process as if you were working with the entire material, in this example, with data from ten interviews. Nevertheless, be aware of the benefits of conducting the analysis in stages, for example starting with the first four interviews, using this to adjust the course of interview focus and recruitment based on what we learn along the way. Read more about preliminary analysis and subsequent rounds of analysis later in this chapter.

In this project, the goal of the analysis is to approach knowledge about the participants' *symptom concerns* (not their medical history, life course or nutritional status). In the example, the researcher's *preconception* is characterised by many years of clinical experience with patients with such digestive complaints. In this project, the researcher's theoretical ambitions and expertise are quite moderate, but nevertheless contribute to situating the project and focusing the analysis (Malterud 2016, Guassora, Reventlow, et al. 2022). The researcher is informed by *theoretical perspectives* on "explanatory models"—professionals' and lay people's explanatory models for how disease occurs and develops (Kleinman 1980).

Four-step analysis with laundry as a metaphor

The analysis consists of four steps: (1) obtain an overall impression and develop *preliminary themes*, (2) identify *meaning units* and organise them into *code groups*, (3)

split each code group into *subgroups* and conduct analytical abstraction by developing an empirically based *condensate* from each subgroup, and (4) rework each code group into analytical paragraphs using the subgroup condensates to synthesise *the result categories* that constitute the main results (see Chapter 12) (Malterud 2012b).

Most methods for thematic analysis start by taking a broad and open approach to the material (Graneheim & Lundman 2004, Braun & Clarke 2022). In STC, on the other hand, we initially develop a quite small number of preliminary themes and code groups that we develop further. The process of abstraction, once the data has been coded, with the conception of an empirically based condensate for each of the subgroups, is also distinctive to STC. Below, I describe how this is carried out in practice.

An everyday metaphor (laundry) concretises the review of the four steps of analysis. We start by imagining a pile of dirty clothes to be washed and sorted. The clean clothes are then to be placed in a chest of drawers. The chest of drawers is flat-packed and must be assembled, and the drawers can be optimised for different types of clean clothes. Each dresser drawer is labelled to indicate what is in the drawer. We revise this label as we see what fits in each of the drawers. Finally, we will sew something new from the sorted contents of each drawer. The new textiles will also be given names. Finally, these will be displayed at an exhibition. The names will serve as a concentrated and abstracted understanding of the meaning and content of the new textiles.

The raw data are the audio recording from the first four interviews (the laundry where the washing starts). In the transcription process, the raw data are cleaned (putting the dirty laundry through the washing machine's programme for colour washing). We start the analysis process with a large pile of dry and freshly washed laundry in all colours.

If this sounds strange to you, you will understand more as you read on, and even more when you encounter your own data hands-on.

1. *Overall impression—from chaos to preliminary themes*

In the first step, we familiarise ourselves with the material. We read the transcripts to get an overall impression and develop some (5–8?) preliminary themes that somehow express something about the participants' symptom concerns. At this stage, we work actively to temporarily set aside our preconceptions and theoretical perspectives, to be open to the overall impression. However, we do not set the study aim aside, and concepts from the project's substantive theory (here: explanatory models) remind the researcher to attend to the lay perspective. We also actively try to put aside what we already think we know about symptom concerns among patients with irritable bowel syndrome.

The interpretation is already underway, and for now, it is the bird's eye view that counts. If the analysis is to be feasible and meaningful, the data material must not be too extensive. The work at this stage can be done in an armchair or on a sofa. We can take notes as we read, but otherwise we should primarily form impressions at this stage and resist any urge to systematise.

Once we have read everything, we ask ourselves what *preliminary themes* from the text may suggest about different types of concerns that digestive problems may arouse in participants. 5–8 themes are feasible—10 are always too many. Unlike most thematic analysis methods, this approach does not begin with numerous codes to review and summarise later. We return to the laundry and take a quick look at all the garments—check what we have in the pile of clean laundry and start considering which main groups are useful for further organisation. We can sort by type of garment (socks, underpants, T-shirts shirts, blouses and jumpers). Or we can sort by who owns the garments (Eve, John, Martin, Anne, Christine, Elisabeth). It is also possible to sort by colour (red, blue, yellow, green or purple garments). Which sorting principle is best depends on what these piles of clothes are meant for. If we are going to make rag rugs later, we might choose colour sorting, while the laundry that is returned into the chest of drawers in the children's room is sorted by owner.

Browsing the data will provide new impressions, ideas and a basis for interpretation. In creative and inductive analysis, preliminary themes rarely match the paragraphs in the interview guide. If preliminary themes are too similar to the starting point, we may be pursuing our preconceptions rather than proceeding towards new patterns. In STC, we prepare a list in which the preliminary themes are each given an interim name, such as

- something dangerous
- rumbling
- socialising
- inflammation in the body
- how will it go?
- stress

The preliminary themes are neither results nor categories. These concepts have not yet been developed through interpretation and systematic reflection. They represent only a first inductive step in organising the material, suggesting provisional answers to the study aim. Examples of superficial analytic strategies can be observed in articles where only this step has been accomplished. In the presentation of the results, we then revisit the same themes as headings, often followed by lively quotes. However, if your goal is to apply a relevant and robust method, a great deal of interpretive work remains after this first step. The analysis method will help you navigate through a structured review of the material in several steps.

2. *From preliminary themes to code groups and meaning units*

Each researcher then drafts a brief list of preliminary themes and meets with the small research team to negotiate shared and divergent interpretations. It is by no means certain that the most important matters are what you agree upon. That is why it pays to spend time discussing our understanding of the preliminary themes we have set up, and how they can best be expected to shed light on the study aim. We will then reformulate the terms we first came up with, agreeing on 3–5 revised themes that form the basis for *code groups* in this step of the analysis. Ten code groups are always too many and invite superficial analysis with meagre results.

Now we are going to organise the part of the data that proceeds to close reading. We put aside the remaining, which is not included in the analysis. We start by reviewing the data line by line to identify, organise and sort *meaning units*. These are text elements that could conceivably shed light on our study aim; therefore, we now differentiate between relevant and irrelevant text. All text is systematically reviewed line by line, so that we do not just include what seems most compelling.

We are now sitting at our desks or keyboards. Imagine that our empirical data are freshly washed and dried laundry (the meaning units). We will now sort the laundry, removing what cannot be used for the purpose, while the remaining should be distributed in the drawers of the chest of drawers in a way that is constructive for further work with these garments.

For the next level of analysis, we concentrate on meaning units—text elements that carry knowledge about one or more of the preliminary themes from the first step and thereby express something about our study aim (different aspects of symptom distress). A meaning unit is delineated by meaningful content, not by volume or responses, usually including approximately 2–8 lines.

When we harvest and sort meaning units, we have the code groups in mind. Marking the meaning units in the text, we also begin to organise and systematise them. Using the code groups as a guide, we select chunks of text. According to their content, they are now labelled with a *code*—a tag that brings together meaning units that have something in common into code groups. This is called *coding*. In coding, we aim to organise all included meaning units by the different ways in which they articulate content related to the study aim. At this point, we prioritise and establish a manageable number of code groups (3–5?). Ten is always too many, even here.

Coding can be compared to sorting the garments we have approved for further use. These will be placed in different drawers in the new chest of drawers. We start by assembling the flat-packed dresser, knowing that we will have to adjust the system of drawers over time. If the chest has too many drawers, we will lose the overview, and sorting will be blurred. First, we label the drawers with the tags (codes) that we have agreed upon as names for the code groups. These are developed and revised as the data gives us input and ideas. As soon as we start sorting, we realise that it is useful to further elaborate and refine the intuitive classification that the first version of the code groups represents. Perhaps a code group appears to entail two or more separate phenomena, or perhaps some code groups deal with different aspects of something that are actually the same thing. Or perhaps the data are pushing us towards a new code group.

For example, in our project about symptom concerns in irritable bowel syndrome, we sort what we initially called "rumbling" into the code group "socialising", because the participants describe rumbling as something that worries them in social situations. Perhaps the code we originally chose is not sufficiently specific to delimit what we are looking for. Instead, we can reinterpret what we initially labelled "something dangerous" to "serious illness".

Now we also consider whether our codes include phenomena of roughly the same class. The content of each code group will eventually form the basis for accounts of symptom concerns that in one way or another have something in common. Still, the code groups must become increasingly distinct and durable—they ought to be mutually exclusive and differentiate text that deals with different phenomena. This process is related to Constant Comparison, a procedure from Grounded Theory (Glaser & Strauss 1967).

During coding, with the study aim, preconceptions and theoretical perspectives in mind, we discard phenomena that stand out as foreign elements and differ significantly from others. Using the laundry metaphor, we can say that socks, underpants, T-shirts, blouses and jumpers represent different forms of clothing, but we do not include tablecloths or bedclothes.

In our example, we decide to proceed with code groups that all represent different aspects of concerns about the impact of the symptoms on the future ("serious illness", "socialising", "inflammation in the body", "how will it go?"). "Stress", on the other hand, appears as a foreign element alongside these.

We stop and wonder how such a tablecloth can sneak in among socks and blouses, revealing that this indicates how preconceptions about causality had sneaked into the first stage of the analysis. We remove this matter from further analysis because it does not say much about symptom concerns, which is our study aim. Such choices may readily be reported continuously in the *decision trail*—an important tool for recording choices in an inductive analysis (see Chapters 6 and 10). Without tracks, it can feel insurmountable to reverse the process, even when you are not completely satisfied.

A gradual transformation from theme to code and on to *revised code groups* means that we change the original sorting principles flexibly in accordance with what we learn in the face of data. Again, only when the researcher takes three steps forward and two steps back is it possible to capitalise on the growing insight gained from proximity to the material.

We imagine that we adapt the conceptual framing of the drawers in the chest of drawers as we see what finally belongs in each drawer, with corresponding changes of labelling along the way. We also need some blank labels available so that we do not slavishly follow the first and best categorisation principle. Text that does not shed light on the study's aim should not be included, even if it may look interesting.

In our example, we sort the meaning units into the code groups

- serious illness
- gradual social isolation
- spread to the rest of the body
- deterioration

Along the way in the coding process, text appears that causes us to add a new code group that we call

- inheritance

When we establish new code groups during this stage of the analysis, we return to the text we have already reviewed, so that we now include, for example, all meaning units with text about symptom concerns related to parents or children. Such a process gives access to conceive of something new and elaborate it further in a systematic way. It is therefore crucial that our empirical data remain of a manageable scope. In this example, the preliminary analysis has 40 pages of transcribed text, while the final material, which in this project originates from ten participants, may amount to 100 pages of transcribed text.

You may code one and the same meaning unit into several code groups. However, if there is a lot of double or triple coding, this indicates that your codes are not sufficiently distinctly targeted. In this case, it may be worth taking a few steps back and considering whether some of the code groups ought to be merged or reformulated. Again, the decision trail is an important tool for reflection and learning. Each of the codes and code groups contains many different nuances and can be further sub-grouped. With other analysis methods, this is done as part of the coding process. However, it can be easy to lose the overview, and in STC such strategies belong in the third step of analysis.

In practice, the coding process can be accomplished in many ways. Personally, I prefer scissors and paper to prevent a linear process. If you use digital tools, remember that the computer program performs neither interpretation nor analysis, but only assists you in organising the text. Software is not an analysis method, just a technical device for organising data.

Some software tools may also draw you into logics of analysis that are not compatible with the STC process or even with the Big Q (see Chapter 4).

Coding involves systematic *decontextualisation*, where parts of the text are removed from their original context. On your way from raw data to preliminary themes in the first stage of analysis, and then from themes to code groups in this stage of analysis, it can be helpful to look back from time to time to identify the hidden rules you used to establish the code groups, and what criteria you chose to include or exclude meaning units in each code group. It is not always easy to grasp this clearly, but it is easier if we admit that we probably follow a tacit logic, perhaps without realising it. This logic represents our definition of the codes.

Along the way, we may find that we have included very few meaning units in some code groups. We then consider whether these belong in other code groups, or perhaps, on reflection, do not count as meaning units. Other code groups can be so voluminous that it is appropriate to split them up. However, we should still exercise quite strict moderation regarding the number of code groups (3–5) for interpretation and analysis to contribute to the development of a few convincing, durable and original result categories expanded through your analytical text (see below and Chapter 12). The alternative could be a superficial analysis with fragmented results.

We may reflect upon our code groups and the phenomena and concepts they signify. Have I organised a pile of clothes? What do I really mean by socks? Feel free to use the decision trail to enter preliminary definitions of the codes as they eventually appear. If you do not manage to put this into words that you can share with yourself when the coding is complete, you are unlikely to convince the reader that this was a substantial and clear unit for sorting and organising meaning units. Nevertheless, do not waste too much time on discussing inclusion or exclusion of the single meaning unit. Such decisions are closer to everyday life than to laboratory research.

The contents of the code groups are still not results, just bundles of meaning units that you have organised and sorted. Several stages remain in the analysis process, involving interpretation, abstraction and synthesis of what will count as relevant and robust knowledge with transferability to situations beyond where we originally collected our data.

3. Abstraction—from code groups to subgroups, each affording a condensate

In our fictional study, we have now reduced the empirical data to a selected corpus of text, consisting of meaning units organised into 3–5 code groups that may lead to new and valuable knowledge about the kinds of concerns digestive symptoms can cause. In the third step of analysis, we will now interpret and abstract data by creating condensates from subgroups through a systematic process.

The process in this step of the analysis is unique to STC and does not appear in comparable thematic analysis methods for thematic analysis. Feel free to re-read this section a couple of times as you work through this step of the analysis process. If you are already familiar with STC, you may also spot new elements here.

Each code group represents a drawer in the dresser. Each drawer contains many different garments, and the process in the previous step of the analysis has ensured that each drawer differs from the other drawers so that we can distinctly notice the difference, both by looking at the labels and when we open the drawer. In this analysis step, we begin to sew together the old garments in each drawer as a basis for our new creation that will eventually be exhibited. Every single garment will be assessed in this process.

We pull out a drawer and place all meaning units from this code group on the table. Later we will return to the other code groups.

First, we split the meaning units from this code group into 2–3 *subgroups*, each representing a key aspect of this code group. In practice, I do this by laying out all the meaning units from this code group on the table and sorting them, like a jigsaw puzzle. We consider which meaning units express something about roughly the same thing, and which thereby together constitute a subgroup. You need to decide what main aspects of this code group the data best describes, though without investing time in naming it. Do not create many subgroups—again, this runs the risk of losing the overview. In the code group "serious illness", there may for example be texts about cancer, bowel obstruction or ulcerative colitis.

In what follows, we will concentrate on subgroups and how we conduct analytical, empirically based abstraction from the meaning units they each contain. From here, we will follow a distinct, systematic procedure to develop a *condensate*. The condensate will become your working note as a basis for the articulation of results in the fourth and final stage of the analysis process. Imagine that we are sewing together old garments that will eventually become the front and back of the new creation. If you choose to drop or reshape this analytic element, you should not call your analysis STC.

The condensate is a text that presents our abstraction of the sum of the participants' voices about what we gathered in the actual subgroup, for example, concerns about death. From this subgroup, we systematically go through every single meaning unit and collate contributions to a condensate text that we build up and edit in logical order. Ideally, we start with a strong and expressive meaning unit and build up with text from the other meaning units around this text. When multiple meaning units in this subgroup express similar ideas, we choose the expression that best reflects the related texts, without repeating the other ones. In other words, each individual meaning unit is assessed as of whether it brings something new. Nor are we going to list the meaning units one after the other or to draft an intuitive summary. Abstraction through condensation is a more specific procedure, intended to capture and co-edit all relevant nuances of the actual subgroup's contributions to a coherent expression capable to elucidate the study aim.

We write the condensate in the first person to remind us that we now will speak for each of the participants, preferably roughly in the language they used during the interview. We try to be as close to the text as possible, incorporating expressions from the participants and avoiding theoretical terms that we have brought with us from earlier. We review every single meaning unit in this subgroup and decide whether it can be included, or whether, on closer examination, it does not provide text for the condensate. Perhaps it fits better in one of the other subgroups or code groups, or perhaps it is removed from the analysis because it does not contribute anything relevant to the study aim.

In this way, the content of each of the subgroups within each code group is abstracted and condensed in the form of a text in which we co-edit the expressions from the meaning-bearing units. We review the entire empirical material systematically, while asking ourselves what the condensate can communicate about the problem. In other words, the condensate is not an intuitive summary, but a text that you have designed and edited according to a specific procedure.

From the subgroup on cancer within the code group "serious illness", we might develop such a condensate:

> I can't let go of the idea that it's really cancer. Regardless of what the doctors say, I know that this is something more serious than nerves. My uncle also had similar problems, and he died of bile duct cancer. Cancer is a terrible disease—every time my stomach inflates, I get scared of how this will end. My father died suddenly on a mountain hike—it's much better than being addicted and in pain for the rest of my life.

So, this is not a quote, but a working text that compiles, recaps and abstracts what has been congregated in this subgroup, with clear traces of all included meaning-bearing units, carrying the words and concepts of the participants. Note that I do not use quotation marks here.

Next, we select a "golden quote"—an authentic quote that illustrates what has been abstracted above, for example:

> "As much pain as I'm in, it can't possibly be anything other than cancer. It's certainly not psychological."

Sequentially, we review the other subgroups in the same code group, developing condensates from these. We then repeat with subgroups and condensates from the other code groups. Again, we take the opportunity to revise the code groups as the subgroups pass on to us with new insights about the study aim.

4. *Synthesis—from condensates to analytical text and result categories*

In the fourth step, we put the pieces back together, *recontextualising*. We will now *synthesise* and articulate the result categories with their corresponding analytical text (see Chapter 12), presenting our main results. Here we will practice emergence (see Chapter 1) by further developing the complexity, combining the individual parts (from meaning units via condensates) into new insights, processed as analytical text (Smith 2010). The synthesis must be communicated in a way that is trustworthy and respectful to the participants' accounts. At the same time, you raise the text above a descriptive level, taking responsibility for analytical interpretations proceeding towards new knowledge. In the preceding steps, we have dealt with detached pieces of text. Now, we must also assess whether the results still constitute a relevant and robust description from the context where they originate.

Our synthesis conveys to the reader how our interpretations answer our study aim. In turn, we open each of the drawers in the chest of drawers. For each code group, we retrieve what we sewed together in the previous step of analysis as condensates from two to three subgroups. For each code group, the condensates will now be finalised as a new garment, where all the usable old garments have been recycled. First, we review and elaborate the knowledge from each code group towards result categories with analytical text.

We rework the subgroup condensates from each code group to synthesise two to three major aspects of each result category, presenting them as analytical paragraphs under a shared subheading that conceptualises the result category. In the analytical text, we tend to use expressions that originate from the meaning units, but not in the form of a series of quotes. Now we write in the third person, because the researcher's role at this step is to act as storyteller with an interpretive mission.

In the results section, I do not give subgroup paragraphs specific subtitles to prevent misleading detail levels and unnecessary fragmentation. Sometimes, it happens that peer reviewers request a table to present the analytical process. However, with STC, such tables present a misleading, static view of the analysis. Therefore, it may be necessary to reject such a demand. Yet, at this stage of the analysis, I must still consider what each of the subgroups contributes in terms of analytical text for the result category that the code group with condensates from the subgroups will now be developed into.

For example, an analytical text about cancer concerns might look like this:

> Many participants said that they thought a lot about whether their symptoms could indicate cancer. Several mentioned that it was difficult to understand that abdominal pain of such intensity could be harmless. A 42-year-old woman had recently watched a TV programme that emphasised the importance of contacting the doctor when her bowel movements changed. She herself had suffered from intermittent constipation and diarrhoea for the past ten years but felt that her doctor had downplayed this. In our material, several of the participants told dramatic stories about family and friends who had been diagnosed with cancer after a long period of suffering. Stomach cancer was perceived as particularly serious.

This analytical text from the synthesis of one of the subgroups conveys a selected, relevant aspect of one of the result categories in our research project, which is about concerns about serious illness. The synthesis is an abstraction that conveys commonalities with variations from several unique stories that we have compiled and abstracted through analysis—not as a continuous chain of individual meaning units. Still, we may sometimes let one participant speak. The quotes illustrate specific nuances of the results presented in the analytical text. While writing, it may turn out that some subgroups are not sufficiently rooted in the material for it to be possible to make such a summary and must therefore be deleted. Similarly, we repeat the procedure for the subgroups within each code group.

We will now create an appropriate name for the new garment we have created, based on a well-chosen selection of the old garments. Although the names of the *result categories* are rooted in the original themes and codes, they must establish conceptual development from the analysis process. Renaming each of the result categories (with analytical text and quotes from the subgroups in this code group), we develop a short, self-contained designation of the most important results, recalling in short form what we came up with ("what is the name of this?"), which is an outcome—something else than what we wanted to investigate. It is well worth the effort to spend time and thought on this last part. A distinct, short version of this can be regarded as a micro-condensate.

But the analysis is still not yet complete. We need to validate the results—the analytical texts and the names of the result categories—against the context from which they were extracted, recontextualising the results with the empirical material. Feel free to read the original transcripts to be reminded of what was said. We should not expect all parts of our analytical text to be linkable to each individual participant, but we should stop if we realise that we are trading with interpretations, descriptions or concepts with uncertain anchoring in the raw data. This validation is not reported in the article.

To challenge our results, we also look systematically for data that contradicts the conclusions we have reached. If we notice that some participants have contributed very little text at all, we should raise critical questions. However, there is nothing unusual or problematic about some participants making particularly rich or controversial contributions—we simply take this into account when we discuss transferability. Although we do not emphasise numbers and scope in qualitative studies, there are differences between knowledge that is rooted in large parts of the material and knowledge that mainly originates from one or a few participants.

Analysis also includes an assessment of what we have come up with, compared to existing research. Emphasise new and valuable results rather than confirming the results of others. In the example above, the researcher should reassess their literature search and see if similar results have already been presented by others. If this is the case, the relevance of the results is weak, and a new round of analyses can be considered.

Inductive logic and iterative process—three steps forward and two steps back

Analysing empirical data with STC rests on an *inductive* logic that safeguards subjectivity and uniqueness (Gatens-Robinson 1986, Sandelowski 1996). Even if we maintain a steady course as we navigate through the forest, the trip only becomes exciting with an open and flexible view of which paths can provide the best views. Theoretical perspectives also contribute to insights that may sharpen focus and adjust the course (Guassora, Reventlow, et al. 2022). New and valuable knowledge is perhaps best established in unfamiliar terrain. But then it is important not to get lost in the forest.

In this way, analysis is a challenging balance between rigorous procedures and creative power. We often must take a few steps back to consider alternative paths. If we stay on a predetermined course, we run the risk of ending up in a deductive dead end pursuing our preconceptions, perhaps out of a small q misguided positivist loyalty to the starting point (see Chapter 4). Furthermore, in such cases, we may neglect the impact of the empirical data. Therefore, this is not a constructive strategy when you aim for new and valuable knowledge rooted in subjectivity. Some describe their project in humble terms as descriptive or exploratory, which can also lead to a risk of deficient analytical courage.

Iteration means repeating something many times. Doctors know that reiteration of prescriptions means that they can be used several times. An *iterative* process is characterised by movement. In qualitative analysis, this has the specific meaning in that we do not take two steps forward and two steps back, but rather three steps forward and two steps back. We do not move mechanically and linearly but stop to invite reflection. In this way, we may spot new patterns that refresh our interpretations. But an iterative process can also lead to a lack of momentum and be used to justify untidy processes, sometimes associated with a procrastinating writing block.

Knowing the path we have taken allows us to understand and share substantial choices in the analytical process. To arrive at our results, we must also follow a relevant and robust procedure that we can account for, so that we return to the previous interpretive position if that seems more productive than where we are. In other words, this is not the free approach method. With systematic procedures, the analysis method can serve as support for creative theory-informed interpretations and empirically based abstractions, without the results becoming random opinion or narrow local knowledge, and we can maintain an overview and strengthen intersubjectivity and transferability (Malterud 1993, 2001b).

The analysis must be open for questions we did not realise we could have asked and suggestions for answers to these. We must ensure that there is sufficient flexibility to make room for emergence (see Chapter 1)—that we perceive and develop patterns and combinations that were not initially obvious. If the analysis has led to surprises, we have seen something we did not know before—this is an excellent sign. With qualitative analysis, several valid interpretations can exist concurrently. The study's aim and the theoretical perspectives provide support and context for interpretations that can yield the most relevant results (Guassora, Reventlow, et al. 2022), and a systematic approach contributes to a robust framework and intersubjectivity. It is therefore important not to be locked into a perception that the analysis is or should be a linear process that can be presented as a table (see above).

Figure 11.1 illustrates the differences between a deductive analysis following a linear process without deviations (top), compared with an inductive, iterative analysis (bottom), as suggested by STC. When we move our interpretive focus back and forth between different parts of the empirical data, the opportunities for emergence—where we establish something new—are greater than if we try to collate everything that has been said into themes we brought with us initially. In practice, the most important thing is that you do not insist to preserve the main points from the interview guide when it comes to data development and analysis. Then you will easily stumble into your preconceptions.

Stepwise analysis and subsequent analytic sequences

Stepwise analysis during the data development phase, preferably before the formal analysis phase has begun, enhances the possibility to sharpen the project's focus and study aim. This will also support an overview of the material. Stepwise analysis prevents "the 1000 page problem" (Kvale 1996), where the researcher never manages to complete a proper analysis of a large, confusing and partly irrelevant material. Stepwise analysis is particularly relevant for projects based on individual interviews,

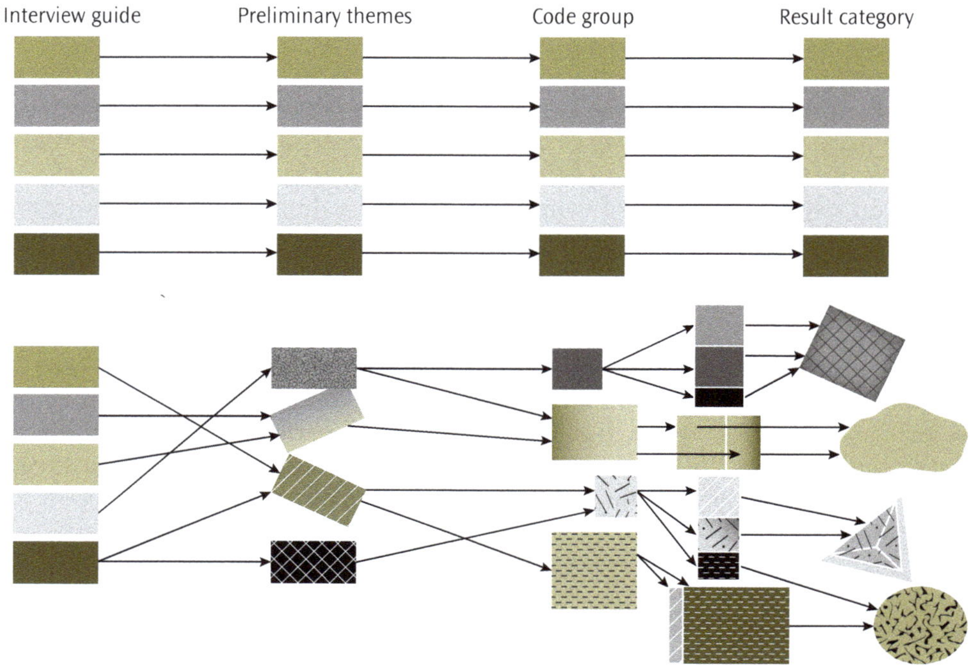

Figure 11.1 Analysis from interview guide to results with inductive logic (bottom) or deductive logic (top) (from Malterud (2025))

though often unnecessary in focus group studies. Here, I describe how you can do a stepwise analysis in STC. If you choose a different thematic method, you may consider how to transfer some of the principles so that you can pass on the benefits of such a strategy.

In the first preliminary sequence of analysis, you carry out step 1, step 2 and partly step 3 as described above. In a limited amount of data, you can establish preliminary themes, develop code groups and harvest and sort meaning units. In addition, you can make a tentative assessment of possible subgroups within each code group, but stop there. If you proceed with STC, abstracting the content of the sub-groups as a condensate, you may risk shutting down further creativity in the process during preliminary analysis. Instead, take a close look at your code groups and subgroups and consider how your sense can contribute to useful adjustments for further data development. You may also want to alter the study aim somewhat because you see traces of other interesting aspects in your material that you would rather choose to pursue.

Once you have conducted several interviews, you are ready to start the next sequence of analysis. Follow the procedure for step 1, reading the new data to reconsider the code groups established in the first sequence of analysis. You can leave the old material at rest now, until you have decided whether new relevant patterns are being generated or whether the initial code groups require modification. In step 2, the meaning units in the new material are reviewed. These are added to the meaning units that you harvested and sorted in the previous round of analyses. You use the revised code groups as a basis for sorting. You then complete the analysis by organising subgroups and developing condensates in step 3, and finally synthesis and analytical text in step 4.

If you are seriously in doubt as to whether your empirical data provide sufficient material for new and valuable knowing, you can close the process for the time being without finalising the analytical text. The decision trail is a helpful support for taking a step back in the process. With the replenishment of new data, you can then go straight to the condensates, strengthen and adjust these and proceed to synthesis with the preparation of analytical text, see for example (Schaufel, Nordrehaug, et al. 2011). The repetitions in such a stepwise analysis may seem unnecessarily meticulous. However, this kind of systematic approach provides support and rigour as we gradually work our way towards an increasingly focused problem, where it becomes clearer what we want to know more about. In this way, the project's IP may be strengthened, and data can be utilised even better (Malterud, Siersma, et al. 2021).

Detailed procedures or creative interpretation—yes please, both

The more intuitively the analysis is carried out, the more difficult it is to understand (reflexivity) and communicate (intersubjectivity) what you have done. The procedure description for STC demonstrates a comprehensive and time-consuming procedure where analysis is not an impressionistic and private matter. In that sense, it gives a correct picture of qualitative analysis not being something you do in passing. Nevertheless, many researchers experience that STC provides a clear and detailed compass that strengthens the project's progress and feasibility.

Some would argue that content and meaning are overridden by structure and proceduralism in this way. There can be many reasons for choosing other analysis methods, and this is a relevant argument. The details are included here to give the novice a concrete and practical starting point where approaches, procedures and metaphors demonstrate how the assumptions can be put into practice. The experienced researcher can move more freely through the material without losing control of the process, but novices and experts alike need to conduct qualitative analysis in a systematic yet open manner.

Nevertheless, qualitative analysis is not a technical or mechanical practice, but a strategy characterised by the creative and informed management of subjectivity and interpretation. Even if the analysis is carried out 100% methodologically correct and accurately reproduces the participants' stories, it is not at all certain that this will lead to appropriate research with new and valuable results (see next chapter). There are many examples of qualitative studies that are instrumentalised when the methodological aspects take precedence at the expense of knowledge development. This is called *methodolatry* (Chamberlain 2000) and is not a direction encouraged by STC.

Many paths to the goal—thematic analysis, phenomenology and beyond

STC is one of several quite closely related methods for thematic analysis (Graneheim & Lundman 2004, Braun & Clarke 2019, 2022). There are also other strategies for analysis beyond thematic analysis. Feel free to choose another method if you are not comfortable with the assumptions and approaches of STC, rather than modifying or excluding elements that you do not like or understand. However, if you refer to STC, the reader will expect that you have followed the prescribed procedure.

Although Giorgi's psychological phenomenological method of analysis was an important inspiration for STC (Giorgi 1985), STC is not a phenomenological analysis method. For STC, social constructionism (Berger & Luckmann 1967, Smith 2010) is a more appropriate philosophical basis (see Chapter 2), not phenomenology (Kohak 1978). I share the phenomenologists' assumption that subjective experiences are valid knowledge. Still, with STC, we do not immerse ourselves in the lifeworld as a fundamental perspective for analysis. However, whilst there are some similarities, there are important differences.

In step 1 of the analysis with STC, we try to tone down our own experiences so as not to drown out the voices of the participants. This attitude is related to the phenomenological concept of *bracketing*, which means that the researcher sets aside their own experiences. With STC, we emphasise the recognition and significance of the researcher's point of view as a prerequisite for situated knowledge (Haraway 1991, Steier 1991). We do not, however, consider it desirable or possible to maintain such an analytical distance throughout the project.

The phenomenological method seeks *the essence* of the object through gradual reduction. With STC, we do not explore essences but are more concerned with subjectivity as diversity. In line with social constructionism, we imagine that a phenomenon can appear in different versions, depending on perspective.

A resemblance between phenomenological analysis and STC is nevertheless that the analysis should describe the most relevant aspects of the phenomenon we are investigating as accurately and carefully as possible, including relationships to other phenomena. In other words, we are concerned with the context of subjectivity, which by the way also applies to most qualitative methods.

Compared to other methods of thematic analysis, STC offers affordable and feasible premises for the analysis, particularly by limiting the scope of preliminary themes, code groups and result categories. The method favours projects with limited amounts of empirical data, ensuring appropriate IP, and encourages creative interpretations supported by inspiring substantive theories rather than descriptive reproduction of what participants have said. The process of empirically based abstraction by condensation described in step 3 is a specific prerequisite for conducting STC, different from for example the more theoretically based abstraction of Thematic Reflexive Analysis (Braun & Clarke 2022). This type of condensation can be demanding to understand and learn, but it makes the approach to abstraction, synthesis and transferability significantly easier and clearer and represents a systematic approach that can otherwise be difficult to maintain and report.

CHAPTER 12

What counts as a result—and what does not?

The outcome of the analysis is the reward and the proof of delivery from the knowledge development of the project. Your results are intended to convince the reader that you reached a provisional conclusion with knowledge that contributes something new and valuable. It is distinctly different from where your colleagues finished and you started, and thus a fruitful starting point for further elaboration and application. With the results, we transmit our interpretations and conclusions as evidence to be peer-reviewed, published and shared so that others can assess validity and relevance for theory and practice. The results section is the core of the article or thesis, with the introduction, methods section and discussion demonstrating assumptions and reflexivity. Presenting results with a potential impact for colleagues and patients requires scientific, methodological and literary expertise. Therefore, the research process must, from the outset, involve an understanding of the demands placed on where we are heading—what we will share at the end. This is about more than technical writing skills.

Why this question must be asked

It may seem obvious that the result is what we read in the results section of an article or a thesis. Still, even technically sound studies can leave readers questioning the authors' actual contributions. As a supervisor, researcher, peer reviewer and opponent, over the years, I have read many articles and theses presenting qualitative studies. I am concerned about an increasing tendency towards important flaws in what is presented as results. This may be due to deficient understanding of the researcher's mission in qualitative studies, where the researcher is an explorer in a previously unfamiliar terrain.

This challenge has become particularly clear to me in my pursuits of qualitative metasynthesis, in which we identify, interpret and summarise the results of qualitative primary studies on a specific matter (see Chapter 18). Qualitative metasynthesis uses

DOI: 10.4324/97810037860´6-14

the evidence from prior studies as empirical raw data to be elaborated, summarised and synthesised in the analysis. In my experience, the results sections or summaries of qualitative primary studies meant for inclusion may contain disappointingly little raw material for analysis. The studies in question may be of poor scientific quality, even though they have been conducted in accordance with the most rigorous checklists and published in high-status journals.

Such concerns are warnings about much more than problems with raw material for metasynthesis, namely a potential lack of shared understanding of what a qualitative study is supposed to provide. With weak, unclear or self-evident results, the contributions of qualitative studies to the knowledge base become unconvincing.

Some of these shortcomings are so pervasive that they deserve a note in an introductory book like this. For the novice, it is particularly important to avoid flaws in the development and presentation of results that will jeopardise the scientific quality of a study that otherwise requires a lot of effort. Here are some ideals, concepts and recommendations, while specific advice on implementation follows in the next chapter.

The common thread

The analysis shall link the research question and the results. As a researcher, I am responsible for developing a clear common thread between the questions that follow from the project's study aim and the conclusions we present at the end. Without clear questions, we will not get clear answers, and without a well-developed study aim, we will never be able to develop results with an impact. The common thread will reflect the project's internal validity (see Chapters 3 and 21). To navigate creatively through the material while maintaining a steady course towards fresh answers or questions, we need a sufficiently clear sense of what we are exploring.

Our results also must make obvious that the researcher is well-informed about the literature in the field and substantiate how and why we come up with something that supplements, challenges or deviates from what is already known. For many years, the British Medical Journal has asked its authors to answer these two questions:

- What is known from before?
- What does this study add?

If your results do not provide a good answer to the last question, it may be due to incomplete analysis or insufficiently focused study aim.

Conceptualising result categories

This chapter is not intended as a manual for writing academic articles—that follows in the next chapter. However, it may be helpful to get to know some concepts in this non-fiction literary genre that can sharpen your attention as you prepare to share your results. This is about the format and content that is required and expected in a journal article or a thesis. Here we concentrate on the article format, but the terms below can be used in all kinds of presentation of qualitative studies.

In a journal article, there is not sufficient space to present plenty of results, without running the risk that the presentation becomes meagre and superficial. Hence, we should select and refine carefully what we want to render at the finish line. Even in journals without word restrictions, in the results section, it is a splendid idea to prioritise only your most important messages, presented for example in the form of two to four *result categories* (some call these "themes"). Result categories do not emerge from nothing. They convey your interpretation of selected, relevant answers to various aspects of the study aim—*what this study adds.*

The results section of your article starts with a short, overarching introduction where each of the result categories is briefly announced and summarised in advance of their more detailed elaboration below. Then follows the presentation of your result categories as subsections, each of them consisting of (1) a subheading, (2) an analytical text with a couple of paragraphs and (3) a quote illustrating each of these paragraphs. These are three different text formats with different missions and significance.

Let us start with the *analytical text,* because it communicates the substantial outcome of analysis and is the core of the results section and hence also the article. This is where you put forward your interpretation of what each of your result categories entails, i.e. your main answers to the question you raised in your study aim. Do not insist or argue. For each of the result categories organised as subsections, you may present a couple of main aspects (referring to the laundry metaphor as "2–3 shades of green"), each of these followed by an illustrating quote.

It may be tempting to subdivide even more, but then your results will easily appear fragmented and blurred. Be brave: decide upon your major results and let the minor ones go. In this way, your message will become sharp as well as nuanced, instead of thin and widespread. Your analytical text should therefore be prominent and be allocated most of the space in the results section. Do not waste space or words elsewhere in the article which can be better utilised for results.

Sparse or inadequate analytical text provides weak results that may indicate an unfinished analysis or a lack of understanding of the task of analysis. Sometimes we see results sections representing nothing but a rough code tree, often with subheadings verbatim transferred from the interview guide. In such cases, the content probably presents knowledge that is already *known from before*, perhaps as assumptions from preconceptions, theory or literature searches. Such a situation may be due to unfortunate loyalty to the project's starting point, based on the small q notion (see Chapter 4) that stability in the process is best. But it may also come from a blurred understanding of what kind of phenomenon a result is supposed to be. If so, the researcher wastes the opportunity to develop and share results from a process where associations and digressions can emerge and be digested and disciplined through a rigorous strategy.

The subheading for each main result category can be used to concentrate and articulate the results of the subsequent analytical text, preferably by means of some apt terms or concepts that abstracts, integrates and names what follows. These subheadings convince the reader that the analytical work has cleared up ambiguities, obviousness and overlaps. Here we have the opportunity to prepare a micro version of what we came up with—giving this result category a name which tells what it is all about and signifies that a fresh message. Presenting the result categories as "thematic emergence" gives the reader the impression that the author was waiting for something to emerge, without any real analytical effort (Varpio, Ajjawi, et al. 2017). This is different from emergence as an active process, as described in Chapter 1.

Subheadings that only tell what we investigated (such as The doctor-patient relationship, Being taken seriously, Lifeworld, Family, and Challenges) give a vague and unfinished message about what the subsequent analytical text may communicate. As a reader, I accept that these concepts were relevant before and during the analysis, but I want to see more clearly what was added by the analysis itself through the interpretation of the empirical data.

In a study of relationship counselling in general practice, for example Berge develops these three result categories to describe the doctor's role: (1) general practitioners (GPs) in a facilitating role, not on an assembly line; (2) navigating the 'elephant in the room'; and (3) GPs as biomedically competent life witnesses (Berge, Brekke, et al. 2024). In another study on the experiences of medical staff with video support in contact with callers to the emergency number (113), Idland develops these three results categories: (1) change in dispatcher's perception of the patient and the situation; (2) reassurance for the dispatcher; and (3) worries about increased time consumption and the possibility of unpleasant images (Idland, Iversen, et al. 2022).

Selected *quotes* serve to illustrate aspects of each aspect of outcome categories. Well-chosen quotes can be successfully used to flesh out the analytical text. But many researchers overload the results section with quotes, overshadowing their analysis. The analysis is not complete when the reader is presented with detached, random elements of raw data or uncommented series of quotes. The quotes are neither results nor do they serve as proof that the results are true. They should therefore be given limited space and significance in the presentation of the results.

What is not a result—and why?

Mention of the obvious and trivial in everyday life often appears in interviews and transcripts as part of a text where the focus should otherwise be on what we want to explore. But in a qualitative study, our task is to highlight and prioritise interpretations that can tell us something about our study aim that we did not know in advance—what does this study add?

Our mission is not to provide a complete account. Even with issues that we perceive as important, perhaps even such as basic conditions for healthcare quality, we do not currently need scientific studies to establish that patients want to be taken seriously by the doctor, that eye contact is important for good dialogue and communication, or that recognition can feel important to patients. We know this from experience, logic and professional ethics. However, results from a qualitative study with a more specific study aim and analysis can take us further, for example from treatment groups for women with chronic muscle pain on how recognition is concretely translated into clinical practice (Steihaug & Malterud 2002).

Results from qualitative studies sometimes amount to little more than repetitions of insights that have already been thoroughly documented elsewhere. This is not necessarily plagiarism or textual similarity but indicates perhaps that the author has not sufficiently familiarised themselves with the landscape before the study was initiated. Such presentations of results may also be an expression of professional modesty—a fear of embarking on interpretations and abstractions that may challenge the empirical material by involving the researcher's personality in the analysis, or a belief that our results will be truer if they agree with what others have found. This is a misguided small q attitude to subjectivity (see Chapter 4) —it is precisely the researcher's unique position that can enable interpretations that enhance fresh insights.

However, the researcher may also think the topic is so important that the results deserve to be repeated, perhaps with the disclaimer that this is only a descriptive or exploratory study. In that case, it would have been a better use of resources if the researcher had instead utilised existing evidence to go further, for example when it comes to nuances in palliative care with palliative sedation (Schaufel, Førde, et al. 2024).

Sometimes the common thread is so indistinct that we can barely see it. The results may be interesting reading, but the project's study aim remains unanswered. In such cases, the problem may have been insufficiently elaborated from the start (Alvesson & Sandberg 2024). An appropriate substantive theory can help to sharpen the focus so that the analysis leads to result categories that are sufficiently independent, coherent and diverse with a synergy effect (Malterud 2016, Guassora, Reventlow, et al. 2022) (see Chapter 20). In the article on GPs negotiating sick leave, for example, theories of the street level bureaucrat's dilemmas were used to identify strategies that included (1) alliance-building from the patient's perspective, (2) rapid return to work as the main goal and (3) input from other actors to find alternatives to sick leave (Lipsky 1980/2010, Nilsen, Malterud, et al. 2015).

It is also possible that the empirical data contained so many exciting clues that the original starting point became less thrilling. Perhaps the dialogue in the interviews indicated that the patients' experiences pointed in other directions than originally assumed, and that this became more relevant than what we initially wanted to investigate. Such experiences can form the basis for creative analyses that open new avenues. For this to result in scientific knowledge, the original problem must be critically reflected upon and reworked. This is not a forgery of premises, but may offer a further elaboration of the study aim.

Finally, there are articles from qualitative studies where the author's preconceptions and theoretical perspectives dominate the results section without proper utilisation and interpretation of empirical data. The results are supposed to be neither a mirror image of the preconceptions nor the theory—if so, there is a lack of reflexivity, interpretation and analysis. Feel free to read many qualitative studies from other authors before you get started yourself. Do not hesitate to ask yourself: Was this new and valuable to me? This will give you an impression of both strong and weak results, and you can decide for yourself how to make the best of what you have.

In this chapter, I have presented some ideals that may seem unattainable to the beginner. But striving towards a goal while learning along the way is not, in itself, problematic. By showing clearly what is new (in the results section) and what is old (in the introduction and discussion), we offer the reader insight into our path through the analysis from empirical data to the results. You can read more about how to handle this in practice in the next chapter.

CHAPTER 13

Writing your study—the craft and the joy

In the final stage of the research process, we summarise, synthesise, discuss and communicate what we have investigated and interpreted. In medicine and health sciences, scientific reporting mainly takes place as journal articles. The journal article has its own formal requirements, often discipline-specific. Such requirements sharpen our concentration so that we focus on the message and the study's strengths and weaknesses. This is when we will find out whether the work is well-connected and has a sufficiently clear common thread. The writing process in a qualitative study can be challenging and demanding, but it can also be a creative and integral part of the analysis work. Here we will see how this is done in practice.

Format and outline

Before starting the writing process, you identify 3–4 relevant journals you want to submit to in order of priority. Articles are often first rejected, then more or less revised and resubmitted to another journal. Read the guidelines for authors carefully so that the rules of the game do not come as a surprise. The maximum number of words or characters is an imperative framework condition, and you also need to know whether this number includes the entire text or whether abstract and references are excluded from the count. Where this is not specified in the guidelines, it is advisable to consult previously published articles in the journal.

Do not believe that your project is so important and comprehensive that you need to use twice as many words as normal. Instead, take the journal's limitation of scope and words as a positive challenge to sharpen the message, expose what is new and valuable, and peel off the rest, without dismissing documentation and credibility. Some journals accept more words than the normal standard for a fee. In that case, carefully consider if this is truly necessary and if you have tightened your text well enough.

The completed article starts with an introduction that logically leads to the study aim. This is followed by a description of the design, method and sample, and then come

DOI: 10.4324/9781003786016-15

the results. The results section is the core of your article (see Chapter 12). This is where your interpretations are synthesised and staged in a convincingly readable manner, clearly anchored in empirical data and theoretical perspectives. The article terminates with a discussion of the results and process, followed by a short section of conclusions or implications.

In the medical publishing tradition, this formula is summarised in the acronym *IMRAD*, which is an outline with a fixed order: Introduction, Method, Results, And Discussion (Sollaci & Pereira 2004). Check in the author's guide of the actual journal whether the abstract should be structured with fixed paragraphs (most common) and whether the different sections of the article should be organised in a specific way or with a specific designation.

Researchers from disciplines beyond medicine and health research often question the practice of presenting a qualitative study in a framework with a limited number of words and with a structure that requires an editorial distinction between results and discussion. One answer to this is that anyone who wants to contribute to knowledge development must learn the rules of the game. We do not change medical knowing by publishing our results in a social anthropological journal. Another answer is that the medical form requirements can contribute to better focus and strengthen the dialogue with peers who are familiar with other research methods. Be mindful, nevertheless, of the small-q trap (see Chapter 4), which requires careful balance on your part.

The article's requirement for concentrated communication represents a positive challenge to the researcher, who in this way must distinguish between big and small, important and unimportant, and prevent redundant verbosity. At the same time, these requirements enable us to be more attentive to whose voice is heard in different sections of the text. In the results section, the participants' voices, as interpreted by the researcher, should be clear. In the discussion, the researcher is visibly present with reflexivity and comments.

In the writing process, I do not start with I (for Introduction), even though the final text will do so. In my experience, the writing work can be facilitated if you follow this order:

- **Results** are the core of the article—start here.
- **The study aim** is the question that the results elucidate on or provide an answer to—conveyed in short form via the article's title.
- **Method** presents the approach we employed to shed light on this issue.
- **The results discussion** highlights what is new and valuable compared to existing knowledge and evaluates alternative interpretations.
- **The methodology discussion** section reviews the strengths and weaknesses of the research process—are the results developed with relevant and robust tools?
- **The introduction** presents the project's specific platform, which may have become clearer after you have discussed the results.
- **The list of reference** is supplemented during writing and carefully reviewed at the end.
- **The abstract** is the very last thing you write—only once you know what the article is actually about.

What knowledge did your analysis add—Results

The previous chapter dealt with ideals, concepts and recommendations for understanding the task and skill of presenting results. Here we will look at how this can be done in practice. With the synthesis in the final stage of the analysis process, we are well underway with the text communicating the outcome of your project. If we continue drafting the article from this starting point, we can maintain our focus on the empirical dimension of the project—what data development, interpretation, abstraction and analysis have contributed towards evidence. If the analysis was carried out using Systematic Text Condensation (STC) (see Chapter 11), you can take the analytical text from step 4 of the analysis process as your starting point.

Take this opportunity to carefully consider what is new and valuable, and how this can best be highlighted. The aim is not to keep the analytical texts "clean" and pristine—on the contrary, we will now gently edit and arrange them so that patterns and categories from the interpretation come sharper into view. In the writing phase, we often reorganise the results section somewhat, but we must not become such keen editors that we discard the systematic approach provided by the analysis method. For STC, it is best to maintain analytical text from subgroups intact as much as possible. If you now start chopping this up into small pieces and moving them around, you dismiss the connection to the systematic analysis.

Your edited results should still be clearly rooted in the empirically rooted interpretations and patterns that you developed through the analysis. Also when using analytical methods other than STC, it is equally important to preserve the traces of the analytical process—you should not erase everything during the writing phase in an excessive editorial zeal. Remember that this is non-fiction writing, not fiction. Feel free to use the decision trail for progress notes on recontextualisation.

The efforts of verbalising the subheadings in the results section, i.e. naming the result categories, can be utilised to further sharpen what we have arrived at. Therefore, postpone these until you are almost finished with the rest of the results section.

The results section should leave the reader in no doubt about whose voice they are reading. This is where the knowledge crafted from the empirical material is conveyed. We aim to provide the reader with insight and confidence and share the understanding from the subjectivity processed by our interpretations. There will be footprints of both the researcher's voice and the theoretical perspectives, yet this is not the place for commentary or discussion. If this occurs, it easily becomes ambiguous to the reader who is speaking here (Malterud 2001b).

The IMRAD structure also serves as a valuable reminder to make clear to the reader when the author's preconceptions or theoretical perspectives are being voiced. Is this a text that could just as easily have been written prior to the co-creation of the empirical data? Or are we reading the researcher's meticulous interpretation and synthesis of the participants' voices—text that is clearly rooted in the data and analysis, and that conveys the new insights achieved by carrying out the project?

But results are not communicated as raw data and quotes (see previous chapter). In the results section, interpretations are transformed into analytical text that conveys transferability as evidence at a more abstracted and general level than what applies to the individual participant in the local context. Selected quotes illustrate key points in the text but are not results. If we have several quotations addressing the same issue, we select the one that most clearly gives voice to what we wish to present. *Tables* do not normally belong in the results section, since quotes form a natural part of the text flow and are integrated into the text with the results categories. A table with quotes should therefore not be used to reduce the number of words in the article. The demographics of the sample are a premise and not a result and are therefore best presented in the methods section.

Most of the results section consists of analytical text (see Chapter 12). This text should have a clear connection with the empirical material, in that you refer to specific circumstances supporting your conclusions. Exclude claims that predate the project, such as objectives or hypotheses, and focus only on results supported by data. A strong presentation of results bears clear traces of ambiguities and paradoxes reflecting the complexity of the matters we have explored, while the result categories still are durable, independent and stand on their own. Uncertainties may indicate that the researcher has attended closely to the fact that a case can be viewed from multiple sides at once and has used emergence to develop something beyond the individual parts.

We will not present everything we have heard or seen but will prioritise what best informs our study aim. As a rule, the results will consist of different aspects, nuances or components that shed light on different aspects of the problem. When STC is used as an analysis method, this corresponds to an edited and adjusted version of the analytical text from the code groups with subgroups from the analysis (see Chapter 11). A journal article gives you space enough to give an appropriate presentation of 2–4 result categories. If you have more than this on your mind, you may rather split up the presentation and write several articles or make an even stricter assessment of what is new and valuable.

The presentation of results should be preceded by a short intro paragraph summarising your main interpretations. If you wait with this introduction until the rest of the results text is complete and you have taken the effort to name the result categories, this intro will be easy to write. Put time and energy into drafting this introduction, supposed to present very briefly each of the result categories as the short version of what came out of this project.

It is always difficult to write briefly enough. The proximity that the researcher advances to the participants and the data in a qualitative study creates a risk of the researcher falling in love with the data. You can (rightly) be excited by elegant formulations and well-articulated participants, but at the same time lose the distance necessary to assess what is relevant to the reader and the study aim. But the love of the material should not outweigh the requirements for reflexivity and prioritisation. Metapositions in the form of comments from your supervisor or colleagues can be valuable, especially when you think you have fantastic material (see Chapter 16).

If these were the answers, what is the question—Study aim

In a qualitative study with ample progression, the study aim gradually becomes more focused and specified. The writing phase offers a good opportunity to more distinctly rewrite the question that is answered by your results. The more clearly the study aim is formulated, the easier it is for the researcher and the reader to consider congruence and decide on the study's internal validity—the common thread between questions and answers. A clear-cut study aim also enhances the Information Power (IP) of the project, even this late in the process (see Chapter 7) (Alvesson & Sandberg 2024).

The title of your article should specifically convey the updated study aim—forget loyalty to what you labelled the work packages of your first project outline. Now, the reader's interest should be aroused with a short, adequate explanation of the message. An exciting title will convince the reader that you managed to investigate an issue that interests others and conveys that the research process was forwarded with focus and concentration. The title may distil the project's study aim or most important result in one sentence, for example "The fibromyalgia diagnosis—hardly helpful? A qualitative focus group study about patient experiences" (Undeland & Malterud 2007). Here, a subtitle contributes more soberly by informing about the study's context or design. Previously, it was common to include a quote in the title of the article (Soderlund, Skoge, et al. 2000, Johansen, Holtedahl, et al. 2012a). Such a practice runs the risk of you choosing a catchy quote that may not be appropriate for your result categories. Nowadays, many editors do not want it that way.

Paths to knowledge in this project—Methods

In the completed article, the presentation of design, material and method comes before the results, as a logical expression that this is the pathway to the conclusions. In an article based on a qualitative study, it may be easier to write the methodology presentation after drafting the results. By then, you know the analytical endpoint and can describe the path that led there. This presentation should be straightforward and descriptive, declaring what you did. This is not the place for extensive justifications—those belong in the method discussion, if needed at all. We shall not waste space in the methods section with extensive explanations of the nature or excellence of qualitative methods. We must assume that the qualified reader does not need textbook material.

In qualitative studies, the design and methods are often adjusted along the way—the path is created as we go, and experiences from data development and analysis can lead to changes in the original plan. It is more important that the methods presentation briefly states what we did than giving a point-by-point chronological account of why we chose to deviate from what we originally intended to do. In some projects, such changes are signs of poor planning or inadequate knowledge of the field. This may not be of interest to the reader of a journal article, although such considerations may have a natural place in the summary of a PhD thesis.

However, in projects where the course of the project has provided important insights that led to unforeseen, significant changes in methods, such experiences should be shared in one way or another. The path we have travelled is also part of the knowledge we will communicate, but what is relevant to report can always be considered. It is a matter of taste whether this belongs in the method presentation (descriptive) or later in the method discussion (commenting).

Our presentation of the empirical data shall give the reader an understanding of the design and sources used for analysis. You explain the sampling strategy, perhaps including brief remarks on IP (see Chapter 7) and the extent to which this has been carried out. Our readers need sufficient information about the participants to grasp matters concerning internal and external validity, and to visualise the context in which the study was conducted. It can be tempting to create detailed tables summarising demographic and medical features of the sample. However, this type of participant information increases the risk of breaching privacy assumptions, especially when the sample is small and localisable (see Chapter 25). Understanding the context—including demographics—is crucial but can usually be conveyed at least as well in short textual form, considering carefully what the reader needs to know.

Your text will form the basis for assessing the sample in terms of relevance and external validity. If we choose to use IP (see Chapter 7) to consider the sample's content and scope, we should comment briefly on each of the five dimensions encompassed by this term—it is not sufficient to state that IP was satisfactory. IP comments also require follow-up as a brief consideration in the method discussion (so-what?). Saturation is a concept fundamentally different from IP and is not to be used alongside it (Malterud, Siersma, et al. 2021).

Some projects include an intervention which can also be perceived as a kind of method. When communicating such projects, it is important to distinguish between how the intervention was implemented (*intervention method, clinical method*) and which method was used to describe and analyse the implementation of the intervention (*evaluation method*) (Stensland & Malterud 1997, Malterud 1999, Steihaug, Ahlsen, et al. 2001) (see Chapter 17).

The methodology presentation also includes a paragraph on the analysis. Here we must be concrete and specific—broad labels such as qualitative analysis, text analysis, content analysis, hermeneutic analysis or phenomenological analysis express very little about how you actually bridged the gap between data and results. If you have followed a method that is well described in the literature, a reference to this is usually sufficient. If you do not write anything about analysis, we must assume that you did not carry out any analysis.

Theoretical perspectives are also included in the reporting, partly to situate the context of the study, and partly to support the analysis (Malterud 2016, Guassora, Reventlow, et al. 2022). Therefore, your choice and use of theory should be made explicit in the article. When using theories that are widely known in our academic community, keywords and literature references are sufficient. A sentence or two in the introduction followed up in the discussion may be enough to invite the reader to go to the reference. If the theoretical perspectives are new, unfamiliar, marginal or controversial, you can provide a more comprehensive presentation of the most important principles or concepts, preferably as a separate section (Slåtten & Malterud 2024). Read more about theoretical perspectives in Chapter 20.

How can our results be interpreted—Discussion

Writing out the results invited us to consider the reflexivity, relevance and validity of our study. In this phase, we notice weaknesses and limitations due to our methodological choices, and we prepare for consideration of the impact of this on our interpretations and conclusions. The point is neither to conceal nor deny the challenges, but to use the discussion section to demonstrate how the validity and scope of the knowledge have been examined and assessed by those who were closest to the process (Stige, Malterud, et al. 2009).

The discussion section of the article gives you an opportunity for critical self-reflection. The discussion is usually divided into three separate sections: (1) results discussion, (2) methods discussion (often called strengths and limitations) and (3) consequences (and implications). However, traditions differ from journal to journal when it comes to the order of the various elements in the discussion section. Personally, I find it most logical that the discussion of strengths and weaknesses of methodology comes before the discussion of the results, but the opposite is often the case. You should therefore check the normal order in the journal where you want to publish. In articles where theoretical perspectives have a prominent place, it is also necessary to have a discussion section incorporating discussions of interpretations and results, more specifically in relation to the theory. The discussion section often begins with an ultra-short description of the main results—not be a repetition of what has already been written as intro to the results section but as an even shorter version.

In the *results discussion*, you may convince the reader that you know the status of the research field and that your interpretations add something new and valuable. The last point is crucial to whether the editor will accept our article as interesting. Claims that nothing has ever been done in the field before are arrogant. We are supposed to present references dealing with related issues or studies. Remember that there is a lot of research relevant to medical and healthcare issues outside Medline/PubMed, especially from qualitative studies.

In qualitative inquiry, it is more important to make explicit how our study adds nuance to or deviates from previous studies than to point out how it aligns with or supports previous research. Here, you should highlight your most important interpretations and conclusions—not as just another repetition, but in comparison with previous studies. You may write, for example "NN demonstrated xx, while our study extends this understanding by yy", or "MM concluded that zz, and our interpretations specify key conditions under which this applies". This part of the writing process is somehow the final stage of the analysis. If we fail to make clear what distinguishes our results from those of others, and merely confirm correspondence, we must return to the analysis and work through the data once more. From previous research, for example, one could get the impression that general practitioners (GPs) are passive providers of sick leave, while the study on negotiation strategies shows that doctors have several active attitudes to this issue (Nilsen, Malterud, et al. 2015).

Once we have established a convincing and nuanced demonstration of the study's originality, we will discuss the significance of our results, preferably in the context of the field of practice. Here we may create space for some selected alternative interpretations of the results, with logical arguments for why our conclusions nevertheless provide the most relevant answers. Theoretical perspectives can help to highlight further interpretations and nuances. We can put a critical spotlight on the theory that we have chosen, assessing other relevant theories. An ordinary journal article has limited space for presenting such considerations, but in the summary of a PhD thesis, you can leave plenty of room for this.

In the *methodology discussion,* it is also helpful to distinguish between the writing order and from the order in the final article. My recommendation is to write the methods discussion immediately after you have written the methods presentation, while the considerations about method are still fresh and active. In the methodology discussion, the researcher is advised to demonstrate an awareness of selected specific strengths and weaknesses of the chosen design. We will discuss what is the impact of this for internal and external validity, both what we now know as an outcome of the chosen design and sample, and what we still do not know. We will stand by the choices we have made. If, during this consideration, it turns out that our methodological approach has led to serious weaknesses, it may in the worst case be necessary to terminate the project without publication. This kind of hard-won experience can be the price to pay for projects that were inadequately planned.

When discussing methodology, be specific and stick to the selected questions that are at stake in your own project. Do not address general issues such as the relationship between qualitative and quantitative methods or anything else that belongs in a textbook. It is not necessary to repeat or assess all the details of the design and implementation. In the methodology discussion, we look into a few prioritised issues that have been influential here. A project of appropriate scientific quality is often characterised by a methodology discussion that is both as specific as possible and thorough and thoughtful. For example, in the article on GPs' negotiation strategies in connection with sick leave, we discuss how the focus groups' linkage to a course in social insurance medicine may have influenced the interpretations, given that participants were likely to be more interested in such issues than usual (Nilsen, Malterud, et al. 2015).

You may choose to discuss the sample in terms of IP and transferability (external validity) of the results. In addition, we must address aspects of internal validity by clarifying which facets of the phenomenon these methodological choices illuminate, and which remain beyond the reach of this design and method.

You are also expected to give some specific comments on the impact of your own situatedness (see Chapter 5). General statements to the effect that such factors may have had an impact are not very enlightening. In the methodology discussion, the researcher must also briefly summarise their own influence on the process and consider what this means in concrete terms for the outcome. It is a misleading understatement to write that the researcher may have had an influence on interpretations and conclusions— to move the claim beyond a small q level, you must specify more specifically what this means (see Chapters 4 and 5).

At the end of the discussion section, we look ahead and point out some relevant implications of what we have concluded. Do not use this space to summarise the main results yet again. These should be well enough presented earlier. This is where the project's relevance is put under scrutiny. What is the potential impact of our results on medicine and healthcare? Can our results lead to specific recommendations about something that can be changed or implemented? Do our experiences point in the direction of research questions that can provide more answers to the problem? Do we need observational studies from general practice to understand the interaction in discussions about sick leave (Nilsen, Malterud, et al. 2015)? It is not sufficient to write that there is a need for more research in the field—you need to be specific about why and how. A short punchline summarising the consequences of the new knowledge is a suitable way to end an article.

Starting point—Introduction

When almost the entire article is drafted, you return to the start. It should not be necessary to read many paragraphs of the introduction to recognise the main question of the article. Presenting prior research highlights knowledge gaps, providing a clear rationale for this article. The idea of the introduction is not to present everything you have collected or read. Write briefly and concisely—save space and words for the results, which are the heart of the article. You should also consider which part of the reference literature is best suited to the discussion of results (because they provide a basis for comparison of your results) and which part of the reference literature is best suited to the introduction (because they provide premises for the study). Do not paste the text from the original project application here. Since then, you should have sharpened the focus of your project significantly, and this should be clearly reflected in the introduction.

Many qualitative studies in medicine and health sciences arise from personal practice experiences of professionals, leading to curiosity, discomfort or a need for deepening and reflection (Malterud 1990, Johansen, Holtedahl, et al. 2012b, Iden, Ruths, et al. 2015, Jansen, Ruths, et al. 2016). Such motives constitute an important, legitimate part of the preconception and help to determine the formulation of the study aim and design. In a qualitative study, the researcher's preconceptions must be visible, so that the reader can know the perspective from which the knowledge was obtained (see Chapter 5). We need neither a comprehensive biography nor detailed information about events that led up to the research. However, in the introduction, the reader must receive enough information to get a sense of the researcher's situatedness that has an impact on the knowledge to be developed. A sentence or two about the researcher's profession, academic background and personal motivation in relation to the study in question can often suffice. In the methodological discussion of the article, we need a short, concrete follow-up on this—on how (not whether!) this has affected interpretations and conclusions.

Literature references

The literature references give the reader access to the relevant knowledge base for this project. As readers, we expect references from the *empirical* field to be studied (e.g. on socialisation to the medical profession (Good 1994)), references that present *theoretical perspectives* influencing the researcher's interpretation (e.g. existential perspectives (Boss 1979)) and references to *methodology* (e.g. Kvale's description of the semistructured interview (Kvale 1996)).

All scientific journals have their own rules for reference style, which are set out in the journal's author guide. These often specify how many references an article can normally contain, how the references are noted throughout the text, and how the reference list is organised. Most medical journals use variations of the Vancouver style, while other conventions, such as APA style or Chicago, are used in journals from other disciplines.

You can save a lot of work by studying the guidelines for authors thoroughly before drafting the article. Most researchers use digital reference-management tools, with EndNote being the most common. The advantage is that you enter a literature reference once and for all from the internet, preferably directly in the original format, and then the reference style in the manuscript can be changed at the touch of a button. I tend to use "unformatted citations" in the writing process—this provides a suitable overview along the way and is easy to edit. I insert the journal's style after I have finished all other writing. Remember to switch off the "Track changes" function in your word processing programme when you change the reference style, otherwise you will have a mess and a lot of work with all the format changes.

Even when you have downloaded a reference correctly, it is not certain that everything is correct in the end. Therefore, proofread the bibliography carefully, reviewing the specifications of the journal you are opting for. Any changes should be made in your reference library, once and for all, not in the article text. Be sure to delete duplicates—sometimes the same reference appears in several versions. Also check whether references with preliminary indexing (Epub) have been given final status with page numbers and change of year. Many journals also require a DOI (Digital Object Identifier)—a unique number used to identify the references.

Scrupulous accuracy in the bibliography is part of the editorial team's requirements for approving the article, so that readers can subsequently obtain the references. The novice author always needs the supervisor's support with the reference list, both to learn the principles and to check that these have been followed to the letter in the version of the article submitted for review, and perhaps also with assistance to revise references that are out of place.

Articles with an unnecessarily large volume of references are increasingly appearing. You should not display everything you have read or heard about—prioritising references is also an important academic skill. Therefore, make a judicious selection of literature references that you include in the article. When there are many relevant ones to choose from, you preferably pick the most specific, often the most recent. Occasionally, however, an old classic may be your most important source. Look for original articles based on empirical data or for systematic reviews. Choose references that have specific relevance to your project and be careful with general and overarching references that do not really provide information about what you have used them for. Never add a reference that you have not read and check carefully that your application of the reference is appropriate. Web references must always be updated with a recent date before you submit the article—broken links do not give a trustworthy impression. If you are writing an English-language article, you should use a minimum of references in other languages for the sake of your English-language readers. The reader should be able to access everything you refer to.

Core content—Abstract

Only when the article is virtually finished can you write the summary. By then, you understand the article's main points. Many journals or reference databases require set sections for the abstract. Follow this template unless there are obvious reasons to deviate from the rules. You can cut and paste the study aim and intro results from the article text that has already been written. To do this, your results section must be congruent with your study aim (see Chapter 12).

If you struggle to write a concise abstract, your analysis may be incomplete, or your project outcomes are unclear. In qualitative studies, we particularly face this challenge when it comes to providing a short and concise presentation of the results in the abstract. We are more interested in what you found than what you wanted to investigate. If you are unable to express this clearly, it may be useful to take a step back before finalising the article. If you have worked thoroughly on the subheadings and introduction in the results section, you will already have developed clear terms and descriptions for your result categories that can be reused in the abstract.

The writing process

Writing an article always takes much longer than you think. This is true for novices as well as for seasoned researchers. This part of the research process should not be underestimated when planning your project. Putting knowing into words is an important aspect of knowledge development, and your project will suffer if the writing phase becomes unpleasant or burdened by time pressure. Be prepared for every paragraph to be written several times. It is therefore unproductive to put a lot of effort into linguistic details, wording and grammar in the first drafts. If, at the next stage, we choose to delete this page or paragraph, premature fine-tuning will have been in vain. The readability of the final text determines whether we managed to develop knowledge that can be shared with others. Kvale calls this *communicative validity* (see Chapter 21) (Kvale 1996).

If English is not your mother tongue, and you are writing your article in English, you will need language polishing supported by AI or a professional before submitting. You must review the proof carefully to check whether the proofreader (who has usually no methodological insight) has distorted the meaning or terminology. It is also always necessary to run a spelling check in your word processing programme just before submission.

When writing becomes a creative process, subjectivity in interpretation and analysis is enhanced. For this reason, we should not be afraid to include tentative formulations or incomplete reasoning that may provide useful material for further thought by drafting. Much of what is written will not be included in the final article. The supervisor plays an important role in the writing phase unless the researcher is independent and experienced. It is the supervisor who knows the academic rules of the game and can judge what is academically relevant and robust and what is not. A productive division of labour between a novice researcher and a supervisor typically consists of the researcher writing and the supervisor offering feedback. It is easier to both give and receive comments if neither party perceives the draft as a finished product. If the supervisor lacks experience in writing articles from qualitative studies, you should consider including a co-author with such experience.

If you get stuck while writing, it can be helpful to put aside the section that is holding you up for a while. It is better to let the problem rest for a while instead of getting stuck in a dead end where the wording just gets increasingly complicated. Move on to another section of the manuscript or do something else for a while. Then the problem may be solved or resolvable when you return to it. If the symptoms of writer's block persist, it is better to discuss the situation with your tutor instead of sitting alone with a guilty conscience, low production and plenty of "good" excuses.

PART 3

On different forms of design and data

CHAPTER 14

Dialogue across designs—understanding experiences

Conversations are mutually constituted by information exchange and social interaction. With words, we create the reality which we take part in. When the researcher co-creates qualitative data together with participants through conversations—data interaction—the social and cultural context provides a crucial framework. Accordingly, the researcher must comprehend the dynamics between participant and interviewer, the role of subjectivity within this exchange, and the implications this holds for knowing, interpretation and results. In this chapter, we will take a closer look at different approaches and challenges for the development of qualitative data from conversations with one or more participants.

The qualitative research interview

The research interview is a specific kind of interpersonal interaction (Seidman 2019). Interviews with individual participants are also called *in-depth interviews* or *unstructured* interviews. A better term, however, is *semistructured interviews.* It is certainly debatable how deeply it is desirable and realistic to approach in a research interview, and we should not interview without purpose and meaning. We choose individual interviews when we want to invite participants into a time and space that support the sharing of experiences and reflections requiring safety, such as experiences among lesbian couples in maternity care (Dahl & Malterud 2015), or about the needs among relatives of patients with Huntington's disease (Røthing, Malterud, et al. 2015).

We prepare a *list of topics* or an *interview guide* in advance that reminds us briefly what we aim to develop data on. When interviewing adults about growing up with parents who had alcohol problems, we sought to hear how they remembered their everyday experiences, the impact of their parents' alcohol use, and the nature of their relationships with support services (Werner & Malterud 2016a). When the purpose is to find out more about something we do not already know, or to conduct a conversation

DOI: 10.4324/9781003786016-17

that will enable access to new questions about the study aim, the interview guide must not be too detailed, and you do not follow it slavishly. Think of it more as a to-do list.

In qualitative studies, it is neither necessary nor desirable to standardise the interview situation. On the contrary, for a Big Q approach (see Chapter 4), the interview guide is steadily being revised during data development, as the researcher learns more about where the focus should be. This allows the interaction to be adapted to the encounter with the individual participant. Notice that when peer reviewers request the interview guide as an appendix to your article, this can wrongly imply that the questions should be identical from interview to interview.

We obtain our most valuable knowledge when we succeed in inviting participants to share experiences as concrete events, narrated as stories with special impact in a specific case. This approach is referred to as the *critical incident technique* (Flanagan 1954, Bradley 1992). Feel free to ask "Tell me about what happened to this last week...", or "Can you give an example of what you're talking about now?". Otherwise, it is too easy to steer the conversation towards something we already know enough about. If so, we are only travelling within the framework of our preconceptions. Similarly, a conversation may become overly superficial and generalised if participants limit themselves to what they mean in general, or to what most people do in such situations, without being encouraged to articulate their own specific experiences.

Informed consent mandates the research interview to be a conversation in which the study aim is the main topic. Without being aware of this, we run the risk of talking only about loose ends. That is the reason why a qualitative interview should never be unstructured. It is a critical research skill to be sufficiently open and targeted at the same time. It can pay off to keep an open mind and wait curiously when the participant starts to talk about something that might seem like a derailment. The new and valuable knowledge is often found along such sidetracks. Nevertheless, the prerequisite for knowledge development and interaction is that we do not talk past each other—that the participant does not enthusiastically talk throughout the interview about something else than what we meant to explore. Yet, the balance between flexibility and control is subtle.

In semistructured individual interviews, it is essential that the researcher can seek out, investigate and manage subjectivity—both in the participant, in themselves and in the interaction of the interview. Exercise is needed to conduct conversations in which subjectivity is given a valid voice, so that the words convey knowledge about the content and meaning of what we are talking about. Kvale (1996) takes a phenomenological perspective as his starting point when he sets out ideals for the qualitative research interview. The aim is to develop data based on the participant's experiences, with loyalty to their own understanding of their story. According to Kvale, the interview should provide access to knowing rooted in the participant's life world—living knowledge as it surfaces to the person living the life we are talking about. The interviewer ought to create a situation where it is possible for the participant to talk about the connotations and substance of what we are talking about for the person in question.

In the data co-creation, the interviewer must work on themselves before, during and after the interview to best be able to ask naive questions and listen without preconceptions. We should not set conditions for receiving the knowledge that the participant wants to share, even if it is sometimes necessary to ask clarifying questions or change the track. Although the interview must be conducted with an open mind, the researcher should stick to the study aim, so that the conversation is focused and contributes to strong Information Power (IP). But we must also be prepared to understand that the relevant centre of gravity may lie somewhere other than where we initially thought.

The best qualitative interviews leave room for ambiguity. Most human phenomena come with multiple sides, and contradictions, dilemmas and paradoxes may offer important insights that we cannot get hold of when we only go for unanimous narratives. The interviewer should also be responsive to variation and change in stories of process and development, as well as to perspectives that may shift during the conversation. If we are to learn something new from the participant, we must train our sensitivity as interviewers. This is necessary not only to create a safe and confidential space but also for us to hear something we did not know before. If the interview does not yield surprises or knowing that confronts our preconceptions, we may not have listened well enough.

To understand what is being said and what is unfolding, the interviewer needs an appreciation of both rational and irrational aspects of interpersonal dynamics (Seidman 2019). Ideally, the interview should be a constructive experience—not only for the researcher, but also for the participant. In some projects, it may even be an explicit goal that the conversation should lead to new insights, awareness and change in the participant. More often, we are content when the interview gives the participant a genuine sense of contributing knowledge of potential value to others. A special variant of the semistructured individual interview is *the life form interview*, which Råheim used in her project on women with fibromyalgia (Råheim & Håland 2006). The starting point for this method is specific events from morning to evening on the day of the interview and the day before, with supplementary questions about what happened and how it was experienced.

The doctor and other healthcare professionals in the role of interviewer

There are many commonalities between a good medical dialogue and the qualitative research interview. Healthcare workers with experience of therapeutic conversations will recognise many of these ideals from their own practice. Still, this does not imply that the experienced clinician by instinct is skilled at the craft of developing, collaborating and organising qualitative data. There may even be clear contradictions between the research dialogue and the clinical dialogue, in terms of both goals and means.

In the consultation, the conversation is deliberate and goal-oriented, at best directed towards understanding and solving the patient's problem. In psychotherapy, the conversation is a means by which the patient can formulate and reformulate their encounters with themselves and their surroundings. The cultural traditions and professional rules of the game for medical problem solving provide the doctor with experience in a form of dialogue that is directly or indirectly very directing. For the actual purpose, this is not necessarily wrong.

At the same time, it is an underlying premise in clinical practice that the conversation should provide access to the patient's agenda and support the patient in mastering their own life. The general practitioner (GP) has a lot of such experience from diagnostic activities in open, unselected practice, where the problem is often not defined in advance. Such ideals are not similarly suited to research interviews aimed at co-creating qualitative data.

Doctors conducting qualitative interviews must therefore invest time and effort in learning the craft. It is particularly important for medical practitioners to develop expertise in an open conversational style that allows space for associations and digressions, and for the participant's own version and interpretation. At the same time, you need to practise maintaining the common thread from the project's problem. Reviewing audio recordings and transcripts from the first interviews together with the supervisor offers helpful amendments to the interview style. When you transcribe the interviews yourself, you gain first-hand insight into what was said and how it worked (see Chapter 9). Step-by-step analysis (see Chapter 11) also provides opportunities for revising the course of questions and themes.

Healthcare professionals need to cultivate an awareness of how their medical background creates a context for what is said and what is heard (Reventlow & Tulinius 2005). People respond differently when they know the interviewer is a doctor compared to someone who is a social scientist. If the interviewer additionally is also the participant's doctor, there may be plenty of issues that are withheld for strategic reasons, although the trust in a good doctor-patient relationship can also give access to topics that would not be told to just anyone.

An interviewer with a background in medicine and health sciences can never escape medicocentrism—seeing the world through their medical glasses (see Chapter 8) (Kleinman 1995). However, the dominance of medical lenses can be moderated somewhat when the researcher is aware of the drawbacks this can cause in the co-creation and interpretation of data. Collaboration with research colleagues from disciplines beyond health care can help to highlight unrecognised medicocentrism and other professional taken-for-granted entities, thereby broadening the perspective (Reventlow, Overgaard, et al. 2008, Alræk & Malterud 2009, Larun & Malterud 2011a).

Are resource-intensive individual interviews always best?

Individual interviews usually take one to several hours and require peace, quiet and freedom from distractions. Repeated interviews may sometimes also be conducted to elaborate on topics that came up in previous conversations. The qualitative research interview is a type of data development that quickly generates a lot of material, first as audio recordings, and then in text as transcripts. For example, a transcript of a one-hour conversation can represent an estimated 12 single-spaced pages of text. Not all parts of such a text contain the same amount of relevant material.

If we want to learn more about how the patient experienced what happened with the doctor, interview data may provide good access. The individual interview can apparently entail a safer and more sheltered situation for the exchange of sensitive material (Schaufel, Nordrehaug, et al. 2011). On the other hand, the closeness of the one-on-one situation can be perceived as extra uncomfortable if the participant does not feel at ease meeting the interviewer.

Focus group design (see below) may therefore be a good alternative to individual interviews, first and foremost because the group discussion provides a richer interaction arena for data co-creation, but also because a focus group material of strong IP can often provide sufficient data with less extensive effort (Malterud, Siersma, et al. 2021). A dataset of a smaller scale can subsequently create better conditions for appropriate analysis.

Research interviews with individuals or in groups imply the strongest validity for exploration of people's experiences, perceptions or beliefs. By contrast, they provide only indirect information about events and interaction. If we want to explore what happens when the doctor talks with the patient about sensitive topics, it is better to draw on observational data, for example from audio or video recordings (see Chapter 16), rather than interviews (Nessa & Malterud 1998a, Schaufel, Nordrehaug, et al. 2009, Guassora, Reventlow, et al. 2014). Early in the planning stage, we should therefore carefully consider whether individual interviews are the most relevant route to the type of knowledge we are looking for, or whether other designs provide more relevant and robust data for our purpose.

Focus groups—group interviews

Group discussions can also serve as a way to co-create qualitative data (Malterud, 2012). *Focus groups* are a specific strategy for this purpose (Morgan 1993, Krueger & Casey 2000, Malterud 2012a). In focus groups, we use the added value of the interaction between the participants for knowing a different nature than we get from individual interviews. This design is particularly suitable if we want to learn about experiences, attitudes or views in environments where many people interact. Focus group designs were originally developed in marketing, but are now used for different purposes, especially for the development of experience-based knowledge (see Chapter 19) or to investigate initiatives and organisations (Lid & Malterud 2012, Lid, Oppedal, et al. 2012, Ree, Harris, et al. 2014). Focus groups were judged to be the most appropriate design for exploring GPs' negotiation strategies regarding sick leave (Nilsen, Malterud, et al. 2015).

Although there are many guidelines in the methodological literature on conducting focus group studies, there is general consensus about key aspects such as how many groups to include, their size and composition, and how interviews should be carried out (Morgan 1993, Krueger & Casey 2000). Focus groups usually consist of 5–8 participants who talk together for an hour or an hour and a half under the direction of a *moderator*. Audio recordings are used to store information from the conversation. In addition, it is helpful to have a research colleague in the role of secretary. The secretary takes notes from key moments of the mood of the conversation, trying to capture aspects that may not be noticeable on the audio file. Assigning speaker pseudonyms can also be a task for the secretary—it greatly facilitates the analysis when we later know who said what. The secretary does not participate in the conversation. Each group is composed as homogeneously as possible, because we want to emphasise a common basis of experience for the conversation and prevent tensions within the group that could steer the conversation in the direction of competition or contradictions. We can, for example, conduct groups where we gather GPs and home care nurses in separate groups if we want to study these professional groups' attitudes to dementia diagnostics (Waldorff, Bulow, et al. 2001).

There is no law of nature claiming how many groups you need, and the variation is huge among published articles in this field (Carlsen & Glenton 2011). Assessing the sample's IP (see Chapter 7) matters more than attempting to cover every aspect of the issue. The latter is neither possible nor desirable. When the interaction and dialogue in the groups have been productive, 2–3 focus group interviews usually provide data of strong IP, suitable for appropriate analysis (Undeland & Malterud 2007, Malterud, Fredriksen, et al. 2009, Malterud & Ulriksen 2010b, Tollefsrud & Mengshoel 2020, Malterud, Siersma, et al. 2021).

Within a focus group, the moderator takes on a much more directive role compared to an individual interview. The moderator must ensure that the participants have their say, monitor group dynamic processes that can guide the exchange of knowledge, but primarily ensure that the conversation is anchored as concretely as possible to the study aim. The participants must be properly informed about the purpose and organisation of the conversation, so that their expectations are congruent with what will take place. In focus groups with patients, it is particularly important to make it clear, both to yourself and to the participants, that the purpose is not group therapy or sensitivity training, but a shared exchange of experiences for the co-creation of research knowledge.

When the conversation is over, the moderator and secretary often summarise the most important interaction-related key points while the audio recorder is still running. I would, however, caution strongly against making this a preliminary, intuitive analysis aiming to summarise the results. At this point, the researcher is immersed in immediate impressions that differ markedly from the reflexive stance required for analysis. Notes and audio recordings from focus group discussions are qualitative data that must be processed, transcribed, interpreted and analysed before the results become scientific evidence. Methodical examination of the data will often lead to other interpretations and conclusions than what you thought you noticed at the end of the conversation.

It is also possible to conduct group interviews inspired by focus group techniques, without having to fulfil all the recommendations in the methodology literature, for example regarding the number of participants or interview duration. Under optimum circumstances, even a single group interview can provide ample material with appropriate IP (Søderlund, Skoge, et al. 2000, Bjørkman & Malterud 2007). Considerations of IP and validity are particularly important in such designs. If the group interview has too few or too many participants, the conversation may become heavy or superficial. Yet, there is no rule stating that eight participants is always a maximum number. When a discussion group has many members, it can provide a wide range of viewpoints. Still, it is important to set a clear topic and ensure that everyone has a fair chance to share their thoughts. In such situations, we must carefully assess whether statements have been sufficiently challenged during the conversation and refrain from making conjectural assumptions about what people may have meant by statements appearing unclear.

A special variant of the focus group technique can be used for internal evaluation of group-based interventions, such as a programme for experience-based discussions in specialist training for GPs (Lid, Eraker, et al. 2004), or treatment groups for women with chronic muscle pain (Steihaug, Ahlsen, et al. 2002) (see Chapter 17). If we conduct an evaluation session midway through the project, we can learn from the experience and adapt further development of the programme along the way.

Group interviews may also take place after the project's completion to review its feasibility, compare participants' experiences with initial objectives, and gather insights that clarify how the process unfolded (Ree, Harris, et al. 2014, Idland, Iversen, et al. 2022). In such cases, the project manager should not be the moderator. Such a setting will restrain both questions and answers in the conversation. Nor is it beneficial to have the project manager present as an observer. Even without participating in the conversation, the project manager's presence will have an impact on what is said and, in this way, provide some limitations on what kind of knowing this conversation can generate. Be particularly alert to the risk of an echo effect in such contexts, where participants chiefly replicate variations of the project's objectives rather than articulating and interpreting their own experiences. (see Chapter 17).

A focus group design is a rational strategy for co-creating qualitative data, requiring fewer resources than if each of the participants had been interviewed individually. On the other hand, group conversations embody a different type of knowing than individual conversations, because the context is different. It is the study aim that determines what is the most appropriate path to knowing and knowledge. If you want to use this method, you need to read and learn more than what is written here (Morgan 1997, Malterud 2012a).

Enhancing the efficiency of interview studies?

Conducting and transcribing qualitative research interviews is resource-intensive. It can be tempting to outsource parts of this process, either to technical personnel or with artificial intelligence (AI) as a tool. However, gains in time efficiency may come at the expense of subjectivity and reflexivity, with subsequent flaws for the relevant and robust development of new and valuable knowledge (see Chapter 9). With qualitative data, more is rarely better, and reflexivity should take precedence over efficiency. Even if you are a technology enthusiast or adept at delegating, you gain substantially from hands-on participation in the process, working calmly to co-create material that is manageable, accurate and characterised by strong IP. This is the best starting point for proper analysis.

A common beginner's mistake is to decide on the number of interviews, conduct them according to the project outline and then start analysing. This approach entails a substantial risk of producing an overly extensive empirical material with weak IP. Kvale (1996) describes this as "the 1000-page question"—a situation obstructing proper analysis. You can prevent this by establishing material whose composition and size correspond as closely as possible to the study aim, while preliminary analyses along the way adjust the course (see Chapter 11).

In qualitative interview studies, the interaction and dialogue are essential contributions to the project's IP (Malterud, Siersma, et al. 2021). AI-based clinical patient interviews are now being developed for use in mental health services (Li, Zhang, et al. 2023). This is not transferable to qualitative research interviews, where you need to be particularly alert to surprises, questions you did not know you were going to ask, unpredictable courses of events and avoid standardising. A generative dialogue requires proximity to your unique study aim and empathy with those who share their experiences that neither digital tools nor technical personnel can provide. You will therefore achieve the most interesting knowledge if you conduct not only the transcripts but also the interviews yourself (Li, Zhang, et al. 2023).

Gaining hands-on insight by personally transcribing interviews early in the data development process can enhance your interview technique. This allows us to see which questions give the participant the opportunity to tell their story and which strategies do not work as expected. In a study of how patients with life-threatening illnesses thought about dying, it turned out that the first interviews were slow and yielded little (Schaufel, Nordrehaug, et al. 2011). During transcription, the researcher realised that theoretical concepts had stolen too much attention and disrupted the form and direction of the dialogue. Realising these flaws after just a few interviews is preferable to ending up with a large but superficial collection of data following many interviews. AI is not a qualified companion for considering this kind of subtle and subjective interpretive nuances. You can read more about AI in Chapter 23.

CHAPTER 15

Beyond conversation—narratives, unique cases and digital traces

Stories about people's experiences may amount to substantial empirical data for a qualitative study. A good story is not (yet) scientific evidence, but it can enable the development of new insights holding transferability beyond the original context through interpretation, analysis and abstraction. Any story is told and perceived in a social and cultural context in time and space. As researchers, our understanding of the text is strengthened the more we know about the unique context. Narratives with individual stories represent a special type of empirical data, where we need to pay particular attention to coherence and context to be able to abstract and consider transferability. Therefore, let us look at opportunities and challenges when using qualitative research methods to transform an interesting story into scientific knowledge.

Narrative tradition and analysis method

In all cultures, oral storytelling traditions exist in various forms—for entertainment or education, for expressing values and norms, and for exchanging experiences and information. In the literary tradition, stories are referred to as *narratives*. There are many definitions of narratives, but what they share is that a storyteller takes the listener on a journey through time, organised around a sequence of events—*a plot*. In other words, a text, conversation, or story does not automatically qualify as a narrative. Stories about health and illness are important aspects of what people share with each other and are therefore also important elements of humanistic medicine (Gatens-Robinson 1986, Hunter 1991, Frank 1995, Mattingly 1998). This form of knowing has gained increasing prominence, and the concept *of narrative-based medicine* is established as a counterweight to evidence-based medicine. (Hurwitz & Greenhalgh 1998, Launer 2003, Charon 2004). However, narrative medicine is not the same as research with narrative analysis.

DOI: 10.4324/9781003786016-18

Narrative interviews and analysis serve as sources and tools for systematic exploration of the meaning and scope of texts that tell stories (Riessman 2008, Josselson 2011, Frank 2012). *Narrative analysis* of interviews with open-ended, overarching questions may elicit more nuanced information about patient experiences than semi-structured individual interviews with thematic analysis. Analysis within cases from a single or a few participants, for example based on medical history or life course, can offer a substantially different picture than analysis across cases where many different stories are synthesised and communicated (see Chapter 10) (Synnes 2015). Participants normally choose versions of the story that can best concretise and give meaning to what they tell.

Narratives contain roles, structure, temporality and plot, and narrative analysis serves as a tool for examining how these elements shape the story and our understanding of it. A narrative often follows a structure with an introduction, middle section and conclusion, although it does not always proceed chronologically. The ending may be open, ambiguous, or categorical. By linking events sequentially, often around a distinct turning point, narratives illuminate processual relationships differently from biomedical causality (Bakken, Mengshoel, et al. 2023). Narrative analysis puts high demands on reflexivity and considerations of internal and external validity – assessing the soundness of what we have come to understand and the scope of that understanding (Thorne 2009).

Sviland & al use narrative analysis in a case study design (see below) in which data from interviews (group and individual) and written text together shed light on a course of treatment for a single patient with Norwegian psychomotor physiotherapy over eight years (Sviland, Martinsen, et al. 2018). The authors demonstrate how knowing from the data is interpreted and communicated by organising a story with a timeline, highlighting some crucial turning points with an impact on the course of treatment.

The subjective experience is re-experienced when the story is told, thereby creating a new frame that contributes to the experience changing over time. The elaborated narrative is therefore no less true than the original. For the researcher, the primary question is what the story tells us about. The exploration may also include the framework in which the story is told. In the encounter between researcher and participant, a specific version of the story is co-created, characterised by time, place, values, moods and endpoints, with the researcher as an active participant in the development of the story.

From a social constructionist and a literary perspective, it makes sense that one and the same event can lead to different stories, each telling the story of what happened in its own way, with the narrator's version being one of several possible (Iser 1978, Lock & Strong 2010, Eagleton 2011). Therefore, it will rarely be adequate to assess the validity of stories in relation to historical "facts". Such reasoning presupposes an unambiguous event that cannot be experienced in more than one way, and thus echoes the small q (see Chapter 4). This type of gold standard thinking is of little use when exploring people's subjective experiences, thoughts and opinions (Flyvbjerg 2006). For medical and health researchers, the idea that there are many different versions of reality may be unfamiliar. However, such an understanding is equally pertinent to clinical practice. The researcher has other assignments and opportunities to assess different interpretations than the clinician does in a busy everyday life, where brief, still thoughtful pragmatic interpretation is an important way of knowing (Daniel 1986, Gatens-Robinson 1986, Leder 1990, Malterud 2001a).

Good combines a social anthropological and a literary lens when discussing the interplay between narrator and audience in a cultural framework (Good 1994). Using *reader response theory* (Iser 1978), he looks into how people talk about their illnesses. Good shows how stories follow a certain literary regularity, and at the same time stimulate the listener's imagination and associations far beyond the reality they "actually" describe. In this way, narrative theory can help us better understand why a particular story turned out the way it did, in both clinical practice and research (Gatens-Robinson 1986).

Texts for narrative analysis can originate from dialogues in oral interviews, from monologues in written texts or from field notes from participant observation. For a narrative to serve as empirical data articulating the narrator's subjective experiences and identity, the researcher must process the data interaction with caution, or the participant's voice risks being drowned out. In interviews with general practitioners (GPs) about their professional role in relation to cancer patients, for example, there must be room for dilemmas and doubts (Johansen, Holtedahl, et al. 2012a). It is the other person's part of the story that should be prioritised, while the researcher carefully considers the impact of their own role as listener, addressee and participant, and the implications this has for the meaning and design of the text. Stories providing strong material for narrative analysis are characterised by complexity, concrete accounts, the development of a course of events, different voices and rich characters.

The story is the analytical unit in narrative analysis, often with temporality as the most important axis (Genette 1980). A major ambition is to sustain a unified and integrated understanding of the individual narrative (Iser 1978, Kvale 1996, Riessman 2008). In this way, we establish commitment to within-cases analytical perspectives with contextual understanding that anchors the text to its roots. Such an attitude can help prevent unfortunate reductionism in the analysis.

Narrative analysis does not follow fixed procedures of the kind described for Systematic Text Condensation in Chapter 11. For example, we may emphasise theme (what is told?), structure (how is it told?) or performative function (why is this told this way), and which actions are embedded?) (Riessman 2008). Or we can probe the text for what is at stake, how the characters react and evaluate what is happening, or whose perspective we are presented with (Josselson 2011).

Researchers with a background in medicine and health sciences need to thoroughly familiarise themselves with theory and methodology to carry out narrative analysis properly. This section can be a starting point, but you need to read more before you get started. In my experience, other analytic strategies may be more suitable for novices. However, narrative analysis does not differ in any fundamental way from other forms of within-case qualitative analysis. Here, too, the researcher is expected to present the path from data interaction and interpretation towards results with intersubjectivity, so that the reader can understand how the analysis has been conducted and assess the transferability of the interpretations. For this purpose, simply declaring that we have undertaken narrative analysis or explored the participants' stories that we have explored is hardly sufficient —we must do it and show how.

The internet as a source—written monologues

In qualitative interviews, whether individually or in groups, the relationship between narrator and listener is a crucial framework condition. The narrator adapts their story to the listener's response, often elaborating on ambiguities or particularly interesting passages requested by the listener in a kind of negotiation. The dialogical space strengthens the dynamics, validity and Information Power (IP) of the stories being told.

However, *monologues* can also comprise unique narratives that are relevant for research purposes (see Chapter 22). To this end, data development with the internet as a source can be an alternative, especially for research on sensitive issues or vulnerable groups with demanding recruitment. People may prefer to remain anonymous also when they have an important story to share (Bjørkman & Malterud 2009, Synnes & Malterud 2018). For some issues, the threshold for participation may therefore feel lower when the gateway is the keyboard on one's own computer instead of a conversation with a stranger. This can, for example, be a suitable format when we want to know more about how lesbians and gays hide their sexual orientation (Malterud & Bjørkman 2016).

Put a lot of effort into articulating a tempting invitation that sufficiently clearly invites participants to express the kind of stories you want, in the format that suits them best. This type of study needs to be actively publicised in environments where you are sure there are a lot of potential participants. A small pilot study before you start the actual inquiry can, with this design, save you a lot of hindsight regarding recruitment, trustworthiness and interpretations. You design the question as best you can and ask a couple of relevant people for feedback on how they understand the question and what kind of answer they would give. This is an open context that is different from the actual study you want to conduct, and you should therefore not include these results in the analysis (see Chapter 6).

Remember that this design does not allow for *dialogic validation*, where you can ask along the way what the participant meant by what was said. We must accept that monological stories will normally be more superficial, with less scope and greater uncertainty than data from an interview study or an observational study. We also often notice that the texts convey more well-known stereotypes and facts about the issue than can be used to develop new knowledge. Therefore, we must be level-headed about what it is possible to learn about in this way. In return, we receive fully transcribed data in the participants' own language.

Privacy is enhanced when the system deletes the participants' IP addresses so that the texts cannot be traced back. This means that we also must accept the risk of *false input*, i.e. texts from participants who do not belong to our target group. In practice, this type of response will usually stand out so that we can identify it. In such a design, we must avoid placing too much emphasis on individual statements, no matter how colourful or fascinating they may be.

It is a proper investment to put a lot of effort into developing the wording of one or just a few questions that can prompt data with strong IP (see Chapter 7). A pilot round or two, in which you check with relevant test participants whether the question format works and elicits the type of information you seek, can be useful. Take care to create sufficient space for the participant to use their own expression in the response. A line or two rarely yields much benefit. But we should not leave too much space either. If the participant is expected to write a long essay or report, we will not get many answers. Many participants are not used to expressing themselves in writing and get embarrassed by undue expectations.

Therefore, we must accept that several answers give a laboured or rigid version of what people intended to say. Some of the answers may be difficult to understand, and the literary standard is uneven. From experience, material of this kind frequently exhibits standardised clichés and repetition. We should not take this as confirmation of strong recurring themes, but as a recommendation to assess the material critically, considering cultural influences on people's expressions.

When we invite participants in a research project to share their experiences via an internet site, all rules of research must be followed. The principle of informed consent can be achieved by the researcher providing information about the purpose of the project and how the material will be used. This can be done on the project's website, where the study starts. Consent is given indirectly by the participants submitting responses. The project must also be assessed and approved by the research ethics committee or data protection authorities (see Chapter 24).

An online sample of participants is self-recruited and convenience based (see Chapter 7). We need some selected background data for every one of them to assess IP and the internal and external validity of our interpretations. The web form should therefore include a small section with questions about relevant demographics. Such a form is best placed after the story has been told, so that participants do not assume the survey is completed once these questions have been answered.

Monitoring recruitment status is particularly important in this kind of study, with announcements about the project in all relevant channels. If you notice that responses are slow, you need to consider whether you need more data, and if so, make new recruitment announcements better aimed at the target group. The study aim and the IP in the empirical material have an impact on your choice of analysis method. In this design, we do not do stepwise analysis. A check of the texts that arrive can give an indication of whether we are on the right track, receiving data with appropriate IP. Read more about processing qualitative data from questionnaires with open response options in Chapter 22.

Social media as a source of empirical data

Social media (SoMe) provide access to many people's opinions, experiences and ways of knowing. Research projects can be conducted retrospectively, drawing on texts posted before the project begins, or prospectively, where researchers invite participants to submit contributions on a specific issue. Using social media as a source for data development allows insight into the perspectives of participants with relevant backgrounds in real-time, ongoing debates. In addition, the text format in such arenas is often concise and opinionated, and people who express themselves are keen to contribute their views, often also in a research project. In a closed social media group with a specific community of interest, we can find exciting academic discussions deserving further exploration. In this context, it can be a major advantage for recruitment if the researcher is previously known and trusted in the group. For example, in a retrospective SoMe-based qualitative study established from an already completed chat discussion, we explored what motives GPs in Norway have when they choose and remain in general practice (Gronseth, Malterud, et al. 2020). The starting point was a discussion triggered by several statements about challenges related to a national GP crisis and the demanding everyday life of GPs. Without this being planned as research, the thread starter had challenged the group's participants to provide input on why they were still GPs.

Another qualitative study was based on prospective social media data (Malterud, Aamland, et al. 2020). Here, we invited the group's members to post short reports of situations where they as GPs had experienced a risk of compromised patient safety when tasks that normally belonged in hospital wards were shifted to the primary care service without proper resource or competence upgrade.

In the case of prospective social media studies, recruitment can pose a significant challenge. It is imperative to encourage potential participants to enrol, to show enthusiasm in the group when there is progress in the deliveries and to be realistic when you notice that the contributions gradually slow down. It is therefore particularly important to make thorough assessments of IP in the sample along the way and to specifically encourage new input that can promote this.

Also, in the case of SoMe-based qualitative studies, procedures for research ethics and privacy must be properly safeguarded, especially when data are developed from closed groups. Be prepared for this to require some extra effort in retrospective studies—it is by no means a given that the participants in the chat had imagined that the text in the post would proceed to anything other than the discussion of the moment. You must obtain informed consent from everyone who submitted material you intend to use as data. Making contact for this purpose may be demanding when participants have been away from the discussion or thread for a period. Themes with possible research relevance may be found in texts where confidentiality towards third parties (especially patients) is a relevant issue. As a rule, you cannot use that kind of text for research, because the person in question is not available for consent.

When developing and interpreting social media data, you must choose a method for analysis that matches your study aim, with data upholding appropriate validity and IP (see Chapter 7). You must consider and discuss issues related to self-recruited, selective samples, and you must decide whether your interpretations are defensible. Inform participants about the future use of the data and update the group when the article is published.

The medical case story

In the tradition of medical communication, *the case story is* a well-known genre. At the morning report in the hospital, the junior doctor presents an oral summary of the night's medical events to the consultant and senior colleagues. The aim is to keep all staff updated on the department's patients and to support shared assessment and ongoing diagnostic and therapeutic decisions for each individual patient. Hunter Montgomery (1991) reveals the invisible rules of the game that apply to this specific written and oral narrative tradition or sociolect, which governs, delimits and consolidates medical knowing. She demonstrates how the doctor may transform the patient's history into a medical narrative genre that distorts aspects originally emphasised by the patient.

Good (1994) points to the impact of medical students being socialised early into a biomedical, doctor-centred style of knowing, in which this medically inflected version of the patient's history takes precedence as a basis for knowledge. Until recently, the prestigious New England Journal of Medicine, which mainly has a biomedical and epidemiological profile, had a regular column in each issue where a medical history was presented in detail. These stories are not qualitative studies but nevertheless follow a specific informal non-fiction literary genre.

Strong methodological expertise is essential when drawing on such sources for qualitative analysis, interpreting subjective experiences and views transformed and embedded in the narrative. We must also be attentive to the significance of the non-fiction genre doctors employ when documenting patients' status, for example in medical certificates submitted in applications for disability pensions (Aarseth, Natvig, et al. 2017).

In a research context, the case study represents an exciting extreme of inductive logic, where the interpretation and communication of the unique can lead us towards something with significance beyond itself (Sandelowski 1996). We must carefully assess the transferability of the selected case and decide what we want to explore by immersing ourselves in this particular text.

In medical history, we find many cultural clues revealing how both the narrator and the listener lean towards a medical framework. Such a framework may look completely different from the perspective of the patient and the doctor, respectively (Mishler 1984). The patient tells what they think the doctor wants to hear, while the doctor emphasises clinical information that may form relevant pieces of a medical puzzle. Conventions and habits from this genre contribute to a rigid and stereotypical template when reiterating medical stories, where the patient's voice often is not well represented (Aarseth, Natvig, et al. 2016). The patient-centred clinical method involves the GP getting to know the patient's understanding of the situation (Levenstein, McCracken, et al. 1986). This method can also suggest a valuable attitude when the medical researcher needs to shift their focus from "the voice of medicine" to "the voice of the lifeworld" (Mishler 1984).

Case study design

In the medical research tradition, knowledge derived from a unique story is often dismissed. We are trained to believe that $N = 1$ is a small number and may think that transferability always requires large material (see Chapter 7) (Flyvbjerg 2006). Still, we should not forget that ground-breaking discoveries that we take for granted today are based on insights from stories about individual events. In 1848, railway worker Phineas Gage was the victim of an explosion that drove an iron bar through his head. He survived the accident, but for the rest of his life, he was characterised by a serious personality change. The relationship between the injury and its consequences in a person formed the basis for detailed hypotheses about the functions of the frontal lobe (Haas 2001). Sandelowski argues that qualitative methods ultimately concern understanding the unique, and that respect for $N = 1$ is a fundamental prerequisite for this form of knowing (Sandelowski 1996).

In a case study design, knowledge development is based on one or more individual stories or circumstances (Sandelowski 1996, Flyvbjerg 2006, Yin 2009). The Gage story demonstrates the potential for broad validity of knowledge based on unique stories. Still, we cannot take this for granted. The researcher must consider whether, how and why the story accounts for something beyond itself, and pay close attention to the story's source. A story may offer a retrospective account of an event, for instance, when an unplanned, singular experience produces unexpected moments of surprise and new insight that we wish to convey to others.

The medical case study is a typical example of this type of retrospective story. The starting point for a retrospective case study can be patient record notes, test results or autopsy results, while the prospective case study is often based on field notes and audio or video recordings (Guassora, Johansen, et al. 2021).

We can also stage events to create or capture a story, for example by making video recordings of consultations that are later retold and analysed. Observational studies based on a few and selected events can be examples of prospective stories (Nessa & Malterud 1998b, Malterud 1999, Stensland & Malterud 2001, Undeland & Malterud 2008). The casuistic form does not exempt the researcher from systematic development and analysis of data, even though the basic material may vary widely in type and character.

The case study approach imposes substantial demands on the researcher to situate the story within a broader context and to discuss its relevance. (Thorne 2009). In a prospective case study, the premises for the purposive sample will be of great importance. We need to know where the story comes from to understand its impact in a larger context, and the story must have sufficient IP to provide robust data for analysis.

In a case study design, the researcher must explain why this particular story, situation or organisation was chosen as the basis for presentation and analysis and how it appears as *exemplary* (Sandelowski 1996, Flyvbjerg 2006). Insisting that it is an interesting story is a weak methodological argument. The researcher needs to identify and present the aspects of the story that make it worth telling. Theoretical perspectives may support the transferability of a case study design, for example, as Sviland & al discuss interpretations related to bodily narrative identity in an empirical material about a course of treatment with Norwegian psychomotor physiotherapy (Sviland, Martinsen, et al. 2018). In this way, the unique takes on a significance that can be relevant to something more and something bigger.

The retrospective case study is a special variant, where we make a strategic selection of cases from existing material (*corpus*) that may have had a different study aim as a starting point. We outline a problem for inquiry, look for cases that clearly demonstrate what we want to investigate further, and use a relevant analysis method for interpretations and conclusions. For example, a Danish study based on video recordings from general practice later provided material for a case study on the GP's communicative handling of a consultation containing several different issues (Guassora, Johansen, et al. 2021).

Discourse analysis

Discourse means conversation and incorporates written or oral communication. More specifically, the term also refers to a culture's ways of talking about a phenomenon (Foucault 1970). For example, we are talking about discourses on obesity or homosexuality, where language takes on meaning by creating and recreating symbolic power regarding knowledge, politics or history.

Discourse analysis was originally developed in literary studies to investigate the social and cultural functions of living language (Potter & Wetherell 1987). This research tradition is rooted in *semiotics* and *pragmatic linguistics*, which focus on the meaning and consequences of language. We can study the meaning of *signs* and *symbols* (Skagestad 1981), or we can investigate what we do with language through *speech acts* (Austin 1962). In discourse analysis, we are more concerned with the way things are said and done, and the consequences of this, than with the words and grammar (Nessa & Malterud 1990).

Discourse analysis has advanced into a multidisciplinary research tradition that incorporates different strategies and approaches. Relevant adaptations to the field of study and the problem at hand are necessary—for example, a linguist will be interested in matters that can be studied by means of a detailed transcription method capturing every little pause and interruption, while the medical researcher may be more concerned with the social consequences of language actions (Guassora, Johansen, et al. 2021).

Inspired by pragmatic linguistics, Nessa developed a method for transcribing and analysing clinical interaction in general practice (Nessa 1995a). This strategy involves a methodical assessment and interpretation of speech acts in a medical discourse—what is done by what is said—in the transcribed text, which is then condensed into a summary or synopsis. Nessa's method, based on the consultation as the unit of analysis, is an example of a *microanalysis* strategy that is particularly suitable for analysis within cases where a few selected cases are included.

With discourse analysis, we can study medical communication emphasising the meaning of the cultural context—for example, a busy hospital ward (Schaufel, Nordrehaug, et al. 2009)—or with a particular focus on the consequences of referring to a phenomenon in this or that way, for example, when the doctor shares their interpretation of the symptoms with the patient (Nessa & Malterud 1998a). Discourse analysis can also be used to examine how mass media and advertising convey messages about health and stages of life (Hvas & Gannik 2008, Malterud & Ulriksen 2010a).

Furthermore, we can apply discourse analysis as a perspective or backdrop without necessarily conducting a complete, formal analysis. For example, it may be relevant to keep the attention during analysis focused rather on the way things are said in a consultation than on the meaning of the words (Guassora, Reventlow, et al. 2014). A focus group interview provides a rich source of linguistic interaction, where this may be relevant, as does an observational study in which an event is captured through audio or visual recordings.

Just remember that, in retrospect, we have limited opportunities to validate our interpretations of intentions underlying what was said and heard. In such designs, it is particularly important to pay attention to the impact of our own situatedness (see Chapter 5), to avoid interpretations inappropriate for the participants in the actual interaction. Interpretation of the discourse may also be expanded if we interview the participants after we have made a preliminary analysis of the interaction data (Arborelius, Timpka, et al. 1992).

CHAPTER 16

Observation as situated research practice

Interviews and other dialogues and conversations present direct accounts of how the participant experienced something that happened, but we only get indirect descriptions of the actual event or course of events. Conversely, observational data can offer direct accounts of interactional processes and contextual circumstances, while the experiential dimension remains largely inaccessible. Data can be developed from observations in a variety of ways. Such data carries large amounts of information with different types of sensory imprints that are methodologically challenging to organise, interpret and synthesise. The researcher swaps between the overlapping roles of participant and observer. Theoretical perspectives are particularly important to make the researcher's interpretive perspective clear and root the study's situatedness when analysing observational data. Metapositions offer helpful vantage points to support knowing into something more and something different than a private, autobiographical narrative with confined validity and transferability.

Participant observation

Participant observation is a research method originating in ethnographic and social anthropological traditions (Malinowski 1944, Garfinkel 1967, Atkinson & Hammersley 1994). Here, the researcher participates in the study context, investigating the study aim from an insider perspective (Savage 2000, Maanen 2011). Participant observation can be a valuable strategy for the researcher to familiarise themselves with the impact of the cultural context for health issues such as pregnancy, birth, childbirth, childlessness and child mortality, as Blystad did in her study of the Datoga people in northern Tanzania (Blystad 2000). However, fieldwork with participant observation can just as easily take place in domestic surroundings (Gullestad 1984).

In ethnographic fieldwork, the researcher's subjectivity is particularly pronounced in various roles in the field being explored and the data being co-created (see Chapter 5). You must build trust to gain access to your target group, and you constantly move

DOI: 10.4324/9781003786016-19

back and forth between an open attitude and an analytical attitude (see Chapter 5) (Savage 2000). This approach is different than when you go on holiday and seek your own experiences. The role of the researcher is also different from that of the journalist, where the mission is to entertain or enlighten by reporting what they see. In the analysis process, the researcher relies on field notes, photos or video recordings, often supplemented by more or less formal interviews with key individuals.

As a participant observer, I seek positions that can provide access to cultures and conditions that I want to learn more about. My own presence can provide unique, first-hand access to what is occurring in the practice context. An essential prerequisite is to establish an authentic position in the landscape that provides insight into the problem, without disturbing natural activities too much (Mays & Pope 1995a, 1995b, Savage 2000). As a researcher, I aim to use my impressions, experiences and reflections to develop and co-create new and valuable knowledge that inspires confidence in my observations and interpretations. I will not be a spy or investigative correspondent uncovering sensations from a foreign culture.

Participant observation can be a primary strategy for developing data as well as preliminary work to support the understanding of a phenomenon, environment or context prior to research interviews. To perceive what I observe in the role of participant observer, I need a minimum level of insight into what is taking place. If I want to go along with the day-to-day life of a medical centre to approach different aspects of the sick leave process for different patient groups, I must first become familiar with the employees and learn who is who. If I want to enter functions that bring me into direct contact with patients, I may need to understand how the appointment booking system works and know something about the software for the patient record system. If I am going to be present at consultations that involve negotiations between doctor and patient, I must be able to recognise relevant situations arising, and to ensure appropriate privacy protection related to this.

To take on such roles as an outsider researcher, you need acquaintance with the local system and insight into the purpose of its routines and services. The stranger's privilege is to be able to ask the naive questions that can disturb the local *taken-for-grantedness*. This is especially true for the researcher with a different professional background. If the social anthropologist enters the medical centre, we can expect more inventive questions and challenges than if the researcher is a nurse.

On the other hand, the anthropologist's personal learning may overshadow the events the participation was intended to illuminate, or the researcher may end up pursuing questions that were settled long ago. The fact that the researcher is a stranger is therefore not unambiguously necessary or favourable to create new and valuable knowledge (Morse 1994).

For studies in medicine and health sciences, we must also be accustomed to professional ethics in addition to research ethics. Ethical care is particularly important when a participant observer enters a field with vulnerable individuals and situations, for example in a mental health ward (Øye, Bjelland, et al. 2007). We must enact respect for those involved, and the issue of informed consent must be handled sensibly and responsibly (see Chapter 24). To understand the meaning of these experiences for the participants and what they reveal, you need to seek ongoing comments and corrections from those involved regarding what you have seen, heard and experienced.

Stick to the study aim and ask yourself constantly what the experiences inform you about, under what circumstances these narratives are shaped and communicated, and what different meanings they may carry. There are always numerous possible versions of an experience or observation (see Chapter 2). As a researcher, your task is to seek out the positions that provide the most relevant input to what you want to understand more about.

In disciplines such as social anthropology, methodological competence in participant observation is an important element of basic training. Medical and health researchers need to recognise their lack of grounding in this field and seek collaboration and guidance from colleagues with stronger methodological backgrounds when it comes to participant observation. Simply bear in mind that your goal is to develop medical, rather than anthropological, knowledge.

How are observations digested and shaped by the observer?

An outsider researcher is rarely able to fully blend into the environment without disturbing the context. An ambition is to minimise this distraction, which is easier if the researcher can take on a factual role on site. Still, we should not imagine that it is a "natural", pristine situation we explore as a participant observer. In one way or another, everyone will be affected realising that their actions are being analysed by a stranger.

This can be particularly delicate if the setting feels criticised by the guest, or if everyone becomes preoccupied with presenting a glossy picture of reality. In some situations, for example in a conversation between a doctor and a patient, the noise of the third party's presence may be so noticeable that it is a better alternative to use audio or video recordings as observation material (Schaufel, Nordrehaug, et al. 2009). We would unlikely invite a male social anthropologist into the doctor's office to observe the pelvic examination.

Establishing an appropriate balance between participation and observation is not always straightforward, and there are smooth transitions between the roles of *participating observer* and *observing participant* (Walseth, Abildsnes, et al. 2011). In any case, the researcher must consider the experienced knowledge as situated and shaped by the context from which it is drawn and by the eyes and ears noticing what unfolds (Savage 2000). If the participant observer somehow takes on the role of health care provider, this provides access to a different kind of knowledge than by taking on a patient-like role. One is not necessarily better than the other—here we must often take practical considerations into account, and the study aim determines what is most relevant. The researcher should admit that patients will share a different kind of knowledge when the researcher is perceived as a representative of the healthcare system than as an outsider (Reventlow & Tulinius 2005).

In participant observation, the researcher must learn to live with a built-in ambivalence surrounding their ambiguous role. On the one hand, we must endeavour to establish anchoring and identification with the role we are taking on. This involves close interaction with other people, whom we get to know and care about. Loyalty to the environment's explanatory framework and self-understanding quickly becomes a natural part of a role assumed to be as authentic as possible. On the other hand, our observations and interpretations must be subject to critical analysis and situated in metapositions that allow us to see more perspectives than are possible at close range. Nevertheless, the participating observer is not a reporter or microphone stand—the researcher's mandate emphasises interpretations, which are more than a description of the place and the people. The observations are empirical raw data, not finished results, supposed to be developed and co-created further through analysis and synthesis.

Non-participatory observation

The researcher can also collect *observational data* without being present, using material from an event that is intact except for its documentation. From medical research, we have many examples of qualitative studies where dialogues between the doctor and the patient have been analysed using observational data from *audio* or *video recordings* (Malterud 1990, Nessa & Malterud 1998a, Undeland & Malterud 2002, Schaufel, Nordrehaug, et al. 2009, Guassora, Reventlow, et al. 2014, Guassora, Johansen, et al. 2021).

We can also co-create observational data in an action research project from encounters where the participants gather to exchange experiences and reflections (Steihaug, Ahlsen, et al. 2001). Informed consent from the individuals participating in the recording is an absolute requirement for this type of data interaction. Of course, we could imagine a richer and more exciting material if the recording took place in secret, but such an approach is not compatible with basic principles of research ethics (see Chapter 24).

Although the recording equipment initially may be perceived as intrusive, patients as well as health care professionals soon forget that recording is taking place once the event in question is underway. Audio recordings can feel less intrusive than video because they require less equipment and capture a narrower slice of what is happening. However, as researchers, we should not believe that we are recording the "authentic", untouched event. For example, it invariably matters that the doctor seeks to present themselves as a sympathetic professional. In any case, these are less distorted observational data than when the observer is present in the room or when the event is staged for research. Precisely because subjectivity is sought as a basis for knowing for both researcher and participant, such data are particularly unsuitable for collection and processing by artificial intelligence (see Chapter 23).

Observational data drawn from video recordings can illuminate aspects beyond the information from spoken language. This can be particularly useful for the study of bodily expressions and movements (Thornquist 2006, Oien, Steihaug, et al. 2011). If we want to compare verbal and non-verbal communication in the consultation, video recordings provide more robust material than audio recordings (Nessa & Malterud 1998a, Guassora, Johansen, et al. 2021). It can also be easier to get hold of everything that was said with non-verbal expression from video recordings, supporting the comprehension of the conversation. In many cases, especially in projects that highlight verbal interaction in sensitive situations, audio recordings can therefore be just as suitable as material (Malterud 1990, Schaufel, Nordrehaug, et al. 2009).

This does not mean that video recordings are always superior to audio recordings. In many cases, especially in projects that highlight verbal interaction in sensitive situations, audio recordings can therefore be just as suitable as material (Malterud 1990, Schaufel, Nordrehaug, et al. 2009). What matters depends on what we aim to explore, and we should not assume that either video or audio recordings convey the "true" meaning. Video-based material contains such a wide range of data that there is a substantial risk of the researcher losing focus and becoming overwhelmed by detail. Analysing video recordings places substantial demands on the researcher's systematic approach and requires them, in reporting, to make explicit the principles guiding the analytical process (Guassora, Johansen, et al. 2021). Video is not a research method, just a technical device for recording data.

Seeing with observational data

The narrative of any event has many layers, shaped by the storyteller's relationship to it. The doctor describes the course of a consultation in a different way than the patient, even though the two descriptions refer to the same event (Arborelius, Timpka, et al. 1992). An outsider, a passive observer who does not participate in the game, will notice different aspects of the case than those apparent to active participants. The outsider's perspective may offer a certain epistemic advantage, yet it also entails a risk of misunderstanding, whether by perceiving elements of the material differently from how they were originally expressed, or by attributing meanings to actors' expressions that were never intended.

Audio and video recordings with observational data embody information about what happened and can provide appropriate data about interaction. Just remember that such material still gives us limited access to the participants' experiences. When using this kind of material, it is sometimes an advantage to explore the recordings and transcripts together with those who participated in the event, so that we also gain access to the participants' experience of the situation (Arborelius, Timpka, et al. 1992).

This does not necessarily imply that participants must consent to or approve the researcher's analysis and interpretation. Rather, we must consider whether such a joint review adds analytical material or primarily constitutes dialogical validation of audio- or video-based data. These strategies require considerable efforts, and for it to lead to scientific benefit, arguments for the surplus value must come first, as also a rigorous plan for analysis.

The internal validity of observational data is weak when it comes to issues concerning individuals' lifeworld—are we investigating what we actually want to know? What people were thinking, or their underlying motives for acting in particular ways, cannot be inferred from such data. In such cases, an interview study is more appropriate, whereas observational studies entail a focus on behaviour, expressions and contextual preconditions (Guassora, Johansen, et al. 2021).

Field knowledge and field blindness

Fieldwork on home ground can have many advantages, because field knowledge entails an immediate understanding of phenomena that an outsider may be unable to perceive (Gullestad 1984). When we as health professionals conduct a qualitative study in a clinical or system context—their own or someone else's—we can largely benefit from our field knowledge. We know a lot about illness, health and health services, and we have an immediate understanding of many codes that may be incomprehensible to an outsider.

General practitioners, especially in rural areas, gain unique field knowledge about the district and the people in the district after living and working in the local community. Such knowledge strengthens the researcher's interpretations and also provides trust and mutual understanding encountering the participants. On the other hand, much of this field knowledge is *pre-reflexive*—not very conscious or conceptualised. Therefore, it may merge with the researcher's preconceptions in an indistinct way.

Field knowledge will also, often unconsciously, bear the imprint of one's additional roles—for instance, with medicosentrism as a healthcare professional (see Chapter 14). When we explore a phenomenon, a field or an environment that we are very familiar with, we take a lot of matters for granted. This poses a significant risk of *field blindness*, which can result in us only seeing or confirming what we are used to seeing. The particular challenge for the participant observer is to transcend the blinders that actors within the setting have naturally developed around their own self-understanding, and to prevent the analysis from merely confirming existing preconceptions. When we, as researchers, comprise extensive field knowledge, we often share the actors' blinders. The new and valuable knowledge lives outside and beyond these and can be approached by inventive interpretations.

Metapositions—a view from elsewhere

In all types of qualitative studies, *metapositions* offer different perspectives and footholds than what we see when we sit in the middle of something. Looking at myself and the project from a bird's eye view or from the sidelines, alone or with others, can strengthen my ability to adopt attitudes where the questions become as important as the answers (Andersen 1987, Malterud 2001b, 2002).

The participant observer needs breathing space for reflection that allows attention to what colours the observations, the role the observer plays, and the forms of knowing co-created through interpretation. Queries and challenges from metapositions can help articulate limitations and distortions related to preconceptions and field blindness, thereby sharpening the possibilities for a relevant and robust process of knowing.

To see ourselves clearly in the mirror, we need a little distance, although if we are positioned too far away, we see nothing but the rough contours. To support a nuanced account of our role in the research process, metapositions must be actively cultivated to achieve the appropriate distance. In other words, we need to sharpen our ability and willingness to recognise what appears different when viewed from the outside (Stensland 2003).

Metapositions can be established in different ways. Often it involves disturbing one's own sovereignty when developing and interpreting data, perhaps by being open to insights from others, including even harsh comments on the process. Inviting research colleagues from other disciplines into your considerations may lead to surprising comments. We can also establish analysis strategies where every answer is followed by a counter-question. It is possible to switch between roles in time and space, where we can do data interaction and analysis in different places. Theoretical perspectives, preferably practice-based and project-oriented substantive theories, make valuable contributions as metapositions in both research and practice (see Chapter 20) (Guassora, Reventlow, et al. 2022, Malterud, Reventlow, et al. 2024).

CHAPTER 17

Critical and committed inquiry in action

Research, professional development and quality improvement in service fields often involve the development, implementation and evaluation of interventions. Several different, partly overlapping professional traditions and concepts are available for such purposes. With action research, we work for change while at the same time using the process for inquiry, learning and development. Implementation comprises strategies for translating knowledge-based measures into day-to-day practice and for disseminating them across the field. In process evaluation and other kinds of quality improvement, we assess the outcomes of interventions with subsequent reporting. Here we examine strategies for such knowledge development, attending to the shifting boundary between scientific knowledge and operational evaluation data.

From established practice to improvement initiatives

Researchers in medicine and health sciences are often motivated by experiences from their own practice or organisation. We have experienced getting stuck in problems that are difficult to solve, strategies that do not work, or framework conditions that affect our choices and opportunities for action. We want to contribute to improvement and change— first in our own everyday life, then in a broader context if we see opportunities for others to benefit from the intervention we have developed.

Qualitative methods can support research aiming for development, implementation and evaluation of various *interventions* in established practice, such as communicative methods, depression diagnostics or lifestyle interventions (Malterud 1990, Stensland & Malterud 1999, Malterud, Aamland, et al. 2018, Potthoff, O'Donnell, et al. 2022). Transforming subjective experience into valid knowledge is particularly demanding in a field defined by process and change. To do so, we need expertise and tools, as well as a good blend of enthusiasm, creativity, systematics and self-criticism. We also need the support of those around us who will be involved in the change.

DOI: 10.4324/9781003786016-20

No intervention works for everything, and no research method is universally applicable. Various qualitative designs and data sources may be appropriate, such as focus groups, participant observation or analysis of written texts, depending on the nature of the intentions and amendment on the agenda. In addition, we need relevant and robust methods to handle the processes of developing, co-creating, implementing and evaluating the intervention. Along the way, we need to familiarise ourselves with the impact of the context and our personal role in it. This is where chaos can easily ensue. But such projects can also bring significant rewards when you realise that what you are doing makes a difference to more people than just yourself.

You may believe that you are the first to embark on a particular development project, but you never start from scratch. You therefore start by establishing an overview of the existing knowledge base. An appropriate methodology framework will support you in choosing your ambitions, approach and rhythm, allowing you to gather your thoughts and prioritise your efforts.

In this field, you will find many terms that are both commonly used and have a specific methodological meaning. You will also realise that there is considerable overlap between several of the orientations discussed. If you want to stay on course throughout the project, you need to read enough about the different strategies for development and evaluation before the project gathers full momentum so that you can select the one that fits you best and commit to that path. Going off on a tangent here and there creates an untidy understanding of the process that can make it difficult to report progress and lessons learnt, especially if the goal is to advance scientific knowledge.

Experimental designs are often used for intervention studies in medical research. If we want to develop an intervention or contribute to change in a medical context, such designs are conventionally considered the obvious choice. However, qualitative methods allow us to explore aspects of the issue that align more closely with our conceptual and intervention frameworks, particularly when the target of change is characterised by subjectivity and dynamic processes. You will, however, have to defend your choices.

We therefore start considering some limitations of experimental designs for such purposes. This is followed by a brief presentation of action research and implementation research. Both traditions treat evaluation as a central task, and different forms of process evaluation have also developed as distinct subfields. You can easily get lost in terms and methods here. If you are considering this type of project, you need to go to the sources and read more before you start in earnest. Do not tailor your own system from scratch!

Limitations of experimental designs

The *randomised controlled trial* (RCT) is the gold standard in medical intervention studies when we want to measure efficacy, find out whether A is better than B or assess causality. If these are the kinds of questions we want to answer, we should stick to RCTs. In RCT design, we compare the outcome in two groups, with the intervention implemented in one (the study group) but not in the other (the control group).

However, an RCT relies on assumptions that are hard to fulfil when the issue is part of the health service's daily practice. In an RCT, an intervention must be unambiguous, well-defined and standardised to yield scientifically robust results. This design is not suitable when you take subjective experiences as a basis for learning, aiming for dynamic development of the intervention. Attention to outcome measures alone can result in neglecting both the feasibility of the intervention and the contextual conditions that determine its transferability. If the conditions for an RCT cannot be met, we should not invest resources in it.

More than a few hold that the experimental design is a prerequisite for scientific knowledge. This is to confuse ends and means. No scientific method comes with a guarantee of scientific validity. In experimental research, validity depends on adherence to the assumptions and logic of the chosen design. Still, many medical issues cannot be fitted into such a format without making too many compromises. Scientific quality declines when validity and relevance are neglected in favour of reliability—for example, when measuring irrelevant factors or tracking unintended effects (Olsen, Mikkelsen, et al. 2004).

Compromises are necessary aspects of any research strategy. However, methodological flaws must not be allowed to destroy the project's aim and uniqueness to make it more researchable, corresponding to traditional criteria (Olsen, Mikkelsen, et al. 2004). Action research offers a valid approach to the development of scientific knowledge and is often well suited to community and clinical interventions (Malterud 1995a). Such an approach is not an easy shortcut, but on the contrary, a choice that presents the researcher with numerous methodological challenges and benefits.

Action research as a contribution to social change

Action research was developed at the interface between social science research and political activism, aiming for the development of interventions that could contribute to *social justice* (Whyte 1991). The starting point was Lewin's research (1948) on racial prejudice from the late 1940s. In other words, it is not about change on any terms, but about measures rooted in democratic and moral values. Action research involves the transformation of a social situation with a view to improvement, integrated with action, where each phase is intended to learn from the previous one and shape the next (Peters & Robinson 1984, Winter 1989, Malterud 1995a).

Pragmatic and *pragmatism* are familiar everyday terms that are also used in the context of this type of knowledge development. To act pragmatically is to favour flexible and workable responses to concrete problems, without requiring full alignment with overarching norms or theoretical commitments. American pragmatic philosophy, with theorists Charles Sanders Peirce (1839–1914) and John Dewey (1859–1952), affords the theoretical underpinning for action research, i.e. something more comprehensive and specific than the everyday connotation. The starting point is that knowledge is only valid when it can be employed as productive action, and that results and consequences are just as important as purposes and intentions.

Context influences the outcomes of action, and knowing is a relational phenomenon shaped by interaction. Critical theory has been pivotal to this field (Habermas 1984), foregrounding the value-laden nature of knowledge, the need to make values explicit, the importance of democracy, mobilisation and participant involvement, and the imperative to challenge power and powerlessness. The target group is active participants with influence at all stages of the research project. *Participatory Action*

Research (PAR) is a radical tradition with liberation from oppression as an explicit goal (Whyte 1991). PAR involves a high degree of participant involvement, often with community members or patients in the role of co-researchers (Freire 1970, Thesen & Kuzel 1999).

However, there are also more modest forms of action research as a strategy for exploring reflexive practice. Here, knowing is regarded as the reciprocal relationship between action, knowledge development, implementation and improved practice (Argyris, Putnam, et al. 1985, Malterud 1995a). These can also be strategies and concepts relevant to articulate tacit practice knowledge for further elaboration (Schön 1991) (see Chapter 19). Here too, values, context and interaction are key elements.

Action research represents a dynamic strategy based on subjective experiences and perceptions, which are systematically subjected to testing, interpretation, reflexivity and evaluation (Malterud 1990, Stensland & Malterud 1999, Steihaug, Ahlsen, et al. 2001, Oien & Solheim 2015). This differs substantially from experimental intervention designs grounded in a standardised, stable ontology (see Chapter 2).

Action and research hand in hand

Action research brings together *action* and *research*, not least in the surplus value generated by their interplay. (Malterud 1995a). There will be no action research if there is only action or only research. The action part of the project must carry out the planned change by developing an intervention that is suitable for the purpose. The research part of the project evaluates the process by describing, interpreting, analysing and reporting what takes place (the action itself) and what are the outcomes (experiences and results), situating this in the context of prevailing knowledge.

Action and research go hand in hand. Research must learn from action, and action must learn from research. These activities must be grounded in a shared understanding of the project's objectives and application. Action research projects are often initiated by enthusiastic individuals. This creates a (predictable) risk that the action will be prioritised at the expense of the research part of the project, and that evaluation and reporting will be displaced by the project's daily life, constantly making acute demands (Olsen, Mikkelsen, et al. 2004).

But when the aim is to develop new and valuable scientific knowledge with relevant and robust methods, we start by establishing a project outline, securing sufficient resources for the development and processing of relevant data along the way. It is also necessary to set aside time for summarising and reporting towards the end. This always takes longer than you think.

When the evaluation is conducted by someone other than the person with the idea behind or responsibility for the action part of the project, the researchers' need for evaluation data may push forward unintentional or unfortunate distortions of the intervention (Olsen, Mikkelsen, et al. 2004). This is particularly the case when researchers rely on quantitative criteria and outcome measures that are incongruent with the project's objectives, or when the design assumes a stability that precludes development and learning in line with experience. We must therefore see the action and research dimensions as two sides of the same coin.

The action spiral

The action component of the project consists of a sequence of interlinked steps. (Figure 17.1). Here I will present a model consisting of the following seven steps: (1) problem identification, (2) summarising previous experiences, (3) formulating action aims, (4) planning and developing the intervention, (5) describing the intervention, (6) implementing the intervention and (7) redefining the problem (more on implementation research below).

By comparing action aims and experiences, we find out whether there is a need for further improvement. The first turn is a circle, which subsequently typically becomes a spiral via new turns—*the action spiral* (Malterud 1995a). Action research invites us to learn from and take the consequences of the experiences in the project. Systematic compilation of experience with empirical data co-creation is essential for gaining new insights. Our project is rarely completed after the first turn of the action spiral. At best, we have achieved knowledge driving forward action with the prospect of further improvement through successive turns of the spiral.

Along the way, we ensure that each step in the action spiral is anchored in data that provides a basis for interpretation and analysis. You do not try to include everything—it is the study aim that determines what to emphasise most. To describe and analyse both process and outcomes, relevant data inform us about what occurred and how the intervention was designed and functioned. Each step within each turn of the action

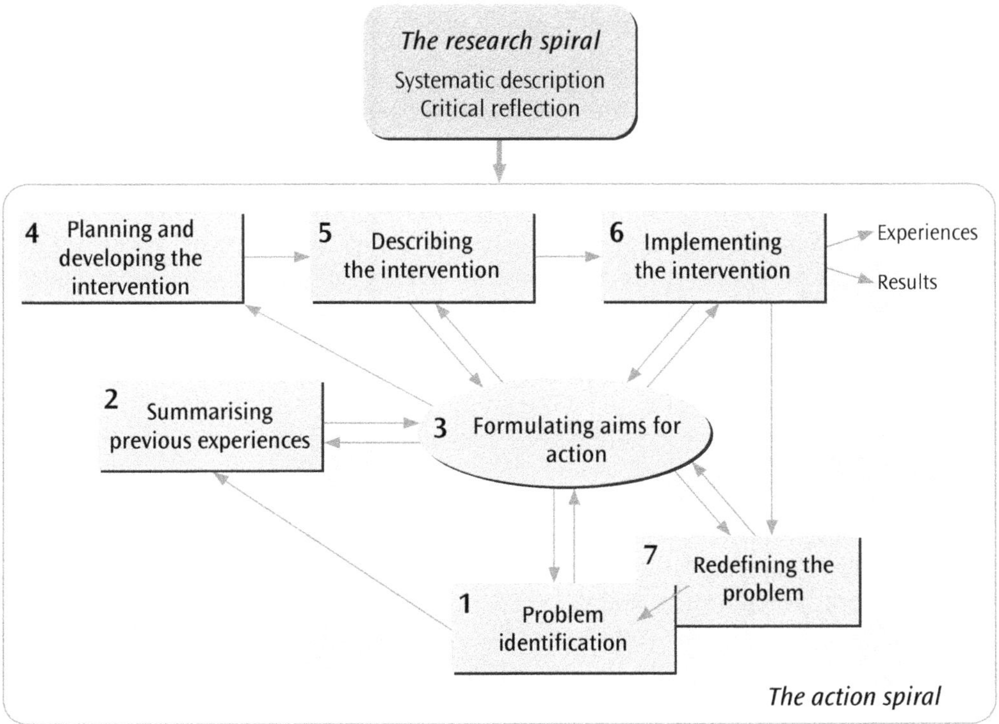

Figure 17.1 Action research with the action spiral and the research spiral (after Malterud 1995a)

spiral gives you a progress plan for the action part of the project, and also a checklist for co-creation of evaluation data (Malterud 1995a).

The process starts with *problem identification* or diagnosis. The project manager and stakeholders review the status and argue why there is a need for change. The problem identification and study aim will always be substantially focused during the process. It is therefore important to avoid an initially fixed and constraining view of the field, to allow new insights to grow as the work unfolds.

We then *summarise previous experiences* of transformation in this domain, drawing on local histories and the roles of key actors in this and comparable contexts, and on relevant theoretical and empirical literature. Negative experiences are just as important as positive ones. Together, these form the basis for articulating action goals—what forms of change are both desirable and feasible? Goal setting sets the trajectory and keeps the direction in view.

Planning and developing the intervention from idea to reality is an important phase, where it is important to spend the time needed. We do not address strategies and tools until this stage, when we begin to consider which actions or interventions might be appropriate. There is always someone else who was there before you. You never start from scratch—literature searches to learn about previous experiences give you a starting point. A common pitfall is to start the action process by designing the intervention. If we do this, we run a serious risk of the action aim being ambiguous, the direction being unclear, the intervention being ill-suited to the purpose, with the evaluation taking a back seat or the stakeholders in the field having serious reservations. Cultivating a new and valuable intervention may be the most substantive outcome of an action research project.

With a clear action goal in mind, we can proceed to grow and present a programme capable of delivering what it sets out to achieve. We perform an intermediate pragmatic validation (see Chapter 21) to assess the potential validity of the program—the soundness of what we have come to understand and the scope of that understanding. Will the intervention turn out to be what it is supposed to be about, and can it be implemented in the actual context? If the programme is also to be applied by others and implemented in a larger context (more on implementation below), we must be able to describe the intervention as a coherent package, with a specification as support for use. Now, it is time to articulate our ideas and present an intervention guide outlining *the preliminary features of the intervention* (Malterud 1990, Stensland & Malterud 1997, Steihaug, Ahlsen, et al. 2001).

Once the intervention programme has taken a form that can be implemented in practice and appears to function as intended, we focus on embedding it in its local context as refined through trial and error. During this phase, we attend to *experiences and outcomes*, considering feasibility and goal achievement (Malterud & Hollnagel 1998, Malterud 1999, Thesen 2001). Stay away from inferences about effect and causality, where quantitative logic and methodology are required. Process and outcome are equal elements of the knowing we want to develop and present. If we have not carried out the preceding steps thoroughly and are unable to explain the intervention and how it is implemented, our results will be of limited interest to others with low potential for implementation. Still, we must not forget that others of course are interested in what we achieved, not just what we did.

The final step in the action spiral is to *redefine the problem*, considering the insights we have gained by moving through the previous steps. We can use this in new strategies for continuing the change work and take decisions about new turns in the action spiral. We can also use it as a challenge to the development of theory and methods in the field in question. Then we return to the first step, fuelled by ideas and experiences becoming gradually clearer.

The research spiral

Evaluation quests imply continuous reflection and learning. We need to develop and co-create empirical data for the systematic interpretation of subjective experience, generating new insights through cycles that unfold into new spirals. Once again, the goal of action defines the study aim, and which methods and data fit the dual purposes of change and evaluation. Action research projects often (but not always) involve qualitative methods, and combinations of methods may also be relevant (see Chapter 22). For example, we can apply modest principles from qualitative evaluation to map general practitioners' (GPs') experiences with a tool for self-evaluation of their own consultations (Lid, Eraker, et al. 2004, Patton 2015). With quantitative approaches, selected issues or results of the intervention can be quantified. In that case, remember that these are not measurements originating from a representative or random sample. Therefore, stay far away from blunt conclusions about scope, distribution, differences and causality. Keep in mind that you cannot comment on the effect of the intervention or causality related to what happened.

Action research creates spaces piled up with organic knowing, processes and interaction. The project manager is an essential agent of change in the field, while also embedded in the very field under study—both participant and observer (Skjervheim 2002, Olsen, Mikkelsen, et al. 2004). Experience from ethnographic fieldwork, especially participant observation, is helpful methodological grounding for the medical action researcher (see Chapter 16). Empirical evaluation data are developed from field notes, decision trail, diaries, documents and correspondence, often supplemented with audio or video recordings. Individual or group interviews with stakeholders and key participants are also relevant sources for data co-creation (Stensland & Malterud 1997, Thesen & Kuzel 1999, Thesen 2001). Researching oneself poses substantial challenges for reflexivity and demands solid methodological expertise (Stensland 2003). A wise and experienced supervisor fulfils an important metaposition.

If the researcher by default collects everything that could conceivably be useful, there is an imminent risk of *data death*. Large amounts of data inevitably lead to chaos and superficial analysis, not preventable by digital support. It is therefore crucial to plan the project with data from purposive samples with appropriate Information Power (IP) to address the prioritised matters while suggesting and achieving the intended change. There should also be congruence—a common thread—between what the data are supposed to elucidate and the type of data. In an action research project, we do not always know in advance what kind of material this will be.

The opposite pitfall is when the researcher collects too little material to substantiate what has been done, or that the material only consists of success stories that support the project manager's best intentions. A general rule is therefore to actively develop and co-create data elucidating reluctancies and negative experiences with an impact on the process and the outcomes. Presenting such data enhances confidence in reflexivity and reveals constraints on the transferability of the intervention.

The *project report* is supposed to tell your commissioner and readers what happened, not what we hoped to happen. In the project report, experiences and documentation should have a distinctly different form and content than the ideals and ambitions of the initial project outline. The text should clearly indicate the sources from which the reported outcomes derive, and it should allow us to discern the contours of actual events through descriptions of experience from the intervention's implementation. You digest, sum up and substantiate your interpretations. The text is not, as in interview studies, made more authentic or trustworthy by a series of catchy or identical quotes.

A relevant and robust plan for evaluation can prevent some of these pitfalls. Empirical data can rarely be generated after events have taken place and must be co-created and organised as they unfold. Furthermore, the evaluation is just as important a contribution to knowing as the action, and sufficient time and resources must therefore be ensured. Just as in the action spiral, the evaluation process is adapted in line with the experiences along the way, while the action to be evaluated changes shape and colour.

Static evaluation designs that rely on standardisation have limited internal validity in action research, where learning and flexibility are central. This is especially pertinent for *before-after designs*, where the effect of an intervention is measured at a certain point in time in relation to the project start. In such designs, the intervention must remain unchanged throughout the process—a precondition incongruent with basic principles of action research and qualitative methods (Patton 2015). Before-after designs are also vulnerable to the influence of contextual influence beyond our control. It can be hard to assess which part of a result originates from the intervention, and which is due to other factors. Imagine we want to run a campaign to influence local people's attitudes to mental illness, measuring attitudes before and after the campaign. If, for example, a TV campaign on mental illness takes place in the middle of the project period, this might be considerably more influential than our programme (Thesen 2001). The plain before-and-after design does not take such circumstances seriously into account and is more suitable for laboratory experiments.

Implementation—from knowing in practice to broader uptake

Knowledge about interventions developed from research is translated into daily operations and spread further out into the field of practice by implementation. Imagine that we developed an intervention programme, perhaps in an action research project. Now we are ready to share it and advance its further development and dissemination. *Implementation research* is a distinct subfield, yet it shares many methodological features with action research. Here, we address the practice of transferability—how others may draw on the knowing generated—and briefly consider documentation and reporting. For disciplines such as social medicine, public health and health services research, this can be particularly relevant.

Implementation processes are always complex and extensive (Craig, Dieppe, et al. 2008). Let us imagine our intervention as a package. We plan to export this package to someone who has ordered it. The recipient expects to find a manual informing them about the scope of use for the content, how it ought to be assembled, and what we do to make it work. It is not a given that the recipient will obtain identical results as we originally did when the programme goes live. But before knowledge from enthusiastic or experimental frameworks is ready for use in practice, many stages of customisation, positioning and dissemination of the initiative remain.

Implementation research is the scientific study of how an intervention is put into practice as strategies, programmes or individual practices (Peters, Adam, et al. 2013). Implementation and implementation research deal with translating what we know into what we do, with close attention to everyday conditions that hinder or enable such processes (Peters, Tran, et al. 2013). This kind of research draws on various roots and elements, including quality improvement (Grol, Wensing, et al. 2005), evidence-based medicine (EBM) (Graham, Mancher, et al. 2011), organisational psychology (Fixsen, Naaom, et al. 2005), evaluation research (Patton 2008) and programme theory (Vedung 1997).

During the implementation process, we tailor a previously tested intervention to the wider context in which it will be implemented. We start by positioning and creating enthusiasm and uptake among users and decision-makers. User training must be quality-assured, establishing the foundation for sustainable maintenance. Implementation research provides the tools to take a closer look at the conditions determining how and whether the implementation is successful. Here, I will present a simple model for *small-scale implementation research* (Malterud, Aamland, et al. 2018).

We are not starting from scratch—our starting point is existing research evidence—our own or others', qualitative or quantitative—that we want to share with others. We seek to implement a knowledge-based *intervention programme* (see Chapter 1) for broader uptake beyond the context in which it was developed. The intervention has already been properly documented in previous stages, preferably with publications in international peer-reviewed journals. In other words, we must first ensure that the intervention is appropriately documented to merit dissemination efforts.

The documentation supporting the intervention may vary methodologically, depending on its type and the problems it is intended to address. Efficacy studies offer an important basis for interventions with a wide reach, such as vaccine programmes or screening services. Such large interventions should not be implemented without confidence that they work. For example, prior to national implementation of guidelines for drug treatment of type 2 diabetes, we will assume that the drugs in question have been tested in RCTs with sufficiently clear results for relevant outcome measures.

However, in domains of clinical or systems practice, implementation of interventions with smaller dimensions than national guidelines may be on our agenda. For example, interaction strategies for use in consultations require different kinds of evidence, with subjectivity as a central premise. In such cases, we are more interested in how the intervention is implemented and experienced than in achieving a standardised result. In such projects, we may plan the implementation of a knowledge-based intervention grounded in a relevant and robust manual for purpose, context and procedure, for example a strategy for home notes for patients with entrenched bodily complaints in the meeting with the GP (Stensland & Malterud 1999).

To transfer the intervention beyond its original context, it must be adapted and piloted to simplify, adjust and test its format and feasibility. At this stage, we familiarise ourselves with the research constituting the intervention's evidence base (Abrahamsen, Lindbæk, et al. 2022). Then we can adapt the intervention for everyday use without losing the core of what has already been documented. We will define the scope of the implementation regarding goals, context and target group.

When the intervention is ready to spread beyond the ranks of enthusiasts, we move on to *scaling*, where we put the adjusted intervention into practice on a small or large scale. First, we must build motivation and alliances with key decision-makers. Then we organise training, quality assurance and maintenance, so that participants experience the intervention as meaningful and can integrate it naturally into daily chores. Piloting and scaling are not one-way phases, but are closely and mutually linked (Malterud, Aamland, et al. 2018).

The *project outline* for an implementation project may include the following elements:

- Problem (identify and define scope)
- Action goal
- Intervention (evidence, adaptation, piloting and procedure)
- Implementation (scaling, target group, finances, motivation, permits, negotiations, training, quality assurance and adjustments)
- Evaluation (experiences and results)
- Final report and recommendations

Conditions for successful implementation

According to Grol, et al. (2005), successful implementation requires systematic, well-planned approach, assessment of whether the intervention is a viable product, readiness of the target group, as well as diagnostic analysis of the target group, context and feasibility. They also list up the needs for strategies to involve the target group in planning, development and adaptation, systematically assessing what needs to change, carrying out the implementation with multidimensional strategies, ensuring that the measures match what needs to be changed, and conducting ongoing evaluation of the process and results. If implementation can fit into existing structures, feasibility and sustainability are strengthened.

Implementation research presents and summarises preconditions and experiences by implementing an intervention in a particular context, preferably with transferability to comparable contexts. A small-scale implementation study from a nursing home in Rogaland, for example, can offer valuable knowledge for the implementation of a similar intervention on a large scale in several regions (Malterud, Aamland, et al. 2018).

As in action research, we must simultaneously address the two different, but intertwined levels of implementation and implementation research (see Figure 17.2). We therefore must plan and carry out a research design with logical coherence and clarification of these two levels. It is just as important to systematically evaluate how you establish dissemination (of an intervention that is itself already documented) as it is to evaluate experiences and results when this is put into practice.

Evaluation researchers distinguish between process evaluation and outcome evaluation (Patton 2015). In implementation research, we use *process evaluation* to study the implementation itself (what happened, what adjustments did we have to make to make

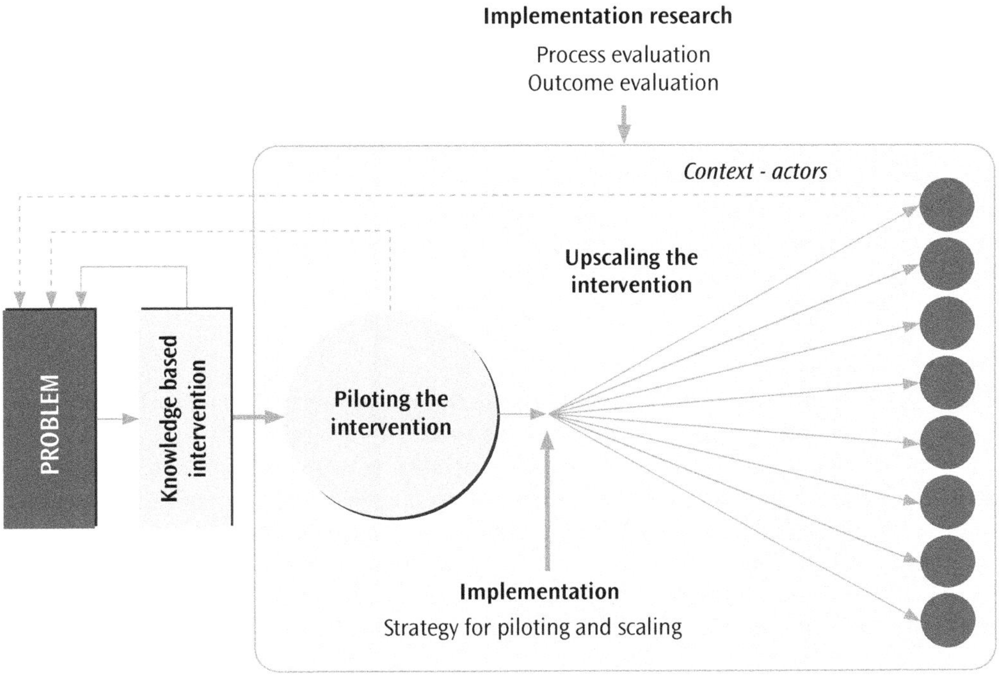

Figure 17.2 Implementation and implementation research (after Malterud, Aamland and et al. 2018)

the intervention feasible, what were the conditions for making it happen, where was the strongest resistance). *Feasibility* studies with a relevant and robust design provide insight into the conditions for implementation and scaling (Abrahamsen, Lindbæk, et al. 2022). *Outcome evaluation* is used to study whether and how we achieved the implementation goal but is less concerned with which specific effect or outcome measures were supported by the intervention in the new context.

Implementation research is not supposed to zero in on the evidence base and prove that the original intervention still works. We are primarily interested in understanding what is required for dissemination and scaling out into the field of practice. In implementation research, process evaluation is therefore a logical prerequisite for outcome evaluation—it does not make sense to investigate whether the implementation was successful without knowing more about the procedures for the intervention and strategies for implementation.

Some key dimensions of implementation success are *coverage* (what proportion of the target group completed the programme) and *intervention fidelity* (whether and how the intervention, as adjusted in the pilot phase, was implemented in accordance with the manual). We also explore conditions for workable implementation—both success factors (facilitators) and resistance (inhibitors) (Fixsen, Naaom, et al. 2005, Grol, Wensing, et al. 2005, Malterud, Aamland, et al. 2018).

As implementation researchers, we address how the intervention is handled through piloting and dissemination, and what adaptations were necessary for the transition from small-scale to large-scale. Subsequently, we may look at the outcomes of the adjusted intervention as it is utilised in implementation on a larger scale. We may later conduct a pragmatic RCT to examine the intervention's effectiveness under everyday conditions. To compare our results with the efficacy demonstrated in the original studies under more ideal conditions, we need to specify how the intervention was configured in our implementation. This is the only way to prevent a "black-box" problem— a situation where we do not know what works (Glasziou, Meats, et al. 2008). However, for implementation research, the study focus should primarily include the dissemination process itself, i.e. the adaptation, introduction, training and maintenance of the intervention in the new context.

Process evaluation

Evaluation concerns making sense of change by tracing what happens when an intervention is put into practice, drawing on systematically assembled material rather than assumption or impression. Above, we have utilised this meaning of the term within specific strategies such as action research and implementation research to assess how living knowledge is developed and disseminated as a contribution to change.

It may also be worth considering an evaluation of a medical or healthcare programme based on action research principles, with a lower level of academic ambition than that of scientific articles or PhD dissertations. In such cases, it may be more imperative for the commissioner to receive swift feedback as a report, rather than waiting for the detailed caveats of a scientific publication. Nonetheless, scientific designs and methods can inform systematic and critical reflection, opening up discussion of the soundness of our understandings and the scope of interpretation and conclusions in community medicine and health services research.

As this is a book about research methods, we do not go far into the field of evaluation research (programme evaluation, qualitative evaluation) (Patton 2015). *Process evaluation* is a methodological approach that shares several points of contact with qualitative methods commonly used to inform public and private policy and decisions on resource allocation. Such a strategy can be applied for all parts of the scale between the development of scientific knowledge and reporting for decision-making purposes. The first format often involves time-consuming publication in peer-reviewed journals, while the second is disseminated as reports with less academic and methodological ambition and a shorter gap between implementation and conclusions. Process evaluation is normally funded by the commissioner (public or private) and is often carried out as contract research, outside universities and university colleges.

The evaluator's role as a participant during the intervention process may be different in process evaluation than in action research, where the evaluator is a well-defined actor in the intervention planning, conduct and implementation. If the evaluator enters the project under conditions that constrain independence, fundamental questions about the framing of problems and measures may be foreclosed. Ambiguity around this distinction often gives rise to conflict among the client, the project manager and the evaluator (2004). Such controversies may arise from differing expectations between the parties about which results count as valid evidence of whether the project has met its objectives and delivered the expected outcomes. Clarifying and negotiating expectations is therefore a crucial starting point for such a project.

Research for knowledge-based policy—an action-oriented pragmatism?

Knowledge from research and evaluation is increasingly requested by politicians and public administration as a basis for decision-making, often in the form of commissioned research with evaluation reports where deadlines are short and quality assessment is limited. *Evidence-based policy* may seem as a contradiction in terms, unless you imagine knowledge as something flowing through a pipe from research to decision-makers, finalising decisions (Oliver, Lorenc, et al. 2014). If so, you risk omitting the impact of values for policy. Weiss (1979) describes the trade-off between ideals and realities regarding the impact of social science research for public decision-making, remarking that there is not always a match between expectations and influence. Similar challenges appear in public health practice (Malterud, Bjelland, et al. 2016). Nonetheless, it is constructive that decision-makers request research knowledge.

An important question for the researcher prior to the project start is whether this specific assignment deserves priority, and which methods are sufficiently relevant and robust to bestow the requested knowledge without too many compromises. Regardless of evaluation framework or academic level, we will encounter certain recurrent challenges when implementing and reporting interventions in the health services that involve human interaction in a social context. When the intervention itself is the focus, prioritisation and reflexivity become decisive factors for the scientific level of knowing in planning, implementation and reporting of the project.

Here, it is neither realistic nor appropriate to describe and analyse every tiny detail. Within this field, you should rather aim to maintain an overview, distinguish the major from the minor, and address selected elements of implementation and evaluation that merit particular attention. We must never lose sight of the practice context and the specific organisation and implementation of the intervention. Any ambitions for a comprehensive research design may therefore rather be replaced with practical expertise in prioritising relevant, pragmatic and selective focus.

Elaborating the evaluation outline, we should preferably be interaction-oriented pragmatists rather than significance-oriented epidemiologists. If we initiate an applied, practical project of this kind by planning an RCT, we risk losing sight of process and context (Peters, Tran, et al. 2013). The process evaluation may rather include a few well-chosen and feasible questions for further dissemination of the intervention in other contexts.

The development of a clear-cut manual for an intervention programme is key to action research as well as implementation research. In implementation projects, we additionally need a tidy account of the adjusted intervention as a prerequisite for further scaling. We need to know how and why assumptions and approaches have been adjusted during the pilot steps, so that we have a realistic image of what is to be implemented further on.

In qualitative research where subjectivity is the point of departure, there is no inherent contradiction in having the same person develop, implement and evaluate a programme. However, in projects such as those presented in this chapter, the researcher is often a keen enthusiast who does not always hold sufficient doubts or reflexivity. It is also necessary to achieve sufficient understanding about the epistemological assumptions for serving as a qualified participant and observer at the same time (see Chapter 1) (Skjervheim 2002). In such cases, we need reflexivity to recognise and challenge our interpretations and conclusions (see Chapter 3). Anchoring the work in robust and relevant analytic methods, adopting metapositions informed by theory, and establishing reference groups or multidisciplinary teams will strengthen both the credibility and the usefulness of what we report.

Echo effect—reproducing and confirming your aim?

Qualitative studies in medicine and health care commonly explore the experiences of participants who have taken part in some kind of intervention, such as a treatment programme for women with chronic muscular pain (Steihaug, Ahlsen, et al. 2001) or the experiences of medical staff with the introduction of video support for emergency medical calls (Idland, Iversen, et al. 2022). To evaluate such a programme, you should, early in the project, clarify what you mean by impact and outcomes, so that data generation and analysis become more than a statement of purpose framed by good intentions (see Chapter 12).

Assessing interventions that we have personally developed or implemented poses distinct methodological challenges, especially when the project involves sustained, close relationships with participants. Your role as the researcher may turn out to be perplexing and demanding when you have vested interests in ensuring that the programme works and that the participants are satisfied. With such designs, methodological clarity is therefore especially important.

With qualitative methods, we acknowledge that our approaches are not suited to assessing programme results in terms of whether, or to what extent, an intervention is effective. Quantitative research methods, preferably with an RCT design, are superior to study the intervention effect, with statistical methods comparing the outcome of those who participated in the intervention with a control group that did not receive this programme (Ree, Lie & al). Still, we can certainly explore impact and outcomes of a programme with qualitative methods. These are subtle but important nuances, with subjectivity and experiences as key concepts to set an analytical course.

A positive challenge is therefore to address subjective outcomes, as experienced and expressed by unique individuals (see Chapter 12). When objectives, measures and evaluations are all shaped by the same person, the risk of an echo effect increases, producing results that just reflect the study aims. As a reader, you may notice the echo when what is reported simply mirrors the project's original objective. In such cases, the results insist that the objective was achieved while offering limited understanding of the conditions that made it possible, and the subjective impact for the people participating.

If I say "The explanation is clear because it is understandable", my conclusion merely restates my premise in synonymous terms. The statement therefore lacks an independent premise and amounts to *circular reasoning*. In everyday language, synonyms may aid comprehension, but rhetorically, this is justifiable because it does not present as an *argument*.

In scientific contexts, by contrast, we expect arguments, claims and conclusions to be supported by *premises* that add substantive, independent grounds. For example, "The programme has promoted a stronger sense of belonging because participants described fresh and specific types of mutual support in their group discussions". By contrast, saying that "The programme strengthened belonging because it increased participants' feeling of connectedness" merely repeats the claim in different words. This latter form of circularity is a *tautology*—a claim that lacks substantiation because it simply restates its own premise.

When participants reiterate a project's overarching goals in interviews, this should not be mistaken for evidence of outcome. Such repetitions amount tautologically (self-confirming) only to an echo of the project goal. What matters is in which ways the intervention gave rise to specific experiences and nuances, not whether participants are able to repeat the project's objectives.

Quite often, this type of intervention is grounded in an underlying intention of how the participants will be affected by the intervention, often with a specific theoretical justification. For example, the goal of the physiotherapy method Basic Body Awareness Training (BBAT) is that patients learn to investigate their own patterns of movement to build awareness and practical understanding of how bodily capacities can be developed and used to meet the demands of everyday life. For a study on patient experiences with BBAT to avoid the echo effect, it must come up with something beyond the patient having established better insight and knowledge about how their own movement resources and potentials can be developed to deal with the challenges of daily life. Here, we expect knowledge presenting different specific aspects of how these goals had been translated into everyday experiences. For example, the results of the evaluation can contribute to nuances of experiences of how patients with schizophrenia experienced BBAT to influence their affect regulation and ability to concentrate (Hedlund & Gyllensten 2010).

Another study presented experiences from a rehabilitation group programme for patients with back and neck problems, where the intervention was designed to enhance participants' positive expectations and coping by communicating that the symptoms did not signify danger (Ree, Harris, et al. 2014). In such a design, an echo effect could easily have appeared in a results section stating that the participants had learnt that the symptoms did not signify danger. Instead, this study documents various concrete expressions of coping, conveying knowledge about how the project's objectives were put into practice through participation in the group programme.

Evaluating such programmes, we should ask how the intervention contributed to positive and negative change (Idland, Iversen, et al. 2022), rather than confirming the participants' statements that the goal has been achieved. Participant statements that echo the researcher's aims contribute little to understanding what was experienced and maybe changed in the project.

CHAPTER 18

Metasynthesis—surfacing prior evidence and creating new knowing

Research should build on the existing knowledge base, irrespective of methodology. As researchers, we should engage with, critically appraise, and extend the insights of those who came before us. Large amounts of research publications are digitally available, but it can be hard to get an overview. Systematic reviews based on the evidence from previous primary studies can lead to new and valuable scientific knowledge, adding to what the primary studies showed. Specific research methodology has been developed for this purpose. Here, we will take a closer look at the principles and procedures for qualitative systematic reviews, also known as qualitative metasynthesis, involving the identification, critical appraisal, analysis and synthesis of evidence from previous qualitative studies.

Sustainable knowledge

Knowledge is a renewable resource, with prevention of waste as a premise. *Sustainable knowledge* implies responsibility for the future with responsible management of today's knowledge resources (Frodeman 2014). We do not have to reinvent the wheel. If we assume that we are starting from scratch and fail to obtain an overview of existing work, we waste research resources and pay little respect to prior knowledge development. We can further develop the distinctive nature of knowledge and realise the added value of the knowledge capital by upcycling and utilising research evidence of appropriate relevance and quality. When scientific rigour is ensured (see Chapter 3), research results from qualitative as well as quantitative primary studies and systematic reviews qualifies as *evidence*.

Review articles, in which the author presents and summarises the scientific literature on an issue, are an established genre in the medical publishing tradition. For a long time, this was a loosely defined format in which the author, at his or her own discretion, prioritised which publications to emphasise. Today, such strategies are known as *cherry picking*.

DOI: 10.4324/9781003786016-21

Specific research methods have been developed for this purpose. Methods for qualitative studies, also known as *metasynthesis*, have some similarities and many differences compared to quantitative systematic reviews. Here, we concentrate on the principles and procedures of qualitative metasynthesis, alongside an examination of how the assumptions and methodological procedures of quantitative systematic reviews were established and came to shape scientific norms more broadly.

To approach an overview of the research literature in a field, we can start by conducting a *scoping review* to "...map the available knowledge in a new and under-researched area. Such an overview can clarify key concepts and identify knowledge gaps and research needs. It can be seen as a preliminary appraisal of the available research literature." (Munn, Pollock, et al. 2022). Scoping reviews provide a description of existing research, but without a critical appraisal of relevance or quality. The purpose is to assess the likely range of published literature, partly to realistically plan the expected use of resources (Arksey & O'Malley 2005, Gough, Oliver, et al. 2017b).

Another type of literature review is a *mapping review*. Such reviews are often used as preliminary work in the planning of major research projects, with an emphasis on effectiveness (Khalil & Tricco 2022), and are often prepared with short deadlines, without meeting all the requirements of a scientific study.

For reviews to be considered scientific contributions in the form of synthesised studies, we set specific requirements for process, results and presentation (Gough, Oliver, et al. 2017b, Malterud 2019b). Surfacing existing research knowledge is carried out with a strategy designed to limit undesirable inclinations in the collection of data, followed by critical appraisal, and finally analysis and synthesis of studies on the actual matter holding appropriate relevance and quality. The search strategy, establishing the project's source of empirical data, is later reported and discussed. The outcomes of the search are systematically scrutinised for relevance to the study aim and the quality of the methods and results. Publications with evidence from primary studies fulfilling these criteria are included for analysis, which may be conducted with different strategies and levels of ambition.

Systematic reviews—a scientific method for research literature summary

A *systematic review (SR)* is the outcome of a synthesis of evidence conducted using established research methods based on the principles presented above *(Gough, Oliver, et al. 2017b). The purpose is to draw a map of the research terrain for the study aim from available evidence of appropriate relevance and quality. The level of ambition may vary, ranging from descriptive summarisation (*aggregation*) to analytical synthesis (*configuration*) (Greenhalgh 1997, Gough, Oliver, et al. 2017b). Both levels require systematic critical appraisal of the included primary studies according to specified criteria.

SR was refined as a method within evidence-based medicine (EBM) when the information deluge gained momentum from the 1990s (Chalmers 1993, Sackett, Rosenberg, et al. 1996). Surfacing with transparent identification, critical appraisal, selection and consolidation of quantitative primary studies was established as methodological prerequisites (Oxman & Guyatt 1993, Lavis, Davies, et al. 2005). The international *Cochrane Collaboration* became a core foundation for the development of scientific criteria for SRs (Liberati, Altman, et al. 2009, Gough, Oliver, et al. 2017b, Centre for Reviews and Dissemination 2025).

These were supplemented by a methodology for standardised critical quality appraisal in the SRs and for assessing the strength of recommendations in guidelines based on the synthesised evidence (Grading of Recommendations Assessment, Development, and Evaluation—*GRADE*) (Guyatt, Oxman, et al. 2008). SR became the methodological gold standard and trademark for answering the question of whether an intervention is effective, thus imposing an argument for standardising the knowledge base for evidence. The SR methodology was gradually extended to incorporate primary studies on diagnostic tests, prevention and psychosocial interventions and health services, in addition to the original focus on efficacy studies for treatment and vaccines.

Today, results from single empirical studies are rarely accepted as a basis for changing practice or guidelines. The assumption is normally that SRs—preferably several—of appropriate relevance and quality confirm the efficacy or benefit through convincing evidence. These are logical assumption, as long as they are congruent with the study aim.

However, many considered the Cochrane medical model inadequate for developing evidence on health and healthcare, arguing that strategies appropriate for efficacy studies needed to be supplemented with other forms of evidence that allow for contextual, political, and ethical considerations (Black 2001, Orton, Lloyd-Williams, et al. 2011, Gough, Oliver, et al. 2017a, Greenhalgh & Malterud 2018). While the EBM movement's evidence hierarchy declared results from randomised controlled trials as the gold standard (Canadian Task Force on the Periodic Health Examination 1979, Cochrane 1989), social scientists put greater emphasis on epistemological congruence—that the method to be used was appropriate for the study aim (Gough, Oliver, et al. 2017a).

In the 1980s, independent of the Cochrane community, a methodological basis was also developed for qualitative systematic reviews involving the compiling, reanalysis and consolidation of evidence from qualitative primary studies (Thorne, Jensen, et al. 2004, Sandelowski & Barroso 2007). As early as 1985, nursing researchers Stern and Harris published an article synthesising the main results from seven different primary studies on women and self-help (Stern & Harris 1985). A few years later, education researchers Noblit and Hare (1988) presented *meta-ethnography* as a method for synthesising qualitative studies. The method was intended for inductive analysis and interpretation (see Chapter 1), not merely as a summary, but with the aim of generating insights that went beyond those of the primary studies.

Meta-ethnography has subsequently been used extensively, also for the synthesis of qualitative studies without a specific ethnographic underpinning (Dixon-Woods, Cavers, et al. 2006, Bondas & Hall 2007a). Gradually, several additional strategies for qualitative systematic reviews have been proposed, sometimes under different names (Pawson, Greenhalgh, et al. 2005, Bondas & Hall 2007b, Thomas & Harden 2008, Barnett-Page & Thomas 2009, Malterud 2019b). Below, these are referred to under the general heading of *qualitative metasynthesis*.

The EBM community has increasingly recognised that syntheses based on qualitative primary studies can make important contributions to knowledge by addressing some of the limitations of the traditional Cochrane format. (Guyatt, Oxman, et al. 2011, Lewin, Glenton, et al. 2013). *Qualitative Evidence Synthesis* (QES) is the term used in this context (Hannes, Booth, et al. 2013). WHO has accepted such qualitative studies as legitimate evidence bases for complex interventions (World Health Organization 2014).

The Cochrane community has also developed *CERQual*, a method comparable to GRADE (see above) for assessing how much confidence we can have in the results of a metasynthesis as a basis for decisions on recommendations and guidelines (Lewin, Glenton, et al. 2015). In the EBM community, quantitative research methods are dominant, which entails numerous challenges and compromises in developing qualitative methodology while maintaining epistemological congruence (see below). (Thorne 2011, Malterud 2019a).

Meta-analysis is a generic term for strategies for pooling quantitative studies with statistical processing of already published primary studies on the same issue, i.e. something more than collating and summarising. The term was first introduced in the late 1970s as a method for aggregating effect estimates from several different primary studies with comparable interventions. With meta-analysis, compiling evidence from many small studies together enhances statistical power and yields a more reliable overall picture, such as in the classic study on the effect of aspirin for secondary prevention of myocardial infarction (Editorial Lancet 1980). Quantitative meta-analysis is conducted as statistical calculations, while qualitative meta-analysis corresponds to what we here call qualitative metasynthesis, with interpretation and subjectivity as epistemological cornerstones. Below we will look at some assumptions and selected approaches for qualitative metasynthesis as a research method.

More than the sum of its parts

Qualitative metasynthesis begins, as in any research project, with the development of a focused *study aim* that is sufficiently open-ended to allow us to identify as much published evidence as possible about the question we want to explore. At the same time, the problem must be sufficiently focused for our metasynthesis to contribute with new and valuable knowledge, as compared to a descriptive exploratory overview or catalogue of what has previously been done and concluded (Gough, Oliver, et al. 2017b, Malterud 2019b). According to Eakin and Mykhalovskiy (2003), the aim of a qualitative study is more like a compass than an anchor, that is often not fully specified until the end of the research process. For example, a qualitative metasynthesis on experiences of chronic fatigue syndrome may start with a broad ambition to find the most and the best qualitative primary studies on experiences among patients, relatives and doctors, while early on in the process it appears appropriate to exclude studies on experiences among children and adolescents (Larun & Malterud 2007).

In qualitative metasynthesis, the results from collated primary studies of appropriate relevance and quality will become the raw data for a new turn of analyses. Through interpretation and synthesis, these studies yield new knowledge about the problem when considered together. Put differently, existing research knowledge (*incoming evidence*) is analysed and synthesised to generate outcomes (*outgoing evidence*) that exceed the sum of the individual parts. This is resonant with what in Chapter 1 was referred to as emergence—processes where simple units are combined, interact and are transformed into something that is larger and different than the starting point (Smith 2010). Along the way, we use a methodology with established procedures to identify, select and critically appraise relevant primary studies, which we systematically collate, interpret and analyse (Dixon-Woods, Cavers, et al. 2006,

Sandelowski & Barroso 2007, Barnett-Page & Thomas 2009, Gough, Oliver, et al. 2017b, Malterud 2019b).

The sociologist of knowledge Alfred Schütz (1899–1959) was situated within a phenomenological tradition. Depending on the analytical level, he distinguishes between *first-order* and *second-order concepts* (Schutz 1962). Taking this as a point of departure for qualitative primary studies, first-order concepts may consist of people's understandings expressed in everyday language, as captured in empirical raw data from focus groups or individual interviews. Second-order concepts are the outcome of systematic interpretations of participants' first-order concepts, often informed by theoretical perspectives. The results of a strong qualitative primary study are closer to second-order concepts than to first-order concepts. In the methodological literature on qualitative metasynthesis, this terminology sometimes appears, but it is not used consistently (Britten, Campbell, et al. 2002, Atkins, Lewin, et al. 2008, Malpass, Shaw, et al. 2009, Saini & Shlonsky 2012, Murray, Turpin, et al. 2015).

As a contribution to understanding the levels of interpretation in qualitative metasynthesis, I therefore start by sharing my understanding of this terminology for our purpose here:

- *First-order concepts* are the raw data from the primary studies (not available to us when conducting a qualitative metasynthesis).
- *Second-order terms* are the results from the primary studies, as the author has summarised and interpreted empirical raw data (available from the publication we have identified, critically appraised and included).
- *Third-order concepts* are the endpoints of qualitative metasynthesis (where we as authors have collated concepts and results from the included primary studies and developed a synthesis from these).

We head for an *interpretive synthesis*, in which the evidence from existing research is further processed and analysed using relevant and robust methods to generate new and valuable knowledge. This differs from a *descriptive synthesis study*, which is limited to summarising and reiterating existing knowledge (Walsh & Downe 2005, Saini & Shlonsky 2012, Thorne 2015, Gough, Oliver, et al. 2017b, Malterud 2019b).

Literature search and critical appraisal of relevance and quality

The results (incoming evidence) from the primary studies that we ultimately include for interpretation and analysis (heading for outgoing evidence) are our empirical data for qualitative metasynthesis. Methodological principles and specific procedures for this type of data development differ from data co-creation in a qualitative primary study, where data can be, for example, transcripts from semistructured individual interviews. In qualitative metasynthesis, the sample of included primary studies is neither random nor representative. Nor is it a purposive sample, as we often assume in a qualitative study (see Chapter 7). It rather resembles a convenience sample from the endpoint of a systematic and transparent process with a method developed specifically for this purpose. This procedure and its underpinning present some profound epistemological challenges that we will return to later in this chapter.

In the first instance, we obtain an overview of what has already been published on this or related issues. A clear and well-thought-out study aim helps to steer a steady course along the way and prevents the metasynthesis from simply becoming a replication of general material that adds nothing new (Sandelowski 2012, Alvesson & Sandberg 2024). Planning and conducting a systematic literature search should prevent undesirable inclinations in the selection of studies included for analysis. The aim is not to end up with a catalogue of the research literature that only confirms our own notions of what is important, like cherry-picking (Centre for Reviews and Dissemination 2025). Nevertheless, we want to establish an open mind for the best possible breadth and variation, but not for the matter of bias and representative selection.

You will need the assistance of an experienced research librarian in setting up and conducting an appropriate search. Booth (2016) lays out three requirements for an effective *search strategy* that should (1) identify relevant hits, (2) not identify irrelevant hits and (3) have sparse keywords, to prevent unnecessary redundancy. To achieve this, you decide which databases, search terms, time periods and publication languages can best identify what will ultimately be included for further analysis—namely qualitative primary studies of acceptable quality and relevant to your research question.

Unfortunately, the indexing of qualitative studies in traditional medical databases is still very inadequate. Experience suggests that relying only on traditional data sources and keywords falls far short of providing a complete or even comprehensive overview of existing qualitative studies. (Grant 2004). In qualitative metasynthesis, we must also be prepared to conduct extensive additional searches, for example by reviewing reference lists in relevant primary studies, review articles or book chapters ("*back-chaining*"), or through contact with colleagues who are adequately updated in the field. However, the greater the degree of intuitive snowballing we do, the greater the risk of undesirable distortions in the material (see Chapter 7). On the other hand, we may then be closer to a convenience sample, which in some qualitative studies may be considered an appropriate strategy.

Organising and critically reviewing hits from literature searches

Once the search is complete, you upload the references you have identified (hereafter referred to as *hits*) to a digital database, such as Excel, which communicates well with the reference management tool EndNote. In this process, the decision trail with your path notes is a crucial tool (see Chapter 6). You will encounter many challenges and choices that you will later need to understand yourself and, to some extent, explain. You must also ensure appropriate precision to be able to complete the PRISMA form (see below), an established a flowchart illustrating key pathway choices. The template prepared by "Preferred Items for Systematic Reviews and Meta- Analyses" (*PRISMA*) can be found here: http://www.equator-network.org/reporting-guidelines/prisma/.

Before embarking on a further review of what you have found, you must consider whether the material is too large (many thousands of hits—perhaps your study aim was not sufficiently focused?)—or whether it is too small (three—perhaps the existing body of research in this field is too limited to conduct a metasynthesis?) In both cases, it is worthwhile to take a step back in the process. Since this is a qualitative study, it is also possible to concentrate on a purposive selection of hits from the search, or supplement the sample, for example from the literature lists in the hits you have already chosen to include (backchaining). Subsequently, you must put considerable effort into excluding *duplicates*—not merely automatically via the reference management tool, but also manually. This will save you an incredible amount of time that would otherwise be wasted effort and the risk of inaccurate slips later in the process.

The next step is *screening* with a systematic review and rough sorting of the material. The aim is to identify, select and *critically appraise* relevant primary studies that you want to include in your selection for summarisation, analysis and synthesis, first for relevance and then for quality (Dixon-Woods, Cavers, et al. 2006, Sandelowski & Barroso 2007, Barnett-Page & Thomas 2009, Hannes & Macaitis 2012, Gough, Oliver, et al. 2017b, Malterud 2019b).

Do not be discouraged when the first overview discloses hundreds of irrelevant hits, but few hits that look interesting. Even with a thoroughly prepared search strategy, your search will contain a substantial proportion of hits that are miles away from what you intend to research. We can call this *contamination*. This reflects the SR methodology, which many assume is most reliable when employing fine-grained search strategies with the aim of identifying all available evidence.

It is almost impossible to create effective exclusion criteria without overlooking primary studies you would like to include in the list. Along the way, you assess your results, refine your search for relevance and report your revised selection criteria as path notes in the decision trail. On the other hand, a more selective and efficient approach involves excluding a substantial proportion of hits at the first screening stage based on titles and abstracts. Remember to record which inclusion criteria you choose (Centre for Reviews and Dissemination 2025).

Transparency in this process can be strengthened by having more than one person screen and prioritise references, and by using digital tools that support systematic procedures and overview in the review. The sampling strategy presented above has many features in common with the requirements for a complete or *representative* sample in quantitative studies (Malterud 2019a).

For qualitative metasynthesis, I challenge the objective that the search should be comprehensive and reproducible (Tong, Flemming, et al. 2012, Booth 2016), as if we are envisioning an ideal where we can and should find 100% of what is there. If so, we are approaching strategies indicative of the small q, i.e. approaches that lie on the edge of what we would consider qualitative research methods (see Chapter 4) (Malterud 2019a). Still, these ideas and procedures are firmly established as essentials, for qualitative metasynthesis as well. We must therefore adhere to them to some extent, while at the same time taking a self-critical attitude to the compromises this entails.

By systematically reviewing (screening) all hits with a view to our study aim, we will weed out contamination and concentrate further on references with potential relevance to our study aim—*candidate articles*. Along the way, we must consider the (perhaps unarticulated) criteria we use for inclusion and exclusion, and feel free to revise these along the way. This must always be logged, preferably as path notes in the decision trail. This process requires multiple actors—not merely for consensus, but because the task is large and involves subjective judgments that benefit from brief discussions. Often the title of the reference will be enough; sometimes, we also need to look at the abstract. In this step, we do not read full-text references.

The candidate articles are then reviewed again—first for *relevance*. Now we download the candidate articles, and the basis for appraisal is at least the abstract and most often the full text. An excessively large sample of primary studies makes the task unmanageable and increases the risk of superficial analysis and synthesis. To be on the safe side, it is better not to include too much. Digital tools can be helpful to keep track of the screening process, such as https://www.rayyan.com/, which is widely used. Candidate articles that are considered relevant are subsequently subjected to a critical quality appraisal according to set criteria. Here, we appraise not only the methodological quality but also the quality of the results presented, which will become our raw data for further analysis and synthesis. The fact that published primary studies have previously been assessed and approved by peers is not sufficient.

There are many alternative checklists for qualitative studies—some of these are discussed in Chapter 25. For qualitative metasynthesis, the Consolidated criteria for reporting qualitative research (*COREQ*) (Tong, Sainsbury, et al. 2007) or the Critical Appraisal Skills Programme (*CASP*) (2023) are often proposed. A checklist developed for systematic reviews (with both qualitative and quantitative primary studies) from public health research may also be relevant (Harden, Garcia, et al. 2004). But such checklists, intended for all types of qualitative studies, to the project's particular design or methodology and therefore face well-founded criticism (see Chapter 25) (Braun & Clarke 2024a).

Popay, Rogers and et al. (1998) recommend that the quality appraisal of the results from candidate primary studies should also include indications of proximity to social context, flexible design, whether the results derive from purposive sampling with relevant descriptions, sustainable data and theoretical grounding. Even if these points are not included in the checklist you choose to use, they are useful contributions to the overall critical appraisal of incoming evidence. When you get to analysis and synthesis to develop outgoing evidence, you will realise the importance of this.

I find it difficult to recommend helpful alternatives that can be used for appraisal of whether the studies have been conducted with relevant and robust methodology. Moreover, a central difficulty in qualitative metasynthesis is that existing checklists focus on technical quality rather than the strength of the results, which may lead to the inclusion of studies that are technically sound but with limited Information Power (IP).

Ensure that your decision trail reports reliable information about the critical junctures during the review process, using the PRISMA form as a starting point (Centre for Reviews and Dissemination 2020).

In this example (Figure 18.1), the first search round yielded 834 hits. After discarding 329 duplicates, we screened 505 hits for relevance (Fosse, Schaufel, et al. 2014). Of the 72 candidate articles that remained after screening, 52 articles were excluded after critical appraisal of relevance in full text. After quality appraisal, 14 qualitative primary studies were finally included (Fosse, Schaufel, et al. 2014).

You have now established the sample of data that constitutes incoming evidence, but analysis and synthesis have not yet begun. To obtain an overview of the included primary studies, you compile a *table* in which you organise the most important features for each of the studies, with columns for e.g. year of publication, country, relevant characteristics of the study population (such as age, gender or disease duration), number of participants and design (such as focus group or individual interview). You may also consider

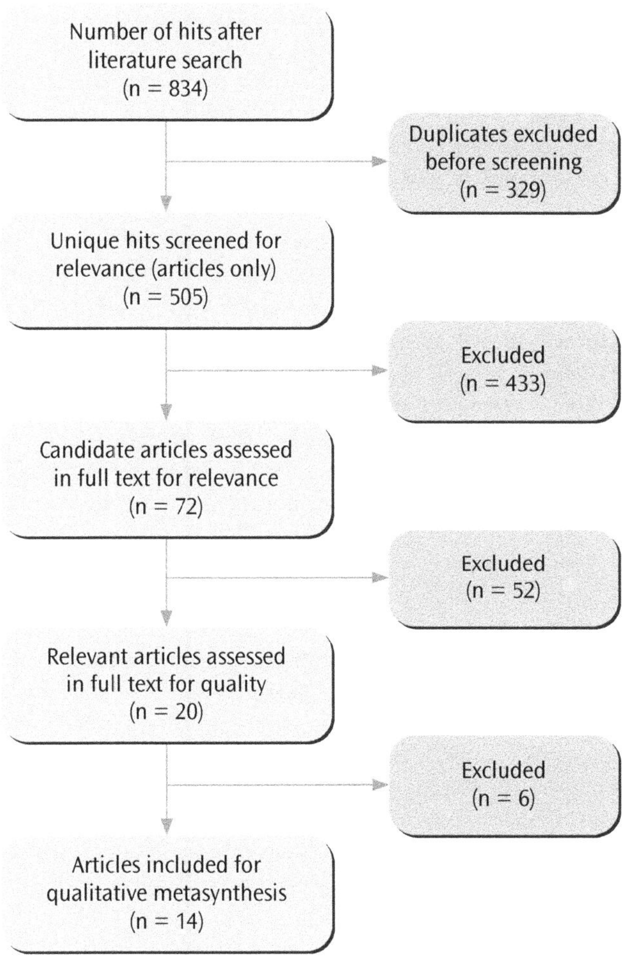

Figure 18.1 Literature search flow sheet

Source: Adapted from Fosse, Schaufel et al. (2014)

including the main results with strengths and weaknesses in such a table, which should give you an overview of the material you are working with (Gough, Oliver, et al. 2017b). However, your table quickly becomes confusing and loses its function if you add further information. Do not try to enter text from the articles in this table.

The table may reveal possible inclinations and gaps in your sample. You must take this into account in your analysis and synthesis, and it must be discussed in your article. For healthcare systems research, it is particularly important to assess the impact of interventions and effects in services where framework conditions are very different from your own.

Considerable methodological diversity may appear in your table, for example with focus group studies, observational studies and document analyses. Some say this is like analysing apples and pears, with differences that interfere undesirably with interpretation and conclusions. I would rather say that methodological diversity strengthens the

IP of the metasynthesis, provided, crucially, that the researcher has expertise in several different qualitative research methods.

The text in the results section from the included primary studies and its second-order concepts constitutes our data for interpretation, analysis and synthesis towards third-order concepts as outgoing evidence in qualitative metasynthesis. This is different from a quantitative meta-analysis, where we use a standardised method to calculate statistics across the primary studies (Pearson 2004).

However, even when methodological rules are strictly adhered to, the results of qualitative primary studies may be poorly developed or inadequately presented. (Eakin & Mykhalovskiy 2003), both in the abstract (which often only tells what was investigated, not what the results were) and in the results section itself (see Chapter 12). For qualitative metasynthesis, strong empirical data are found in primary studies that present new and valuable knowledge through comprehensive, well-founded and thought-provoking interpretations. Atkins et al found that primary studies with descriptive results provided limited useful raw material, while studies with vivid presentations of results based on thorough interpretation and analysis gave more substantial contributions to the metasynthesis (Atkins, Lewin, et al. 2008).

Analysis and synthesis

A great advantage before embarking on qualitative metasynthesis is previous experience of analysing qualitative data from one or preferably several different primary studies that you have conducted yourself. As in any qualitative study, you start by critical appraisal of whether your empirical data (here: the results or incoming evidence from the included primary studies) encompasses appropriate IP (see Chapter 7) to justify conducting analyses. Unfortunately, we will probably realise that many qualitative primary studies, even if they are published in reputable scientific journals, may have weak methodological quality and—perhaps more alarming—meagre results sections that are difficult to process further.

For example, if you end up with two or three included qualitative primary studies, it is better to lower the level of ambition and summarise these by recounting the main results, without organising them more extensively. This is called *narrative metasynthesis* (Greenhalgh, Thorne, et al. 2018) (not to be confused with narrative analysis, see Chapter 15). If you have material with appropriate IP, for example at least ten primary studies with results presenting new and valuable knowledge, you can proceed with analysis, synthesis and further knowing towards third-order concepts.

Analysing the material involves transforming incoming evidence—the result texts—into outgoing evidence—your synthesis—and must be carried out with the same requirements for critical, systematic reflection as in all kinds of qualitative analysis. Notice that inadequate reporting of the analysis method is a recurring problem in published metasyntheses (France, Ring, et al. 2014). It is therefore crucial that you choose, learn and follow an established method. There are many paths to the goal (Thorne, Jensen, et al. 2004, Bondas & Hall 2007b, Sandelowski & Barroso 2007, Barnett-Page & Thomas 2009, Malterud 2019b). Many choose thematic analysis, as we are perhaps familiar with from a primary study with our own empirical data (Thomas & Harden 2008, Malterud 2012b, Braun & Clarke 2022). Other alternatives are meta-ethnography (Noblit & Hare 1988), which is widely used and presented in more detail below. Critical Interpretive Synthesis (Dixon-Woods, Cavers, et al. 2006) and Realist Synthesis (Pawson, Greenhalgh, et al. 2005) are also relevant alternatives, but both analysis methods require more social science expertise than is common among medical and health researchers.

Ytterhus et al. conducted an SR of Norwegian studies (both qualitative and quantitative) on the daily life experiences of children whose parents had chronic illnesses or substance abuse problems (Ytterhus, Hafting, et al. 2024). 729 hits were appraised for relevance, 83 articles were read in full text, and 23 articles were included for reflexive thematic analysis (Braun & Clarke 2019) after appraisal of methodological quality (Harden, Garcia, et al. 2004). The synthesis showed how children maintain relationships through practical tasks, how children experienced emotional ambivalence when their own needs were set aside, and the importance of support from at least one important adult when the environment otherwise often reacted with silence (Ytterhus, Hafting, et al. 2024).

Metasynthesis is distinct from secondary analysis of qualitative data collected for other purposes (Dixon-Woods, Agarwal, et al. 2005). You must decide which level of interpretation you want to use in the analysis—whether you choose to develop a descriptive summary with second-order concepts, or whether you—preferably—aim for an analytical synthesis with the development of third-order concepts (Thorne 2015, Gough, Oliver, et al. 2017b, Thorne 2017). Both strategies require critical review and appraisal of the included primary studies. Synthesis extends beyond mere summarisation and reiteration. The analytical option is the most challenging, but also offers the greatest potential for new and valuable knowledge.

Meta-ethnography

Educational researchers Noblit and Hare were the first to develop and present a method for synthesising qualitative studies. *Meta-ethnography* formed the basis for qualitative metasynthesis and is still the most widely used method for analysis and synthesis. Noblit and Hare presented concrete descriptions of analysis strategy and perspective (translation, metaphors) and different levels of analysis (reciprocal analysis, refutational synthesis and lines-of-argument). Here we will briefly review the main principles and concepts of meta-ethnography (Noblit & Hare 1988, Thorne, Jensen, et al. 2004), both as originally presented and translated into current practice (Malterud 2019b).

The method includes a detailed description of underlying assumptions, concepts and approaches. The authors emphasise meta-ethnography as an inductive method grounded in the interpretive paradigm. The researcher's interpretation of the results of existing research should lead to something different and something more than the results of the primary studies, and context is a crucial condition for understanding. To use this method for qualitative metasynthesis, you ought to go to the original literature, preferably supplemented with thorough close reading of some articles where this method has been used and published (Noblit & Hare 1988, Larun & Malterud 2007, Malterud & Ulriksen 2011, Dahl, Fylkesnes, et al. 2013, Fosse, Schaufel, et al. 2014).

The heart of the matter in meta-ethnography is to take a stand as to how the main results of the included primary studies relate to one another in the ways they were interpreted and presented by their authors (France, Ring, et al. 2014). Noblit and Hare (1988) provide us with two core concepts for this purpose, both of which have a different and more distinctive methodological meaning than in everyday speech.

The first of these is *metaphor*, which is used here for main expressions and notions that the authors of the primary studies themselves have used in analytical texts when communicating their results. Early in the review of empirical data (incoming evidence) from the results sections, we will therefore identify this type of second-order text element that may have sufficient scope and impact to sustain the core interpretations and support emergent insights. This is called *metaphorical reduction*.

The second concept is *translation*. In meta-ethnography, synthesis involves using metaphors from the results to translate the results of qualitative studies into one another. We will compare concepts that address the same thing and transform them into a fresh, unifying third-order concept that sheds light on the problem through an inventive understanding of our interpretations. Then, based on the translation, we return to the empirical material and develop a new and vigorous description of the content of this concept, which will grow to be the analytical text in this metasynthesis.

These two core concepts will make analysis and synthesis feasible, with intersubjectivity and validity properly safeguarded.

Since 1988, a lot has happened when it comes to literature searches, qualitative research methods and systematic reviews. The specific process of meta-ethnography therefore takes a different course in today's research practice, still maintaining the original ideas and understanding of the method.

Noblit and Hare outline a seven-step process—a systematic procedure that it is possible to follow, explain and discuss. In Table 18.1, I present the analysis steps with my elaboration, which, using Noblit and Hare's own terminology, we can describe as a translation to today's research reality (Noblit & Hare 1988, Malterud 2019b).

Noblit & Hare recommend that, early in the process, we decide on a principal level of analysis and synthesis. In *reciprocal analysis*, we mutually translate different metaphors for related phenomena into each other and develop more abstracted concepts. This is the most common level. In *refutational synthesis*, the emphasis is on contradictions in the material. We can also develop *lines-of-argument*, where we develop a logical connection between different main results and third-order concepts (Larun & Malterud 2007). The latter requires rich and complex data with strong IP, and we should not embark on this without the empirical basis being sound.

Meta-ethnography was developed as a method long before the computer technology and search strategies of our time were available, with presentation of synthesis based on two to four studies. Nor were qualitative research methods developed in the same way at that time as they are nowadays. Today, many people question the term "ethnography" in this context (Dixon-Woods, Cavers, et al. 2006, Major & Savin-Baden 2010), because the method is not limited to the social anthropological tradition and participant observation. For metasynthesis from medicine and health sciences, it may therefore be more useful to incorporate the most important principles from Noblit and Hare than to argue that this should be ethnography in the prevailing sense.

Regardless of the analysis method, the aim of qualitative metasynthesis is to contribute to an expanded understanding of a problem through *upcycling* and systematic interpretation and synthesis of available incoming evidence. The purpose is not to test existing hypotheses or repeat and confirm existing knowledge. It is not always easy to write the introductory section of the article without anticipating the results from the analysis, so look for examples of published articles in which this has been done well.

Table 18.1 Meta-ethnography—the seven steps then and now. After Noblit and Hare (1988)—from Malterud (2019b)

Steps	*Noblit and Hare*	*My elaboration—implementation in practice*
1	Getting started	Articulate study aim and search strategy, write project outline, conduct literature search
2	Decide what is relevant for the study aim	Review the hits from the literature search, develop criteria for inclusion, exclude duplicates and hits whose title or abstracts do not fulfil the inclusion criteria, appraise candidate studies in full text, establish a sample of included primary studies, prepare an overview of these
3	Read the studies	Thorough reading of the included primary studies in full text to localise the results from the primary studies that constitute the empirical data for metasynthesis, and to obtain an overview of themes and metaphors
4	Determining how the studies are related	Data extraction in which the empirical data are organised in a matrix where relevant themes and metaphors from each primary study are listed in vertical columns, starting with a rich index study
5	Translating the studies to each other	Systematic examination, extraction and organisation of text segments with related themes and metaphors across studies in the horizontal rows of the matrix, emphasising similarities and differences in expressions and conceptual use
6	Synthesising translations	Review each horizontal row to develop an overarching translation which embraces all themes and metaphors, expressed as a new concept that provides fresh, unifying third-order concept with an original understanding of the results
7	Expressing the synthesis	Elaborate and justify the meaning of the expressions from the synthesis that are reproduced in the new translation and write analytical text for the results section of the article

Because the empirical material—the results sections from the primary studies—usually constitutes a very heterogeneous material, based on different methodological approaches—we face several challenges when synthesising and developing third-order concepts using relevant and robust methods. If you are referring to Noblit and Hare, you therefore need to understand, apply and demonstrate specifically how you have carried out metaphorical reduction and translation. Ultimately, presenting a synthesis that offers enough new knowledge to merit readers' interest is always challenging.

Qualitative metasynthesis and EBM—an epistemological mismatch?

Systematicity and transparency are key criteria for the scientific rigour of all types of research methods, both qualitative and quantitative. The same two principles apply to EBM, as conceptualised by the Cochrane community (Noyes, Booth, et al. 2019) and the Joanna Briggs Institute (Porrit, Evans, et al. 2024). Thus, we could imagine that qualitative metasynthesis—a systematic review of qualitative studies—would be a natural meeting place for these two methodological traditions. This is true, but there are also many important differences because of the two different paradigms and epistemologies that these two scientific traditions are rooted in (see Chapter 2) (Thorne 2011, Malterud 2019a, 2019b).

With qualitative metasynthesis, we face fundamental epistemological challenges that require reflexivity, methodological competence and more than a few pragmatic compromises (Petticrew 2015, Wong 2016). Academic competence implies not only that you master the craft of methodology, but also that you know and can pay due respect to the epistemological assumptions underpinning different research methodologies. Although qualitative metasynthesis is a qualitative research method, many of the established technical rules for this method have strong positivist premises (Popay, Rogers, et al. 1998) with concepts such as facts, completeness, independence, representativeness and objectivity, indicating a need for alertness regarding the small q (see Chapter 4). Here I will briefly mention some of the compromises that entails epistemological challenges (Malterud 2019a):

The inherent goal for the literature search, review and selection strategy is to establish a *complete sample* (the "haystack") where the systematic review leads to independent identification of primary studies to be included in the analysis and synthesis (the "needles in the haystack"). This is different from purposive sampling, which is otherwise standard in qualitative studies (see Chapter 7). Moreover, the idea of independence conflicts with the understanding of subjectivity and interpretation as key foundations for developing, analysing and interpreting data using qualitative research methods (see Chapter 1).

The analysis should bridge the gap between the study aim, empirical data and results. In qualitative studies, second- and third-order results and syntheses are developed through explicit interpretation, with the researcher as an analytical instrument rather than as someone uncovering meanings inherent in the data (Kvale 1996). When metasynthesis is carried out as a descriptive aggregation, often with an emphasis on homogeneity and correspondence (Lewin, Glenton, et al. 2015), the outcome may be a comprehensive catalogue of data without interpretations and synthesis informed by assumptions about flexibility, variation, diversity and contradictions (Thorne 2015) (see Chapter 5).

Transferability of the results from a metasynthesis cannot be assessed independently of purpose and context, no matter how appropriate the methodological approach was conducted. On the contrary, considerations familiar from qualitative research methods of validity (pragmatic and communicative), and reflexivity regarding the study's position in a larger landscape, should be more determinative than ideals of universal evidence, given the correct procedure (Britten, Garside, et al. 2017, Thorne 2017).

These examples are clear indications of the *small q* challenges and underscore the need for particular vigilance. (see Chapter 4). Sometimes, however, we choose to accept some compromises. In such cases, it is particularly important to remain alert to expectations and demands that reflect pronounced epistemological incongruence rooted in positivist premises. Such challenges will arise at all stages of a qualitative metasynthesis, through planning, implementation and—not least—peer review. A typical example is the PROSPERO database, where protocols for systematic reviews must be registered https://www.crd.york.ac.uk/prospero/. This database is customised for quantitative systematic reviews but is unfortunately poorly suited to qualitative metasynthesis.

It is therefore useful to include (at least) one senior researcher who is thoroughly familiar with qualitative research methods on the team, who can argue in favour of sound choices in confrontations with reviewers or colleagues from other research traditions. You can read more about qualitative metasynthesis here (Malterud 2019b).

CHAPTER 19

Between tacit knowing and research evidence

In clinical practice and other parts of the services, knowledge beyond research-based evidence is developed and applied. *Clinical knowing* builds on the investment that we bring with us from education and experience, a knowledge capital that is strengthened over the years with interest from learning, reading and encounters with people. Such knowledge may concern matters such as technical procedures, interpersonal interaction or organisational processes. The tacit *practical knowing* must not necessarily be transformed into scientific evidence from qualitative or quantitative studies. However, as much of this knowledge is grounded in subjectivity and interpretation, qualitative research methods can bestow ideas, concepts and frameworks that enable us to understand, articulate, discuss and share practice-based knowing. Such methods can also support reflection on what aspects of practice may be made researchable and how this can be achieved. Terminology within this area is ambiguous and non-standardised, which is also reflected in the presentation below.

Intuition, or tacit knowing with its own logic?

Within biomedical practice, the hypothetical–deductive method is widely treated as the default model for problem solving and decision making, beginning with the formulation of a hypothesis that is subsequently put to the test. Aligning with this logic in medical diagnostics, relevant differential diagnoses can systematically be eliminated based on a probability-based decision tree—an *algorithm*. Such logical assumptions represent technical rationality and deductive logic (see Chapter 1), developed for a stable and predictable ontology with standardisable conditions that can be relevant and necessary in many medical contexts.

Clinical knowledge and knowing, on the other hand, includes uncertainty, subjectivity, complexity, individualisation and dialogue. In practice, we combine multiple knowledge sources of different types and quality. These are not always compatible;

DOI: 10.4324/9781003786016-22

furthermore, they are not easy to account for, often applied to complex problem-solving within short deadlines. This type of decision-making pattern is frequently referred to as *intuition* or *the art of medicine*—terms that have a somewhat magical and sacred quality about them, entailing perhaps unnecessary protection against transparency and critical reflection. Another point of view is, however, to argue that clinical knowing and the associated knowledge are based on a particular logic deserving exploration, validation and articulation. Within knowledge-based practice, the terms clinical or experience-based expert knowledge are established and recognised (see Chapter 1).

Polanyi focused on the *tacit dimension*, which is pre-reflexive unarticulated knowing—when we know or know more than we can put into words (Polanyi 1983). In healthcare, we have many examples of tacit and embodied *practical knowing* from diagnostics, treatment and prevention, in the form of, for example bodily knowledge (being able to stitch a wound), relational knowledge (knowing a patient through a long life), pattern recognition (recognising a typical rash) or familiarity knowledge (assessing a dying patient). Gatens-Robinson suggests *phronesis*—a term used by Aristotle to denote the capacity to exercise practical wisdom and judgement (Gatens-Robinson 1986). She argues that this approach is more appropriate than algorithms and hypothetical-deductive methods to understand and apply the logic associated with subjective judgement of medical issues in unique situations.

Much of this constitutes professional practice knowledge that is unspoken and taken for granted—we tend to act in these ways either because someone has demonstrated that this is how it should be done, or because experience has taught us that it is effective in achieving its purpose. Polanyi (1983) described this as a unique and dynamic activity—something that we do (knowing as a verb), as opposed to something we find or discover (knowledge as an object). How can these concepts be developed further to support our understanding of clinical knowing?

From reflection-in-action to reflection-on-action

Donald A. Schön (1930–1997), urban planner and philosopher, developed his theory of practice knowledge based on Polanyi's ideas about tacit knowing (Schön 1991). Schön shows how the practitioner exercises tacit knowing as *reflection-in-action*. Without deductive pre-planning and through an unarticulated, reflexive conversation with the situation, the practitioner translates complex issues into a workable format. The opposite is *technical logic*, which we are familiar with from Skjervheim (2002) and Snow (1959), among others.

An extensive experience base (examples, images and actions) is the raw material for conducting judgement-based assessments and decisions in practice. Schön shows how this forms the basis for recognition (seeing-as), where analogies to previous successful or unsuccessful problem solutions point the way to unique solutions. Judgement and individualisation are linked to skills learned from experience and mastery, not to theoretical knowledge (which has a higher status). Medicine and law are mentioned by Schön as disciplines where such a distinction between different forms of knowledge is particularly vibrant.

Reflexivity (see Chapter 3) provides a starting point for understanding and further development of tacit practical knowing. Reflection and critical discussion of what happened, with a particular focus on one's own participation in the situation and the conditions for this, can bring forward new modes of knowing leading to new and valuable knowledge. In an emergent process (see Chapter 1), it may be possible to sense a course of action and put it into words, especially in interaction with others who share similar experiences. In this way, reflection-**in**-action can be transformed to *reflection-***on***-action*, where experiences are shared, discussed and further refined. Schön does not paraphrase much on this last term. Others have subsequently used it as a gateway to the systematic description and analysis of practice knowing in which the practitioner's awareness for decision-making processes and actions is enhanced and put into words.

Surfacing tacit knowing in learning and professional development

Knowledge-based practice (see Chapter 1) is often presented as a triangle in which knowledge from research, patients' values and experiences, and experience-based expert knowledge are assigned equal weight (Sackett, Rosenberg, et al. 1996, Sackett 1997). However, although these three sources of knowledge represent different value bases and areas of application, scientific evidence has (implicitly) been assigned the highest status, with the right of way in the development of guidelines and decisions for the health service (see Chapter 18).

With qualitative research methods, we can develop evidence about both patient perspectives and experience-based expert knowledge. Many of the references in this book originate from qualitative studies with patients, relatives or healthcare professionals about, for example, symptom experiences (Steihaug & Malterud 2008, Larun & Malterud 2011a), encounters with the health service (Røthing, Malterud, et al. 2014, Werner & Malterud 2016b), general practitioners' (GPs') strategies in consultations (Nilsen, Malterud, et al. 2015, Guassora, Johansen, et al. 2021) or ethical dilemmas from practice (Lid & Malterud 2012, Guassora, Reventlow, et al. 2014). When such studies present new and valuable knowledge with relevant and robust methods, recognising the experiences of users and clinicians, the yield may be comparable to knowledge developed with users or clinicians without research experience in the role of co-researchers (Malterud & Elvbakken 2020).

Making experience-based expert knowledge tangible presents greater challenges than exercising it. To do so, we need metapositions and tools for foregrounding and sharing where the subjectivity of practice knowledge is recognised (see Chapter 16) (Malterud 2002). The aim is not to verbalise or make science out of all tacit knowing, but to create opportunities for critical reflection on potentially relevant matters for professional development and learning. In this way, tacit knowing can become more robust and strengthen its status as a legitimate element of knowledge-based practice (Malterud 1995b, 2001a).

Today, such exchange takes place as professional supervision or dialogue between groups of colleagues, where the senior or expert shows the way and articulates the basis for assessment, actions and interpretive logic. Reflection on practice—*situated learning*—as everyday practice in a safe environment (Lave & Wenger 1991) can create learning environments for junior colleagues. Creative research-based strategies for this purpose, with articulation, analysis and implementation also of the tacit knowing of clinical practice, should be encouraged. Relevant substantive theories (see Chapter 20) can help to conceptualise and sharpen focus, not only in research but also in clinical practice (Malterud, Reventlow, et al. 2024).

Can experience-based expert knowledge become evidence?

Focus groups can establish conditions for interaction in which healthcare professionals articulate and share practice experiences from clinical and grey knowledge areas, for example when it comes to strategies for conversations in GP surgeries about alcohol use (Lid & Malterud 2012). It is more difficult to gain access to tacit knowing about cognitive processes and interpretation strategies for complex symptom pictures under high uncertainty in clinical practice. These are medical challenges where the GP has extensive experience but a limited knowledge base (Malterud & Kamps 2021). Relevant theories from other disciplines can offer new perspectives and fresh concepts for previous medical taken-for-grantedness, such as the theologian Lonergan's understanding of knowledge as subjective interpretations, which we can use in clinical knowledge to support the subjectivity in analysis of diagnostic decision-making processes (Engebretsen, Vollestad, et al. 2015, Malterud, Reventlow, et al. 2019) (see Chapter 1).

Much remains to be done in terms of empirical studies using qualitative methods. We may start with a basic assessment of whether the study matter can be translated into empirical data that is relevant and robust, and whether the vital elements of what we are investigating will survive interpretation and analysis. Prior to this, we can try to articulate the problem in some way and make it accessible through text, for example via reflection on practice and situated learning, with no other ambitions than to establish proximity and dialogue with the problem itself. Frequently, we have to acknowledge important clinical challenges as not being researchable, even with qualitative methods (Malterud 1995b).

Researching yourself—introspection and observational participation

In a project about patient perspectives, it may seem counterproductive to assign healthcare professionals the role of participant observer. The clinician will not be able to adopt the patient's perspective. However, when the study aim is about experiences, perceptions or attitudes of healthcare professionals themselves, critical and constructive self-reflection may be an appropriate path to knowing and knowledge (Malterud 1990, Stensland & Malterud 1997, Thesen & Kuzel 1999, Rudebeck 2000). Such strategies may represent a particular type of participant observation (see Chapter 16), which may be better described as *observational participation* or reflexive introspection. For example, Mengshoel (2024) uses autoethnography with narrative analysis to structure her own retrospective accounts on the development of physiotherapy for patients with rheumatoid arthritis.

Such strategies have the potential to facilitate knowing about the logic and the silent processes that underlie clinical behavioural patterns, such as the routes of the diagnostic process when traditional algorithms do not provide an adequate description of a decision-making process (Malterud 1999, Malterud, Reventlow, et al. 2019). We may start with introspection and put words to tacit knowing from clinical practice. Thereby, we can transform reflection-**in**-action into reflection-**on**-action, addressing experiences and concepts that can be shared with colleagues and, to some extent, further elaborated towards research evidence, for example in a focus group study. It is crucial to consider whether these experiences can be converted into empirical data that align with observations and can be shared as knowledge. In this way, we can learn more about, for example how the doctor's vulnerability plays a role in medical encounters (Malterud, Fredriksen, et al. 2009), or what considerations the GP emphasises in the meeting with patients who want sick leave (Nilsen, Werner, et al. 2011).

Observational participation involves many methodological pitfalls that can jeopardise the possibility of developing scientific knowledge. The proximity to the material may imply that I lose the capacity to recognise alternative interpretations, negative conclusions or skewed effects of my own positioning or behaviour (Savage 2000). It is also a risk that I immerse myself in issues or perspectives that become so private that the knowledge is of no interest to anyone but myself. The outcome may also be knowledge that is less new and valuable than expected from a research project. If the study aim is to develop and explore a clinical strategy or intervention, the researcher's enthusiasm may overshadow an analytical attitude. Therefore, such a research strategy requires methodological expertise, experience and human maturity. A wise supervisor can provide good anchoring.

If we plan to research ourselves, it is particularly important to establish material documentation in the form of empirical data. Even when subjectivity is at the centre, fleeting memories and impressions are not necessarily the best resource for data providing appropriate Information Power to the analysis. We need tangible data from audio or video recordings or field notes that build metapositions for the researcher, to make the reader understand that interpretations and conclusions stem from more than wishful thinking. Empirical data allows other researchers access to the material and can thus contribute other perspectives than those you are able to see yourself. The point is intersubjectivity, rather than fact checks. It is useful to involve others in the analysis, even if the aim is not interpretation agreement. An alternative to an empirical study may be to prepare a theoretical review of the problem (Malterud, Reventlow, et al. 2019).

Thorough consideration of the contextual preconditions shaping experiences and results is an intersubjective prerequisite that allows readers to assess the soundness and scope of what we have come to understand. Such conditions can change over time in this type of project, often because of the knowledge developed along the way. It is the researcher's mission to identify, reflect on and communicate the framing and prerequisites of the knowledge, often in very concrete detail, for example how long the consultations took in a project about the development of a clinical method intended to change the conversation between the doctor and the patient (Stensland & Malterud 1997). Altogether, this is about developing strategies that enable the researcher to shift smoothly between participation and observation, and to look at themselves from within, besides, or beyond. Appropriate metapositions are particularly important as tool for reflexivity in qualitative studies where the researcher is the observing participant.

PART 4

Theoretical and methodological questions revisited

CHAPTER 20

Theory situates interpretation, focus and abstraction

Our most important source of knowing in clinical practice and health services is everyday life, which encompasses experiences, ideas, conversations, observations, interpretations and insights from multiple angles. But empirical data are neither fact nor truth. They constitute a vital material foundation for knowing, but for further development of scientific evidence by abstracting our interpretations, more is needed to enable transferability of new and valuable knowledge. Theory may seem perplexing to a researcher with a biomedical background. Still, appropriate theoretical perspectives inevitably have a place in qualitative studies, adding value by situating the project, placing interpretations in a broader context and contributing to metapositions and reflexivity. Such pursuits must overcome the theoretical silence of traditional medical research while being particularly tailored to the ontological domains of health and illness.

The biomedical ballast—taking facts for granted?

A qualitative study in medicine or the health sciences may vary in its level of theoretical ambition (Malterud 2016). Novice researchers often begin descriptively and empirically and progressively advance towards a more seasoned understanding of theoretical perspectives that may enhance analytical clarity. It is, however, discouraging to read an article from a qualitative study where the researcher claims that theoretical perspectives were not applied. In such cases, the researcher chooses not to consider the impact of their interpretive gaze, while relying on implicit theories that remain neither acknowledged nor articulated. It can also be due to beginner's modesty or misguided positivist small q respect for data as "facts" (see Chapters 1 and 4).

Compared to the social sciences and humanities, medical curricula do not offer much introduction to philosophical assumptions, methodology or theoretical perspectives. The same applies to varying degrees to other health science educations. The medical professional culture is still largely rooted in a positivist understanding of knowledge as objective, generalisable facts and a notion of theory as an accumulated mass of

DOI: 10.4324/9781003786016-24

knowledge ensuring an accurate representation of reality (Høyer 2008) (see Chapter 2). We are trained to take many basic assumptions for granted, without understanding the need of making these conditions explicit and consider their impact for knowing (Guassora, Reventlow, et al. 2022).

Nevertheless, regardless of methodology or discipline, the researcher draws on theoretical perspectives to frame the problem, guide development and selection of data, interpret it and present results (Reeves, Albert, et al. 2008). When theory is implicit, unconscious or unarticulated, an essential prerequisite for intersubjectivity is missing, namely recognising and communicating the project's situatedness and the researcher's path through the research process. By scrutinising and acknowledging our own position, we can enact and demonstrate reflexivity and open ourselves to new perspectives.

Many health care professionals find it demanding when knowledge learnt in their undergraduate education is put to the test in the field. Reality does not appear as unambiguous and predictable as we have learned. As healthcare professionals, we are constantly faced with situations that require judgements and decisions under a high degree of uncertainty, encountering sick people who are as different as everyone else. Algorithms and logical reasoning from evidence-based medicine that merge silently with judgement and experience are transformed into clinical knowledge aiming to function reliably and feasibly in encounters with individuals (Malterud 2001a, Thorne 2015). Tacit knowing (see Chapter 19) is the practitioner's resource to sort out complexity in everyday life (Polanyi 1983, Schön 1991).

Novice researchers from clinical practice or health service systems quite often response with uncertainty and distance when the question of *theory* comes up on the research agenda. Many seem to prefer to describe "reality as it truly is", rather than acknowledge the assumption that reality may appear in multiple versions depending on how empirical data are interpreted. They complain (often rightly) that theoretical texts are difficult to understand, and they do not always recognise the significance of other researchers' thoughts with potential to open doors of insight. But theory is not the opposite of practice—on the contrary, theory is a tool to sum up statements about the world (Alderson 1998, Pope & Mays 2020, Guassora, Reventlow, et al. 2022).

Multidisciplinary collaboration can lower the thresholds to the theoretical field for researchers from medicine and health sciences, and searching for theory from social sciences, psychology or the humanities may often pay off. Reading tips from a colleague from another field may facilitate fresh understanding of our study aim more than a traditional literature search, providing an overview of empirical evidence but not very much about frameworks and concepts for understanding. Still, some warning may be given: theory established in disciplines beyond health care is not always appropriate for the development of medical knowledge.

Furthermore, the function of theory may be very different in applied, practice-based research compared to social science or humanities. Research in latter disciplines often aims to develop or discuss theory, or to put an existing theoretical frame of reference to the test in analysing the material (Smith 2010, Guassora, Reventlow, et al. 2022). Medical and health researchers should not pretend to be social anthropologists, literary scholars or philosophers (Leder 1990, Sandelowski 1993, Thorne 2014, 2025). In our domains, the aim of research is rather the development of knowing that can make a difference for patients and healthcare professionals. This practice-based ontology requires epistemological congruence (see Chapters 1 and 4), implying that theoretical perspectives must be clearly and specifically tailored to the phenomenon under study.

In medical research, theoretical perspectives primarily serve as a basis for the researcher's reflexive articulation of situatedness, as a source of inspiration and as a toolbox for shaping a focused and precise study aim, offering constructive ideas and concepts (Sandelowski 1993, Thorne 2014, 2025). We cannot escape the theoretical commitments inherent in a qualitative study by referring to a general medical standpoint or a patient-centred approach, nor by claiming that we simply let the participants' voices speak for themselves (Malterud 2016, Guassora, Reventlow, et al. 2022). Instead, we can actively consider how theory may most beneficially support knowing about health and illness.

Empirical data connects our explorations with phenomena that we can interpret, recognise and challenge. Data are not facts, with inherent, undeniable meaning, just as theory does not always provide the answer. The researcher's mandate as an interpreter in the face of subjectivity presupposes an awareness of the project's context and location. The impact of situatedness is something that we must learn and practice, coming from an academic discipline dominated by biomedicine and epidemiology (see Chapter 5). Without a minimum level of theoretical commitment, your understanding of the assumptions underpinning qualitative methods remains weak. Well-chosen theories enhance and sharpen qualitative analysis, refine subjectivity and support conceptual elaboration, enabling you to develop something new by situating knowing in a wider context.

Pragmatic validity—usability

Ultimately, the validity of knowledge depends on whether it can be used for something—that it comes with consequences and can make a difference for someone. Kvale (1996) refers to the usability of knowledge as *pragmatic validity*. Without potentials for coming into use, the validity of knowledge is limited to a small space at the very edge of reality. Pragmatic validity is then weak. Pragmatic validation, closely tied to relevance, occurs after research is closed and demonstrates whether and how the knowledge was used. When we read about general practitioners' (GPs)' strategies for negotiating sickness certificates, we cannot tell whether this insight will change practice without exploring processes that provide insight into such changes (Nilsen, Malterud, et al. 2015).

Nonetheless, we should always consider pragmatic validity in advance of a project by asking ourselves whether others have already answered the questions we intend to ask, or whether new answers will lead to consequences within the context of the problem. The usability of the knowledge is also determined by external validity—to which contexts outside the study situation may the results maintain transferability (see Chapter 7). In action research and implementation research, with an explicit ambition for change, a demand for pragmatic validity is particularly important (Whyte 1991, Malterud 1995a, Thesen & Kuzel 1999). Pragmatic validation is also an approach to retrospectively assess whether the knowledge delivery fulfils the requirement of relevance, and at what level.

Pragmatic validity is not limited to *applied research*—i.e. knowledge development that is to be immediately translated into action. We can also talk about pragmatic validity when it comes to *basic research*. This is research that aims to develop a theory or method, for example when Nessa's transcription method is applied in later studies of doctor-patient interaction (Nessa 1995a, Undeland & Malterud 2008, Schaufel, Nordrehaug, et al. 2009). If the knowledge developed in our project is not later taken up or used, its pragmatic validity is weak. Communicative validity is also a necessary but not sufficient condition for pragmatic validity. We cannot use something we do not understand or have not heard of.

At this point, researchers from medicine and health sciences may experience a conflict of interest. The format required for the project to gain recognition in the academic community may be at odds with the format that facilitates practitioners and administrators to translate knowledge into action. Knowledge-based practice is an important ideal for the health services. But original scientific publications are read by a limited readership, with practitioners as a minority. The researcher who wants both scientific recognition and practical use must therefore aim for dissemination through more channels than scientific publication to achieve the intended pragmatic validity.

Hypotheses

It is neither possible nor appropriate to erase the human imagination (Morse 1994). There is no research method in which we as researchers start with a blank slate when we enter the field and create and encounter the empirical data. We inevitably bring internal images of the field shaped by the questions we hope to explore. At the same time, we can strive to take responsibility for the impact of our preconceptions, enabling a methodical interpretation of where we are and what we see and hear.

Hypotheses are inner images of what we expect to encounter in our data. They may be explicitly formulated as statements or exist as more or less unconscious notions. During the development, organisation, analysis and synthesis of empirical data, our hypothesis guides our gaze and determines what we see. If we put a question mark behind the hypothesis, we have recognised a problem that we can explore and elaborate on to a study aim. The hypothesis precedes the project, as an assumption underpinning the questions we ask. In quantitative research designs, statistical procedures are used for *hypothesis testing*. Hypothesis testing is traditionally based on principles where the researcher articulates their question in reverse form as a *null hypothesis*. The results will display the probability that the null hypothesis can be rejected.

In a qualitative study, we would rather develop a hypothesis than test it (Pope & Mays 2020). A subtle source of error will grow when my preconceptions, through my unacknowledged hypotheses, distort the knowledge that the field should offer, without me noticing it. In a qualitative study, I therefore need to familiarise myself with my hypotheses so that they are not allowed to suppress my empirical data. Then, there is room for hypotheses—even in an inductive research strategy. The decision trail (see Chapter 6) can be a useful tool for recognising, grounding, reassessing and dismissing hypotheses. It can prevent us from simply looking for confirmation of what we have always believed and thought and instead help us to change track and approach new and valuable knowledge.

Nevertheless, we cannot deny that some level of *hypothesis testing* also takes place in a qualitative study, even if the procedure is profoundly different from that in a quantitative study. We are constantly comparing our observations with what we have previously imagined, consciously or unconsciously. Particularly when the researcher has experience and in-depth field knowledge, much of the research will consist of systematically developing data where the researcher initially recognises some contours. We only develop creative knowing to the extent that we are willing to let empirical data challenge and elaborate on our hypotheses and experiences, above all with the support of relevant theoretical perspectives. In a qualitative study, we put our preconceptions into question by making them visible, while at the same time endeavouring to challenge and transcend our hypotheses. To capitalise on the interpretive potential created at the meeting point between empirical data and theoretical perspectives, we must systematically seek data that either complement the picture or challenge our ideas. This is where pertinent theoretical perspectives can offer valuable guidance.

In a familiar terrain, we do not notice the unknown paths unless we are actively looking for them. You can enhance the latter by introducing *counterhypotheses*. A counterhypothesis embodies the opposite of the discovery you expect to make, according to our hypothesis. By creating counterhypotheses, you establish active metapositions and take a step to the side to get out of your own circles (see Chapter 16). In my own project on women's unexplained health problems, for example, I discovered how an unconscious hypothesis about psychosocial explanations constantly steered my gaze in a narrow direction. I therefore established a counterhypothesis that such ailments were due to a hitherto unrecognised vitamin deficiency (Malterud 1990). The purpose was not to test the counterhypothesis, but to use it as a reminder that knowledge may rest elsewhere than where I think.

In a qualitative research project, a counterhypothesis serves a function somewhat analogous to that of the null hypothesis in quantitative studies. Both are meant to encourage a falsification attitude, preventing empirical data from serving to confirm the truth or superiority of preconceptions (see Chapter 1). But the counterhypothesis is not meant to cancel subjectivity.

Procedures for handling counterhypothesis and null hypothesis are essentially different in qualitative and quantitative studies. The null hypothesis is used to assess the plausibility of the existing alternatives, while the counterhypothesis is meant to prevent blinders and narrow-mindedness, while enhancing reflexivity and diversity.

Scientific theories at different levels

In everyday language, a theory is a hypothesis, an idea or a speculation—something we do not know but believe or think. A *scientific theory*, on the other hand, is a consistent and well-founded set of assumptions that can be used to predict or explain a phenomenon or relationships between phenomena (see Chapter 5) (Malterud 2016). Different academic disciplines have various definitions of what a theory is. In the natural sciences, a theory is supposed to be predictive, testable, verifiable and falsifiable, while social science and psychological theories are characterised by chains of argument, abstractions and concepts that can be used to understand and explain relationships (Malterud 2016, Guassora, Reventlow, et al. 2022).

Ontology and epistemology from different scientific paradigms rest on different theoretical and philosophical assumptions (Thorne 2014, Pope & Mays 2020) (see Chapter 2). In qualitative studies, theory is particularly important for understanding, interpreting, developing and abstracting empirical data beyond a purely descriptive level (Guassora, Reventlow, et al. 2022). What may our interpretations entail, and which are our arguments for this? Here, theoretical perspectives may be helpful.

For researchers in medicine and health sciences, qualitative studies rarely aim for theory development, as in other disciplines (Thorne 2025). However, some terminology within qualitative methods can contribute to unnecessary confusion, for example when researchers from the Grounded Theory tradition (see Chapter 4) refer to theories in a similar way as others talk about the results of a qualitative study—i.e. as the endpoint and outcome of the project. In applied practice-based research, it is usually more appropriate to draw on relevant theories developed by others (Alderson 1998). Furthermore, please note that presenting results as figures with boxes and arrows does not in itself make them more theoretical.

For qualitative studies, different theoretical levels are available (Pope & Mays 2020). Let us take a closer look at what this means in practice.

To understand the principal assumptions of qualitative research methodology, the researcher needs basic knowledge of *philosophy of science*, particularly regarding the differences between the positivist and interpretivist paradigms and their implications for ontology and epistemology (see Chapter 2). Without such a crucial foundation, you will not be able to understand the meaning of subjectivity, reflexivity, sampling and transferability. Nor will you grasp the role of theory in an inductive strategy, where conclusions are drawn from the unique to the general (Pope & Mays 2020). This applies regardless of whether we use a narrative, phenomenological, ethnographic, pragmatic or constructionist strategy.

Such matters are not always apparent to a researcher with a biomedical background. However, extensive philosophical immersion is not necessary to acquire what is needed. Writing a scientific article, we are not supposed to explain the paradigms and the level of philosophy of science—these are things we consider as familiar to the competent academic reader. Similarly, we do not expect an explanation of the mathematical prerequisites for statistics in an article on epidemiological methods.

Grand theories summarise an overall understanding of large and complex relationships. We are familiar with some of these from medicine, such as theories of psychoanalysis (Sigmund Freud), bureaucracy (Max Weber), systems theory (Gregory Bateson) or basic human needs (Abraham Maslow). In a qualitative study, such theories can help to situate the knowledge, but usually at a level that does not add much to the specific interpretive perspective.

Here I will present three different levels of theoretical ambitions for a qualitative study (Malterud 2016):

- Theory as backdrop and inspiration
- Substantive theory to sharpen the analytical focus
- Committed theoretical analysis.

For researchers from applied practice-based professions, substantive theories hold the strongest potential to give the interpretation process a genuinely theoretical boost (Guassora, Reventlow, et al. 2022, Malterud, Reventlow, et al. 2024). Read more about this further on.

Theory as a backdrop and inspiration

Theoretical perspectives may serve as a backdrop and inspiration for your project without taking on a strong role as an analytical tool. By presenting the theoretical perspectives in which you situate your project, the reader can better understand the choices and priorities you made in the study aim, analysis and interpretations. Although this is a fairly non-committal use of theory, you must choose a theory that in some way adds value to your study aim and become acquainted with the impact of this. It may be sufficient and safe to rely on one theory—if you choose more than one, the impact of the theoretical perspectives can become more superficial or unclear.

One example of how you can do it is a study of sick leave experiences among patients with medically unexplained health problems, in which a theory of marginalisation is presented as a starting point for interpretation (Aamland, Werner, et al. 2013). This provides a self-declaration from the authors explaining that the researchers' understanding of marginalisation had consistent weight in this project, though without giving these perspectives a guiding role in the analysis.

Another example is a study of lesbian women's experiences (Bjørkman & Malterud 2012). Here, Antonovsky's theory of salutogenesis (Antonovsky 1979) is used to account for the researchers' focus on positive coping in a field that has long been dominated by perspectives of misery.

The examples show how we can use theoretical perspectives to consolidate and display the study's positioning and thus indicate a more distinct starting point for the study aim. In this way, our premises can be shared with others, on premises beyond our preconceptions. Such theoretical approaches can be further highlighted in the discussion of the results. Here, the analysis may demonstrate how theory supports elaboration or challenges common assumptions, or how theoretical concepts and perspectives offer new insight into the issues addressed by the material. In this way, theoretical perspectives can complement and challenge the researchers' subject-specific background of experience when analysing the material.

Substantive theory can sharpen the gaze and strengthen reflexivity

Substantive theories represent a level of theory that is close to practice and deals with specific conditions, experiences or activities. Substantive theories are well-suited as relevant and specific tools for the development of new and valuable knowledge in medical and health research (Guassora, Reventlow, et al. 2022). Such theories, often developed in other academic disciplines (psychology, literary studies, sociology, social anthropology, philosophy), can sharpen the focus of problem formulation and analysis and offer thought-provoking metapositions for interpretation and reflexivity, also with empirically based strategies for abstraction (see Chapter 10).

Moreover, substantive theories can also be relevant for the clinician, who every day develops practical knowledge in their encounters with patients (without this being the subject of research) (see Chapter 19) (Schön 1991, Malterud 2001a, Malterud, Reventlow, et al. 2024). Substantive theory can function as a "can opener" by delimiting the field and offering useful concepts, or as a "lens" with a more radical and binding commitment to the construction of knowledge where theory and empiricism meet (Høyer 2008).

In the focus group study on GPs' strategies for negotiating sick leave (Nilsen, Malterud, et al. 2015), we used Lipski's theory of the street-level bureaucrat. The street-level bureaucrat sits between a rock and a hard place and must simultaneously consider both the patient's individual needs and prevailing laws and regulations. The street-level bureaucracy perspective of conflicted interests contributed to the focus of the analysis being directed particularly towards data that dealt with perceived controversies in such an intermediate position (Lipsky 1980/2010).

Another example is a focus group study on teenage girls' experiences of sexual harassment by boys at school (Slåtten & Malterud 2024). Here we used Butler's theory of gender performativity to draw attention to how sexualised behaviour is legitimised and how femininity and masculinity are staged through social and cultural conventions (Butler 1988). With this theory, supported by the concept "gender performativity", we were able to more clearly observe various aspects of unfortunate normalisation practices and to focus on how the boys' harassment was almost considered normal in the school situation.

A third example comes from a study of what young people from families with chronic illness or addiction wanted in terms of support from their GP. Here, Schibbye's theory of recognition (Schibbye 1993), materialising concepts and aspects of interest, provided a very distinct focus for the analysis (Gullbrå, Smith-Sivertsen, et al. 2016).

These are examples of how knowing with subject-specific relevance can be accomplished when apt substantive theories are given a prominent role. They also illustrate how a pragmatic study can be situated in a more committed frame of reference with somewhat stronger theoretical ambitions than when we use theory as a backdrop or inspiration. Interpretation and analysis nevertheless are accomplished with inductive logic, where result categories are developed in the encounter between empirical data and theoretical perspectives, without being predetermined or guided by the theoretical perspectives (see Chapter 11). Here, substantive theories can inform abstraction and thus strengthen the originality and transferability of interpretations and results, in addition to situatedness and reflexivity.

Theoretical specialisation—multidisciplinary collaboration

In multidisciplinary collaborative projects, we can draw on our partners' theoretical expertise by engaging with theories of greater depth. Reventlow, a GP and social anthropologist, used Lakoff and Johnson's cognitive metaphor theory to understand how women establish patterns of thinking about osteoporosis at the intersection of bodily experiences and cultural currents (Lakoff & Johnson 1980, Reventlow, Overgaard, et al. 2008).

Werner, a sociologist, drew on Ochberg's perspectives on how stories create notions of identity and gender when she explored female patients' stories about being regarded as decent human beings (Ochberg 1994, Werner, Isaksen, et al. 2004).

Sviland and Råheim, who are physiotherapists, collaborated with Martinsen, who is a nurse and philosopher, on a project where the analysis of a course of treatment with psychomotor physiotherapy was supported by perspectives from Braatøy, Løgstrup and Ricoeur (Sviland, Martinsen, et al. 2018).

For a researcher with a medical and health science background, there can be much to gain from such collaborative arenas, especially when we maintain the intention that the outcome of our project must be intended and perceived as relevant primarily towards our own peers. Nevertheless, I readily acknowledge that it may be challenging to implement this a theoretical level of ambition for a researcher from medicine and health sciences without any other theoretical background.

CHAPTER 21

Validation revisited—soundness and scope of understanding

To validate is to ask critical questions about the validity of knowledge. Validation addresses the soundness of what we have come to understand and the scope of that understanding. In all research, we need to ask ourselves whether our methods offer a relevant and robust path to knowing with the potential to clarify our study aim. In qualitative research, we create descriptions and interpretations of the phenomena under study, and there are often multiple possible perspectives. But not all of them have the same level of validity regarding our study aim. Validation explores the significance, possibilities, limitations and relevance of the version we finally prioritise.

Pertinent results—new and valuable?

Kvale (1996) says that "to validate is to question". Considering relevance at all stages of the qualitative research process supports assessments of different aspects of *validity*. Reflexivity addressing relevance is therefore a key approach to validity (with these three meta-criteria being interdependent) (see Chapters 3 and 25). Taken together, this is the main road to assess the soundness of what we have come to understand and the scope of that understanding.

In a qualitative study, such considerations cannot be reached by calculations, checklists or yes/no questions. Methodically, we articulate arguments and counterarguments, balancing our interpretations and comparing alternative options. This is reflexivity in practice (Stige, Malterud, et al. 2009). In this way, we can push the boundaries of our own knowing and elaborate a reasoned (and seasoned) view of what our interpretations speak to, what they do not address, and of their transferability. By continuously validating our approach, we can learn from experience as we progress, make use of both opportunities and constraints throughout a flexible process, and adjust our design as needed.

We can scrutinise the relevance of the formulation of the study aim (Is this really what we were wondering about?), the sample (Does this provide a basis with appropriate

DOI: 10.4324/9781003786016-25

Information Power to answer our questions?), data development (What knowledge did the participants given us access to?), theoretical perspectives (Are the concepts and models we are using helpful to understand the phenomenon we want to learn about?), the analysis strategy (What do different interpretations tell us?) as well as the content of presentation (Do our results present clear answers to the study aim?). (Remember, though, that open-ended questions with "how" often yield better answers than yes/no.) And if the answers to all these questions are "ok!", we have not been sufficiently reflexive. In that case, we failed to identify the limitations of our project—as occurring in any research project, and the validation should be recapitulated.

Member check

Claiming that the participants' subjective experiences or opinions are the sources of our results, we must demonstrate that the empirical data and our interpretations constitute a valid link between the starting point and the conclusions. Rather than asking whether participants have told "the Truth", it is more helpful to consider what they are being truthful about, and how our own focus shapes this. The stories people share depend on the context of the conversation, and they might have valid reasons for choosing one version when speaking with a researcher. The same applies to how we prioritise the centre of gravity in an observational study.

Any exchange of knowledge represents risks of misunderstanding. Most mistakes arise when one or more actors fail to realise that they are talking past one another. During an interview, the researcher may therefore regularly assess their own perception with questions such as "Have I understood you correctly when you say that..., or?". This must be an open, not a leading question. Through continuous dialogical validation, subjectivity is used to support, as far as possible, a shared understanding between researcher and participant of the co-created narrative. Such questioning enhances intersubjectivity between participant and researcher and thus in turn between researcher and reader (Kvale 1996).

Some researchers send interview transcripts or drafts of the results section to participants for review and approval. This process is referred to as a *member check*. In this way, ambiguities can be clarified, and the interview may be supplemented with reflections made by the participant afterwards. Reading through the transcript may help adjust linguistic forms and dialect expressions that have been inaccurately reproduced. If we are studying linguistic details, this procedure can be an important corrective. In most other projects, however, participant verification is not appropriate (Goldblatt, Karnieli-Miller, et al. 2011). It is the study aim, and the method that determines which validation procedures are helpful, and a text does not necessarily become more accurate when participants have corrected the transcript.

Moreover, member checking can foster an understanding among researchers and participants that the project is primarily about the accurate retelling of stories. Subtly shaped by positivist ideals and the small q (see Chapter 4), we may forget that it is precisely the researcher's responsibility for interpretation and synthesis that renders a study scientific (Thorne 2009, Varpio, Ajjawi, et al. 2017). In a qualitative study, it is therefore entirely possible to arrive at conclusions that do not correspond with what one or more participants expressed. There are also situations where the researcher's interpretation of the material leads to a different interpretation than the one matching the participant's self-understanding (Goldblatt, Karnieli-Miller, et al. 2011). Personally, I do not normally conduct this form of member check or participant validation.

Decontextualisation during analysis should always be followed by recontextualisation—this means that we must return our interpretations to their original context and reassess their validity within this framework (see Chapter 11). On rare occasions, it may then be necessary to consult the participants again. But the researcher is responsible for validating conclusions.

If participants subsequently dismiss the researcher's conclusions, it may also be because the knowledge is perceived as distressing. It may nevertheless be valid and relevant within the context in which it came from. However, such a disagreement may also come into view if the researcher has constrained the participants' voices with preconceptions and interpretations. If so, the result may no longer be a valid expression of what the participants meant and spoke. If participants recognise and accept the final description of their reality, while that description also offers new insights and even surprises, we may assume that we have co-created valid knowledge grounded in the reality to which it belongs. However, this is not a strong argument in favour of member checking as a validation strategy.

Consensus as a yardstick for validity?

When more people agree that a conclusion makes sense, it becomes more likely to be regarded as valid. For example, projects that develop tools for subsequent use in standardised contexts, for example diagnostic classifications, require a shared and unambiguous understanding of meaning. In such cases, consistency between different researchers' interpretations and results is imperative for validity. However, this does not imply that something becomes truer simply because more people believe it to be so.

Firstly, the collective view of the majority often consolidates cultural prejudices that close off new insights. Imagine a project mapping the living conditions of gays and lesbians, with everyone in the research team taking for granted that there are substantial problems in this study group. Then, the interpretations and analyses give attention to describing and confirming these. In this case, the impact of a consensus assessment may be that evidence about life satisfaction and diversity in the same material is overlooked, thus affording the study weak validity regarding positive aspects of the living conditions (Malterud et, Bjørkman, et al. 2009).

Secondly, broad agreement may indicate that the results are so consistent with existing preconceptions that the project adds nothing new. Controversy, on the other hand, can be an indication of knowledge that challenges old truths and brings forward new and valuable understanding. Consensus and independent judgements are therefore rarely relevant validity criteria in qualitative studies, but a symptom of a small q logic (see Chapter 4).

It is not a given that the scientific quality is weak if one researcher has conducted the analysis alone, or that it will always be better when two or five were together and agreed. On the contrary, exposing our material to diverse points of view and metaperspectives can enrich knowing by adding nuance from different angles. Hence, an analysis team may therefore be purposively composed, emphasising positions of cognition that enhance diversity. With such approaches, the potential gain will be more about negotiations leading towards optimal utilisation of the material's diversity than about the truthfulness of the results.

Correspondence and criterion validity

An essential question in validation is whether the research method adequately makes sense of what it intends to address, and what it claims to address. For the measurement of weight and time, there are *gold standards* with international conventions that we accept as the one and only definition of what we are measuring. We can then validate our measurement method by determining the extent to which our measurements correspond to those achieved by recognised gold-standard criteria. A clearly defined gold standard with specific criteria is necessary for this type of method validation, as it allows us to properly compare our techniques and results. However, social constructs of this kind, grounded in consensus, are not thereby truer than other definitions or claims.

Yet, the more people agree, the broader the *cultural validity* of the phenomenon in question. Across a variety of settings, there is broad cultural agreement on the gold standard. The internet provides information about universal time—an easily accessible gold standard. Standardised instruments and methods are important tools in many types of medical research. Electrolyte measurements from various laboratories are only comparable if their testing methods are standardised to a common reference. Then the method is validated by checking correspondence against a defined gold standard. This is called *correspondence validity* or *criterion validity.* How do the results achieved with the new method correspond to the results we get using the old method on the same data?

Here, the criteria embodied in the gold standard are appropriately specified within a deductive framework, constituting a benchmark for validating another method. Validating the method, we validate the results and their trustworthiness. The interpretation of the results rests with us, and such validation strategies are only appropriate when the criteria are clear, stable and beyond dispute. The prerequisite is that it is logically meaningful and technically possible to check the correspondence.

But a lot of aspects of everyday medical life are characterised by the fact that we do not know enough about what defines and characterises the phenomena we want to study. There are no relevant yardsticks. The same applies to subjective aspects of health and illness, life and death. Correspondence, or criterion validation, is therefore not applicable when exploring problems for which several valid versions of the results are acknowledged (see Chapter 2). Subjectivity cannot be accommodated within the demands of correspondence validity. Therefore, these validation strategies are not suitable for qualitative studies.

Communicative validity—research dissemination

Intersubjective dialogues of process and results allow us to share and challenge the knowledge we have developed (Malterud 1993, 2001b, Stige, Malterud, et al. 2009). Knowledge is valid only within the context it originates from, unless it can be shared with others. The researcher's skills to convey their research also affect the validity of the knowledge. Kvale calls this *communicative validity* (Kvale 1996). If we are unable to tell others what we have done in a way that others understand and recognise, the knowing remains private, and communicative validity is weak.

To resonate with the reader, a qualitative study must be presented in a clear and well-crafted non-fiction form. This is especially important in the results section, which should balance recognition with insight to support new understanding. In a qualitative study, the researcher's academic narrative skills are much more important than in an epidemiological research project, where the results are presented in a standardised form based on figures and tables. Still, a small warning is in order here. Readability is a necessary but not sufficient condition for communicative validity. It does not matter how exciting the author's story is, if the article is short of reflexivity, consistency and intersubjective articulation of a systematic analysis process.

But communicative validity is not only about the results and conclusions of the research project—it is just as much about the process (see Chapter 13). Only when the researcher manages to present the path that has been followed, the reader will be able to understand the versions, interpretations and conclusions that are ultimately presented as results (Malterud 1993, 2001b). Intersubjectivity at the process level is an important condition for qualitative evidence, which does neither imply that the reader would have chosen the same path nor have arrived at the same interpretations. The goal is not agreement but knowing, leading to insight and understanding.

Therefore, we must ask ourselves to whom we address with the knowledge we have developed. Hence, Kvale (1996) recommends the validation question "who". It is in relation to a specific addressee that the communicative validity of the project is put to the test. Communicative negotiations between actors determine whether the knowledge is regarded as valid or not. The novice must be proficient in the scientific language expected by the audience and capable of articulating arguments and conclusions that support trustworthiness. For researchers in medicine and health sciences, this may entail the risk of scientific research ideals spilling over into rhetoric and logic from the small q (see Chapter 4).

Power is a key element in this language game. What counts as communicative validity is determined by who, within the system, has the authority to legitimise knowledge. In the medical academic culture, there is a big difference between the authority of conclusions from published versus unpublished studies. Peer review of an article submitted to a journal represents a procedure for appraisal of the scientific validity of the study. When outsiders with expertise in the study aim and methodology examine the article's relevance, quality and readability, a validity assessment is conducted at a new level. If peers, editors and readers do not recognise the language, message or process, the communicative validity is weak.

This is no neutral, value-free assessment. Communicative validity is balanced against cultural academic norms for scientific quality (Stige, Malterud, et al. 2009), not least against current rules for format, style and procedures. Submitting a qualitative study, the researcher may experience that the traditional medical community of science still does not know or acknowledge the methodological rules of qualitative inquiry. In assessing procedural validity, the distinction between ends and means frequently gets lost (Loder, Groves, et al. 2016, Clarke, Braun, et al. 2024). To make qualitative inquiry intelligible within medical culture, careful attention to the articulation of the research process is essential to strengthen intersubjectivity and communicative validity. It is a waste of time and energy to submit an article for review in a journal that has not previously published qualitative studies. Such journals rarely have peers with appropriate qualitative methodological expertise (see Chapter 25).

How true is true?

Many researchers using qualitative methods move away from the concept of validity in its traditional sense. For example, Hamberg et al. rely on Lincoln & Guba when they propose "credibility" as an alternative (Lincoln & Guba 1985, Hamberg, Johansson, et al. 1994). Based on a social constructionist understanding, there are many different versions of reality that can be valid at the same time (see Chapter 2) (Lock & Strong 2010, Smith 2010). Therefore, the purpose of validation cannot be to prove that we have found the Truth, and certainly not with objectivity as a premise.

It is the latter position Kvale (1996) challenges when he asks for "the validity of the validity question" and which Haraway (1991) calls "the God trick" (see Chapter 5). As a researcher, I am not supposed to establish my conclusions as truth or fact. I must demonstrate that I have reflected upon the internal and external validity and can offer a reasoned indication of their soundness and scope. This applies regardless of whether I use qualitative or quantitative research methods. Therefore, I still hold validity as an important concept for qualitative research methods, provided that it is not attributed a small q narrow, procedural meaning that is more appropriate for quantitative studies (see Chapter 4).

Social constructionism challenges the idea of an "objective" reality, arguing that all knowing and understanding arise from social and linguistic interactions within specific local contexts (see Chapter 2) (Crotty 2003, Lock & Strong 2010). Such perspectives can expand our understanding of diversity and contradictions, but on the other hand, also legitimise a relativism where everything is equally good and true. But the fact that several versions can be valid at the same time does not necessarily mean that any answer or result is as relevant as another (Haraway 1991, Smith 2010). When assessing the validity of a qualitative study, the researcher's mission is to consider competing analytic interpretations and to offer a reasoned judgement as to why, in light of the research question, some results carry stronger validity than others. Only then can subjectivity become a creative resource and an ideal for the development of knowledge about people's experiences of life, health and healthcare.

CHAPTER 22

Combining methods—sustaining philosophical coherence?

Viewing an issue from different angles can contribute nuances and corrective measures, adding fresh dimensions to knowing. Combining different designs, methods or perspectives in one and the same project, we can establish metapositions and develop more comprehensive knowledge than if we explore the field from only one side. But adopting a both-and approach demands considerable care on the part of the researcher. We must clearly demonstrate the added value of how one perspective complements the other, and how the epistemological assumptions have been negotiated. The goal is to enhance diversity, not to confirm precision or facts. Let us therefore look at some concepts and challenges and consider potentially relevant strategies for exploration of an issue from several different angles.

Triangulation

Measurements from different vantage points are used by the surveyor to determine the position of a mountain peak in relation to other landmarks in the terrain. The lines of sight to the summit from various locations form angles to each other and intersect at the point where the peak is established on the map. This is called *triangulation*, with the accuracy of the mapped points as a key objective, grounded in measurable facts.

In qualitative studies, on the other hand, our ambition is rather to develop more vivid or sharp interpretations of what we are studying by obtaining various types of observations or perspectives. The different approaches from different angles are not intended to answer the same questions or to confirm positions, but to enable different questions about the same issue. We seek nuance and diversity rather than the precision and factual convergence that topographic triangulation offers (Varpio, Ajjawi, et al. 2017).

For methodological purposes, it is essential not to confuse these two very different meanings of the term triangulation. For qualitative research methods, Patton presents four forms of triangulation: (1) method triangulation, (2) source triangulation, (3) observer triangulation and (4) theory triangulation (Patton 2015).

DOI: 10.4324/9781003786016-26

Method triangulation may involve the application of both qualitative and quantitative research methods (Teddlie & Tashakkori 2009). For example, Larun wanted to investigate the effects and experiences of physical activity for patients with chronic fatigue syndrome (CFS/ME). She carried out a systematic review of relevant efficacy studies (Larun & Malterud 2011b) and conducted a focus group study on the preconditions for positive experiences and the impact of negative experiences of physical activity in this patient group (Larun & Malterud 2011a). In this way, she gained a broader basis to consider how graded exercise therapy can best be adapted to the individual patient.

Source triangulation draws on data from different sources, for example by combining various research designs or by recruiting participants with different roles in relation to the problem (Oien & Solheim 2015). Reventlow, et al. (2008) explored women's perceptions of risk related to osteoporosis, with data from women with or without osteoporosis, interviewed individually and in focus groups. In a case study design about a course of treatment with psychomotor physiotherapy, Sviland, et al. (2018) developed data from focus group interviews, individual interviews and written text to include more dimensions in analysis, but not to validate the correspondence between the different data sources.

Observer triangulation may involve several researchers, often with different academic backgrounds, participating in the development and analysis of the same empirical material, as when a social anthropologist, a political scientist and a medical doctor jointly explored the impact of conclusions from a series of systematic reviews served to inform policy and practice (Malterud, Bjelland, et al. 2016).

Theoretical triangulation means that we use several different theoretical perspectives in the interpretation of the empirical data. In a study of the everyday lives of children growing up with parents who have alcohol problems (Werner & Malterud 2016a), Goffman's dramaturgical theories of social order (Goffman 1959) were augmented by Smart's perspectives on family secrets. (Smart 2011).

Hence, the concept of triangulation is ambiguous and can be tricky. In the methodological literature, it appears as an established strategy that can nevertheless perpetuate inappropriate signals about ideals that conform better with the surveyor's mission (to measure the truth) than with the epistemological basis of qualitative research methods (to explore subjectivity and diversity) (Varpio, Ajjawi, et al. 2017).

Different perspectives can illuminate contradictions and dilemmas and draw attention to the complexity of a qualitative study. Nevertheless, many articles present triangulation as a mechanical safety net, with an underlying positivist premise that the study becomes more credible and the results more accurate when they originate from multiple sources. Therefore, it is epistemological incongruence when triangulation is used to confirm correspondence validity, where one type of result in an objective reality (see Chapter 21) should match the other type of result as closely as possible (Varpio, Ajjawi, et al. 2017).

Several checklists for qualitative studies insist triangulation (see Chapter 25) (Barbour 2001, Braun & Clarke 2024a). However, you should only plan for triangulation if you have a clear idea of how it may add to your project. Triangulation must not be used as a small q strategy (see Chapter 4), to legitimise qualitative methods on inadequate assumptions. There is no reason to talk to both doctors and nurses if the dialogue between the doctors is the focus of your research question (Lid, Oppedal, et al. 2012). You do not need to conduct focus groups as well as individual interviews if your data offers appropriate Information Power (IP) by using one of these methods (Ree & et al. 2014). Nor should you introduce several theoretical perspectives in the analysis if a theory you know well can sharpen your research question (Nilsen, Malterud, et al. 2015). In other words, more is not always better.

When you frame your design around triangulation, you need to demonstrate how multiple perspectives contributed to new insight. Triangulation can only contribute to the development of new and valuable knowledge if we carry out a distinct analytical integration exhibiting the added value of the knowledge from the different vantage points we have explored. Unfortunately, we often find that this link is missing. Therefore, it may be better to choose other terms if you want to pursue diversity in perspectives and methods.

Mixed methods

Combining qualitative and quantitative research methods within a single project is called *mixed methods* (MM) (Teddlie & Tashakkori 2009, Migiro & Magangi 2011) (Creswell 2022). MM designs can offer opportunities for the exploration of complex issues, for example in a study on HIV testing in three African countries (Njeru, Blystad, et al. 2011). The researchers established very extensive data from a population-based survey (N = 5,689), 34 focus groups and 18 individual interviews. Their analyses documented the significance of, and preconditions for, counselling related to diagnostic tests and raised important ethical questions about voluntary participation. Normally, it is not necessary to plan for such extensive data development. In another study on spinal mobilisation for patients with ankylosing spondylitis, six patients undertook a standardised course of treatment from a manual therapist with effect measurements and subsequent semistructured individual interviews (Mengshoel & Robinson 2008). The analyses indicated that the treatment resulted in better movement outcomes, but also that what the patients emphasised was not always the same as the therapist's assessments.

MM studies are conducted in many different formats, where the different methodological approaches take place in parallel or sequentially. The latter is the most common (Östlund, Kidd, et al. 2011). The qualitative study may precede the quantitative study or vice versa (see Chapter 4), and the balance between the different methods varies depending on the purpose. Whatever the case, you need to clarify your purpose of the combination, for example whether qualitative data will be used to contextualise quantitative data, or whether the purpose is to inform a large quantitative survey (Östlund, Kidd, et al. 2011). If you want to combine to confirm and achieve accuracy, you should rather stick to the quantitative sub-study, to avoid epistemological incongruence (see Chapter 4).

A PhD project may be composed of qualitative and quantitative sub-studies. This affords the candidate a broader and more robust academic competence than projects that rely on only one of these methodological traditions. Such projects are often presented as MM studies. However, for such projects to earn the status of MM studies with appropriate scientific rigour, you need solid expertise, planning and supervision on all the applied methods. Often, it may therefore be more appropriate to refer to the project design as multimethod rather than MM. *Multimethod studies* can provide *convergent* perspectives, where you seek multiple nuances of the same phenomenon, or *divergent* perspectives, where you challenge knowing and interpretations in more complex landscapes. Either way, you need to have a distinct purpose and a plan that explains and justifies the effort also of choosing a multimethod design, beyond a desire to establish a comprehensive methodological competence.

For multi-method studies, a systematic strategy for integrating and synthesising the results from the various sub-studies is also needed to achieve the added benefit. Sometimes, we may spot a project outline presenting the first two epidemiological sub-studies as thoroughly described, while the third sub-study is announced as a focus group lacking a study aim as well as a presentation of design and method. Such examples demonstrate a lack of respect for qualitative methods and indicate that the academic quality and rigour of the third sub-project may be deficient. In such projects, a defensible synthesis is difficult to envisage. The reverse situation, with superficial planning of quantitative sub-studies, is far less common. In the study on spinal mobilisation referred to above, the analysis was accomplished with close dialogue between the researchers responsible for the quantitative and qualitative sub-studies, respectively. Still, they also experienced that appropriate intersubjectivity from such interaction is hard to achieve and convey (Mengshoel 2012).

MM studies involve demanding encounters and confrontations between the positivist and interpretive paradigms (see Chapter 2). The researcher must be capable of holding two conflicting ideas in their mind at the same time and be able to find pragmatic solutions and compromises (Migiro & Magangi 2011). Maintaining epistemological congruence leads to challenges in terms of ontology and epistemology (see Chapters 1 and 4) demanding caution, reflexivity and methodological experiences. This implies especially sampling and transferability (see Chapter 7). In an epidemiological study, we apply a representative sample, while in an interview study, we need a purposive sample. These sampling strategies are based on contradictory logics and can lead to serious flaws in interpretation and transferability if we muddle or conflate the concepts. This kind of challenges become particularly prominent in conducting qualitative metasynthesis (see Chapter 18).

Personally, I find it problematic to combine qualitative and qualitative data and use different analysis methods on data from one and the same material with different assumptions, see more about this below. The simplest solution is to prevent the problem by establishing different samples for the various sub-studies, conducting methodologically sound analyses of different data sets, while putting a lot of effort into the interpretation stage with a distinctive integrative analysis and synthesis.

With MM, the level of ambition for analysis is higher than with triangulation (Migiro & Magangi 2011). When results from different sub-studies in a mixed-methods project are integrated in a methodologically sound way, this can substantially strengthen the results (Mengshoel & Robinson 2008, Creswell 2022). This is not easy, however.

The results of the qualitative and quantitative analyses can coincide, contradict or complement each other (Östlund, Kidd, et al. 2011). Even here, there is a risk of invoking a confirmation logic based on the assumption of a truth validated by correspondence rather than the interpretive logic employed in qualitative studies. Mengshoel points out the importance of regarding qualitative and quantitative methods as complementary, not as competing in an MM project, and of respectful and equal collaboration between researchers with sound methodological expertise (Mengshoel 2012).

In an ordinary journal article, there will rarely be room for the appropriate presentation of several sub-studies and even fewer opportunities to present analyses and syntheses. Structural conditions are more favourable in the summary chapter of a PhD thesis, where the candidate is expected to offer an overall interpretation of what the various results mean together. In such a synthesis, theoretical perspectives will also make an important contribution to new interpretations and to the independent positioning of the qualitative and quantitative approaches (see Chapter 20) (Östlund, Kidd, et al. 2011, Mengshoel 2012). To sum up, the term "Mixed Methods" should be reserved for studies where a genuine synthesis is offered and omitted when the project simply comprises sub-studies undertaken with different methods (Migiro & Magangi 2011).

Questionnaire with open-ended response options

A less ambitious strategy for combining qualitative and quantitative data is to include some questions with open-ended response options in an otherwise standardised questionnaire. In medical and health research, questionnaires are often used for data collection in quantitative surveys, typically with a deductive logic employing predetermined response categories for ticking. Sometimes, a few open-ended questions are also included for free-text responses.

With predetermined response options, the researcher's voice takes precedence because the possible answers have already been decided. Open-ended questions are a necessary, though not sufficient, condition for the participant to give answers other than those already anticipated in questions based on standardised instruments. In large questionnaires developed to assemble quantitative survey data, open-ended questions often appear as appendices or inserted sub-questions. Participants can sometimes qualify a response option through an open keyword field, often marked "other" or "which one?". Responses to such questions can hardly be called qualitative data. They deliver a brief answer within a framework narrowly set by the other response options for this question, without taking advantage of the rhetorical power of a well-articulated question.

Still, *free-text responses to open-ended questions* can under certain conditions serve as qualitative data. For such data to generate scientific knowledge, they must arise from well-crafted, appropriate prompting and be subjected to methodical interpretation and analysis. Open-ended questions can be asked in a questionnaire, but only when we attend carefully to the context in which the question is asked, we will understand how the question situates the knowing (Schwartz 1999). Keep in mind that the remaining questionnaire conveys to the participant a clear indication of the kind of knowledge expected. Open-ended questions easily become leading as a consequence of their position in a context where similar questions have been "pre-answered" by ticking boxes earlier in the form. In the worst case, open-ended answers can operate as a self-fulfilling prophecy that the researcher uses to confirm their preconceptions.

Even with rigorous methodical conduct, such data provides limited IP compared to more robust qualitative data, such as interview data co-created in dialogues with participants. Still, there may be potential for new and valuable knowing. In a study on lower urinary infection, 196 women between the ages of 19 and 97 answered a questionnaire about the prevalence of symptoms (Malterud & Bærheim 1999). The women were also asked to describe their symptoms in their own words. All of them responded—some with just a few words, while others provided extensive and colourful descriptions of how lower urinary infection was perceived and expressed. We conducted qualitative analysis of these pieces of text, with the elaboration of symptom descriptions helpful to enhance the clinical accuracy of the medical history in the diagnosis of cystitis.

Hence, there are several methodological pitfalls and sources of error when we plan for free-text responses as empirical data for qualitative analysis. Unfortunately, when the rest of the questionnaire belongs to a different research logic, this part of the material may be processed by enthusiastic researchers without expertise in qualitative methods. Taking an intuitive look at the responses, grouping them according to themes that immediately emerge, and then presenting these, embellished with selected quotes, is not a qualitative analysis. You can read more about qualitative data from free text responses in Chapter 15.

Avoid conflating the concepts!

Respecting the material's uniqueness, possibilities and limitations is an indispensable condition in qualitative studies, applying to what we can draw conclusions about (internal validity) and what scope we can attribute to the conclusions (external validity) (see Chapters 3 and 21). If, in a sample of qualitative interview data on pelvic examinations, we had found that 8 out of 13 participants preferred the doctor to tell them what was happening during the examination (Larsen, Oldeide, et al. 1997), it would be a grave mistake to say that 62% of female patients wanted this. Furthermore, it does definitely not mean that 38% do not want this.

Conclusions about prevalence and distribution or covariation require answers to standardised questions to a representative sample and statistical analysis. A purposive or convenience sample can never speak to such outcomes, and in qualitative research interviews, we are not supposed to ask all participants identical and standardised questions (see Chapter 14). Furthermore, since we did not ask all participants about their preferences regarding pelvic examinations, we also do not know the views of those who did not respond to this topic. Even if we had asked them specifically, a purposive sample of qualitative data never provides a basis for statistical methods to calculate the likely margin of error for the results and assess their transferability.

Nonetheless, some research projects rely on calculating the extent and distribution of textual elements within qualitative data to generate their results. Quantifying qualitative data is sometimes referred to as *content analysis* or quasi-statistical analytical style. Software programs for qualitative analysis contain modules for counting the number of elements in each code group, which may encourage the quantification of qualitative data. However, selection and analysis need to be epistemologically aligned with the research method, and these approaches fall outside qualitative inquiry.

Numbers and quantitative terms are not taboo in a qualitative study but should be used with prudence. Regardless of the project design and analysis strategy, it can still sometimes be helpful early in the analysis to get an impression of how this particular material is distributed regarding the relevant questions. This can help us to spot patterns other than by just reading the text. If a particular statement can be attributed only to a single participant, it may have a different meaning than if it is something everyone is talking about. Such counts are more useful and carry less risk of epistemological shortcuts, when used for exploratory engagement with the material than when they are used to frame the results. Assessing results where qualitative data is presented in a quantitative format is problematic. Peers asking for quantification of different code groups or result categories, or how many people said what, are epistemologically misguided (Clarke, Braun, et al. 2024)

I would especially warn against cross-tabulations of such data, whether qualitative/qualitative data or quantitative/qualitative data. Qualitative data contains ambiguities, contradictions and overlaps that represent diversity and complexity. Furthermore, qualitative data from representative samples, developed from open-ended responses to a questionnaire, cannot be generalised in the same way as pre-categorised quantitative data from standardised response options. Epistemological incongruence is close at hand if we map open-ended questionnaire responses onto variables drawn from the quantitative items.

If we nonetheless reduce qualitative data to descriptive counts, we run into fundamental problems of transferability and external validity. Where such figures refer only to the particular study context, their capacity to travel beyond it is so limited that their status as scientific knowledge becomes questionable. It is better to recognise this limitation than to claim it as a feature of qualitative methods, whose strengths lie elsewhere.

Contradictions and correspondences

Combining research methods can put forward refreshing advances and nuances to our study aim and overarching analysis. Sometimes, diversity in sampling, data, analysis and interpretive perspectives leads to conflicting answers to the same question. This may indicate that one path to knowledge is less adequate than the other, and that we may have focused on something that did not relate to what we intended to study.

But contradictions can also reveal substantial ambiguities, ambivalences and paradoxes—features that subjectivity in human life is replete with. When confronted with life itself, any theory may demonstrate its flaws. Something may look completely different from the inside than from the outside. Medical and health research requires strategies of knowing that allow the contradictions and complexities of illness and health to unfold rather than be reduced (Pope & Mays 2020). When multiple perspectives produce perfectly consistent results, it is worth asking whether they have been used to their full analytic potential. In qualitative research, methodological diversity yielding identical results does not constitute reproducibility in any meaningful sense (see Chapter 21).

CHAPTER 23

Artificial Intelligence—friend or foe in qualitative studies?

Artificial intelligence (AI) is rapidly gaining ground in society, healthcare and research. For such powerful tools to be of maximum benefit, with the fewest possible undesirable side effects, we must carefully examine the possibilities and limitations. Many are asking how AI can help improve the planning and conduct of qualitative studies in medicine and the health sciences. Let us take a closer look at epistemological assumptions such as subjectivity and interpretation in the face of a technical logic of machine learning from language models. This represents a different context from situations in which AI streamlines routinised processes in the health service.

Artificial intelligence can improve healthcare routines and systems

AI is digital systems grounded in machine learning for the synthesis of existing knowledge that will revolutionise many aspects of medical practice and research (Alowais, Alghamdi, et al. 2023). AI is already being used by Norwegian general practitioners to support routine clinical work, including the transcription of consultations into condensed record notes and the drafting of information and referral letters.

Machine learning represents a formidable potential for streamlining, not least for the power of change in processes and routines where human judgement results in unnecessary delays, ambiguities and reduced outcomes compared to AI's superb, lightning-fast reasoning. Current examples include the enhancement of diagnostic procedures (mammography), personalised medicine (cancer treatment), pharmacotherapy (warfarin dosage), public health (vaccine development) and care of the elderly (portable monitor connected to a call centre) (Alowais, Alghamdi, et al. 2023). Well-known issues associated with AI include unreliability (hallucinations and incorrect references), data privacy risks (sensitive patient information), alienation (reduced human-centred care) and theft (plagiarism of research data and results). (Alowais, Alghamdi, et al. 2023, Yu, Healey, et al. 2024).

DOI: 10.4324/9781003786016-27

AI's strength lies in transforming existing knowledge with *linear logic* into algorithms, predictability and fast processes that can be implemented in medical practice and research. The prerequisite is that a knowledge base about the problem, the intervention, the population and the framework conditions for developing strong, relevant machine learning models already exists. Computing power and digital expertise, a basis for decision-making on the introduction of new practices, funding for this and staff training are also needed.

Many questions must be addressed before AI can be used in everyday health services, particularly in settings where (co-)humanity and subjectivity—alongside instrumental elements—are fundamental to how healthcare professionals interact with people who are ill (see Chapter 1).

Furthermore, challenges also arise in clinical knowing and tacit expert logic that does not quite follow the algorithmic path (see Chapter 19). AI cannot take over as autopilot in medical judgements and decisions in landscapes where non-linear, complex and surprising sidetracks sometimes provide the best strategies for diagnosing and treating the unique patient with complex health problems (Gatens-Robinson 1986, McWhinney 1989, Sandelowski 1996). This is especially pertinent in general practice. Many questions concerning privacy and ethics must also be clarified in practice, legislation and governance.

Epistemological contradiction

The epistemological logic underpinning AI is rooted in algorithms based on probability, prediction and technical rationality. These assumptions stand in marked contrast to the human subjectivity and interpretive judgement that form the fundamental basis for knowledge development in qualitative research (see Chapter 1) (Malterud 2001b, Braun & Clarke 2019). In qualitative studies, reflexivity is a methodologically essential counterbalance to pre-determined deductive conclusions as well as random interpretations. Adopting this attitude allows the researcher to recognise and discuss reciprocal influences between themselves, the focus of inquiry and the context of knowledge development. We explore and take advantage of the distinctively human, such as mental representations, abstraction, volition, tacit knowledge, emotions, empathy, morality, memory, creativity, symbolisation, identity formation and language (Smith 2010).

AI establishes deductive analysis strategies with predetermined categories, testing of hypotheses and generalisation at the macro group level, while qualitative analysis is inductive and interpretive, where interpretation and abstraction of the unique allows for understanding of phenomena with transferability beyond the study context. Subjectivity offers a distinctive potential for creativity in the development of knowledge, particularly suitable for exploring people in their social context.

In healthcare, we often encounter phenomena such as complexity, unpredictability, nonlinearity and social interaction (Malterud, Guassora, et al. 2015). Intersubjectivity, sharing and discussion of the trails that the researcher has followed at all stages of the research process, drives the researcher to identify and communicate the unique and personal basis for interpretation. With insight into their own role, the researcher's subjectivity in fact helps to discipline the interpretations of the subjective through reflexivity.

AI implicates consolidating and summarising existing knowledge. But qualitative methods should develop new questions, rather than confirming old answers. Qualitative studies are of limited value if they fail to demonstrate emergence (see Chapter 1) by delivering something significantly new or contributing to new insights. The most thought-provoking knowledge can emerge where we encounter digression, paradox or surprise that disrupt predictions and previous understanding or unpack an innovative logic. In qualitative analysis, interpretation is as crucial as the data itself. Excessive amounts of data may in fact undermine analytical depth by pushing the analysis towards superficiality. Such conditions are rarely compatible with the machine-learning concept. Machine learning cannot substitute or replicate human subjectivity in the development, interpretation and synthesis of qualitative data—an arena of knowing in which thoughtfulness and reflexivity outweigh production and efficiency.

AI in medical communication research

Menichetti and colleagues investigated how ChatGPT can function as a tool in medical communication research (Menichetti, Hillen, et al. 2023). The authors show how AI can produce simple examples related to the problem at hand, organise empirical data, clean noise from data, conduct informal literature searches and improve the language of scientific texts.

Processing qualitative data was also assessed. Deductive sorting of data with predetermined categories appeared feasible, but an example of analysing qualitative data from a consultation illustrated the risk of banal and obvious results: ChatGPT was asked to summarise the emotional status of an elderly patient with heart failure from a transcript of a consultation with a doctor. After several caveats, the conclusion was that the patient might be feeling anxious or worried and that the doctor needed to empathise, reassure the patient and address the patient's concerns to support the patient in the consultation.

Such results go no further than the principles of the patient-centred method, which is a point long acknowledged in clinical practice. The example illustrates how machine learning can provide a simple compilation of existing assumptions, knowledge and data, but that it takes more to create new and valuable knowledge, especially about subjective conditions. Menichetti et al. also point out the "black box" issues related to transparency, with low visibility and discussion of conditions for the choices that the machine learning model makes in its decisions for the analysis (Menichetti, Hillen, et al. 2023).

Value issues in machine learning

ChatGPT, which was used in the example above, is generative AI that uses Large Language Models (LLMs) to create content itself. The machine's starting point for learning and synthesis is what already exists. Result categories can be generated, but they are inevitably based on existing patterns and classification systems. This logic perpetuates socio-cultural stereotypes of gender, class and ethnicity (Yu, Healey, et al. 2024)—normative issues of great importance in medical and healthcare research and practice.

Attempts are being made to load targeted material to correct undesirable value-based biases in AI, for example to elicit patient preferences related to different treatment options. At the same time, Yu and colleagues point out that LLM process combinations of billions of parameters but still cannot capture all relevant subtle nuances (Yu, Healey, et al. 2024). Their conclusion is that we still need the wise clinician. Regardless of how advanced more recent AI versions turn out to be, they will never be able to upload and assess all aspects of the researcher's preconceptions and situation, including relevant existential, psychological, social, moral and ethical assumptions as the basis for interpretation in a machine learning model. Furthermore, tacit practical knowing (Schön 1991) does not readily lend itself to a language-based learning model (see Chapter 19).

Humanistic medicine—subjectivity in theory and practice

In clinical practice, the doctor is a participant and an observer, habitually at the same time (see Chapter 1). Diagnostic activities involve integration of analytical objectification and sensitive interpretation of multiple, often indistinct clues (Malterud & Kamps 2021), regularly under a high degree of uncertainty (Malterud, Guassora, et al. 2017). The human interaction between healthcare worker and patient on issues related to life and death, illness and health, requests trust, security, fairness, dignity and openness.

To understand and manage symptoms, grief, pain and fatigue, we need knowing to understand the uniquely human person, body and biology, and how this is experienced by the person in question. In the qualitative research interview, empirical data are co-created through mutual exchange between participant and researcher (see Chapter 14) (Malterud 2001b, Braun & Clarke 2022). Therefore, research interviews are not suitable for "streamlining" using AI. Robust algorithms can, in many situations, help the clinician to approach sharper and faster diagnoses. However, subjectivity and nonlinear logic often complement classical diagnostic strategies in the unsolved problems in unselected practice, especially when dealing with complex health problems and multimorbidity. Ruling out important diagnoses rapidly and safely is certainly helpful.

But do not forget that the doctor sometimes solves diagnostic puzzles by taking new and surprising paths, deviating from the obvious main path and discovering fresh threads and nuances for medical problem solving (Malterud, Reventlow, et al. 2019, Malterud & Kamps 2021). This type of logic is not easily transferable to AI. It is about encountering and reading patients in the best possible way, together exploring new ways of understanding illness and health, diagnosis and treatment (Malterud 2001a, Malterud & Kamps 2021). Without an epistemological perspective that explicitly acknowledges the (co-)human and subjective dimensions, medicine risks falling into instrumentalist error (see Chapter 1) (Malterud 2001b, Skjervheim 2002).

AI will never become a human being

AI contributes already in exciting ways to healthcare routines and systems and will in the future beyond doubt present unimaginable advances. Comprehensive strategies for streamlining, organising and sorting textual data from medical practice will be further developed, hopefully with a more appropriate concept than qualitative analysis. Naming this as qualitative analysis is an epistemological incongruity, in the same way that subjective interpretation of numbers can never become statistical analysis (see Chapter 4). Ultimately, the issue concerns the role that subjectivity and (co-)humanity should play in medical knowing, and how humanism can be allowed to occupy a prominent place in medical research and practice.

PART 5

In conclusion

CHAPTER 24

Dialogue and reflexivity rather than checklists for rigour?

Your choice of research method does not ensure scientific quality, regardless of whether you use qualitative or quantitative methods. Qualitative studies vary markedly in methodological rigour, and different qualitative designs and methods will to different degrees be congruent with your study aim. Checklists have been widely employed to differentiate between more and less methodologically rigorous studies. Such strategies, however, also contribute to the instrumentalisation and standardisation of qualitative studies. For qualitative methods to become acknowledged and respected in medical and health research, we must enhance methodological competence, invest in well-designed and feasible studies, and avoid unnecessary efficiency at the expense of reflexivity. Although these qualities cannot be counted or measured, they must be taken into account, preferably within reflexive formats beyond checklists.

Some recurrent challenges

Throughout previous editions of this book, I have emphasised important similarities between qualitative and quantitative research methods at a general level, such as "research", "science" or "evidence". When operationalising these principles and translating them into methodology, methods and procedures, however, the differences resulting from the paradigms and the ontological and epistemological assumptions become particularly clear (see Chapters 1 and 2). Quality criteria for quantitative studies are therefore not helpful for the assessment of a qualitative study. This is especially relevant for sampling, transferability and the researcher's role.

As repeatedly pointed out throughout this book, researchers with a background in biomedical traditions face some recurring methodological challenges that can disrupt the rigour of a qualitative study (Malterud, Hamberg, et al. 2017). This is often due to issues that can be described as the small q or post-positivist authority (see Chapter 4), where qualitative studies are unduly coloured by positivist ideals at the expense of the interpretive paradigm (Kidder & Fine 1987). The explanation may be that the

DOI: 10.4324/9781003786016-29

researcher or supervisor does not have sufficient knowledge or respect for the philosophical assumptions underpinning qualitative research methods.

A strong article with distinct methodological quality addresses an issue that is considered interesting by more people than the author (new and valuable knowledge), developed and formulated using methods that make it possible to explore the issue in an appropriate manner (relevant and robust), and acknowledging subjectivity (congruence between assumptions and approaches). A weak article lacking methodological quality tends to address issues the reader already knows well, presented so generally that the result is little more than trivial repetition, a point Kvale (1996) captures in his question, "Why are interview studies so boring to read?". The strong article presents a judicious selection of the state of knowledge, convincing the reader of the need for this particular study, while the weak article presents the total collection in the reference library. The strong article stages the design and method for data development, interpretation and analysis congruent with the study aim, preferably supported by theory exposing the project's situatedness. In the weak article, the author writes a lot about the importance of qualitative methods, but less about specific choices made along the way and their consequences.

The results section is the scene that most clearly demonstrates the differences between strong and weak quality (see Chapter 12). The strong article presents original and well-defined result categories that are displayed thoroughly, illustrated by a few striking quotes, while the weak article reiterates the author's study aim or preconceptions presented with a number of short paragraphs dominated by quotes. In the strong article, the presentation of results demonstrates that interpretation and analysis were carried out as a systematic process, while the weak article claims general assertions, leaving hardly any trace of analysis. The strong article convinces us of its capacity to add something new and valuable, while the weak article insists that the results are important. A short and distinct methodological discussion characterises the strong article, while the weak article refers to a few random paragraphs from the textbook.

In the strong article, we notice clear signs of reflexivity and intersubjectivity. The researcher's role is open to scrutiny by briefly presenting preconceptions and motivations (Thesen 2001) and by establishing metapositions from which the researcher can reflect on themselves (Stensland 2003). The composition and size of the sample are considered and discussed, making it possible to assess IP and transferability (Larun & Malterud 2011a). The analysis process is exposed for the reader when the researcher refers to and complies with an established method (Idland, Iversen, et al. 2022), while the weak article refers to a method or non-committal concepts that have obviously not been applied. In the strong article, theoretical perspectives are explicitly presented and applied (Reventlow, Overgaard, et al. 2008), making the path from data to results accessible (Dahl & Malterud 2015), while the weak article shows no traces of intersubjectivity.

Here I have compiled and repeated many of the recommendations made earlier in this book and put them into perspective, hoping to expose some poles available as a basis for navigation when evaluating our own and others' research (Malterud, Hamberg, et al. 2017). In other words, it is definitely possible to distinguish between strong and weak. However, these examples are not sufficient for systematic methodological assessment of scientific studies, whether for learning purposes in the role of critical reader, as researcher training in work on one's own project, as academic volunteer work carried out through peer review or in critical assessment for qualitative metasynthesis (see Chapter 18). You need to learn the tools of the trade.

Meta-criteria

Many have raised legitimate doubts about how far scientific criteria apply to the assessment of qualitative studies (Barbour 2001, Dixon-Woods, Shaw, et al. 2004, Buus & Agdal 2013). A relevant argument in favour of a sceptical view is that variations between different qualitative methods require more nuanced quality assessment, including criteria of varying appropriateness (Stige, Malterud, et al. 2009, Braun & Clarke 2024a).

The term "saturation", for example, was developed specifically for the Grounded Theory method (Glaser & Strauss 1967) but has gradually gained acceptance almost as a universal criterion, irrespective of relevance and method, required by editors and peers (Buus & Agdal 2013, Varpio, Ajjawi, et al. 2017, Malterud, Siersma, et al. 2021). Similar objections apply to the term "triangulation", understood as the verification of accuracy through measurement and correlation, which has limited relevance for qualitative studies (Varpio, Ajjawi, et al. 2017) (see Chapter 4).

But the diversity across qualitative methods does not mean that each researcher is in charge to decide on their own what is strong and weak. Reading across the methodological literature demonstrates several overarching *meta-criteria* on which there is considerable agreement. Meta-criteria are ideals that are operationalised in different ways. Following Lincoln and Guba (1985), Hamberg and colleagues (1994) invoke the criteria of credibility, confirmability, transferability and dependability as qualitative parallels to internal validity, objectivity, generalisability and contextual sensitivity, respectively. Pope and Mays (2020), in line with Hammersley (1998), acknowledge validity and relevance as the most important criteria but recognise that operationalising these can be challenging. Relevance can be enhanced through detailed reporting and different sampling strategies. Giacomini and Cook (2000b) emphasise the importance of clinical relevance. I have myself highlighted reflexivity, relevance and validity as key meta-criteria, with reflexivity as a supreme ideal that is practised and reported in many ways (Malterud 2001b).

Thus, there are many views on what is good and what is bad. This has changed over the years, offering a good prospect for further development. Consensus on a common standard is unlikely in this field. Seen from the outside, this may seem awkward. Can you trust a scientific community that cannot even present a unanimous list of quality criteria (Stige, Malterud, et al. 2009)?

However, the development and negotiations of quality assessment can also make an important contribution to a vibrant methodological environment and prevent dogmatism and orthodoxy (Janesick 1994, Chamberlain 2000, Carter & Little 2007). In this book, I emphasise concepts and strategies supporting qualitative inquiry in the sense of the Big Q, that is, premises that offer the strongest possible epistemological congruence with the interpretive paradigm (see Chapters 2 and 4) (Kidder & Fine 1987, Braun & Clarke 2019).

Do the project's results justify the investment of the participants?

Asking people to share their knowledge and experiences implies a mutual understanding that this is worth the effort. This is also an issue for research ethics (see Chapter 25).

The participants' contribution is a gift, and we should ensure that such an investment will lead to knowing that is genuinely useful for some purpose. We do not burden people by asking them to participate in a qualitative study that merely repeats what we already know. Similarly, we must carefully consider how much data we need to explore our study aim appropriately. It is a matter of research ethics to ensure that we do not undertake unnecessarily extensive data development. This can be a waste of the participants' time and trust and will also jeopardise our ability to conduct a thorough analysis. Step-by-step data development and analysis along the way, with assessments of IP from time to time, support the development of empirical material with appropriate composition and size (see Chapter 7).

Planning the project, we situate it in a context of knowing where we credit research colleagues who have previously explored the same area (even if we are not particularly impressed by what they have done or concluded). If a literature search reveals that our study aim has already been comprehensively answered by others, we will either expand on this or create another question that deserves attention. Reviewing the literature clarifies which unanswered questions we want to investigate in the project. As researchers, we rely on other people's time and trust, and there is therefore an ethical obligation to conduct a research project with relevant and robust methods, offering new and valuable scientific knowledge.

Checklists

Critical literature appraisal is an important skill for healthcare workers who are not researchers but professionals who translate scientific knowledge into knowledge- based practice (see Chapter 1). For this purpose, we need strategies providing sufficient critical distance to examine the methodological strength and assess the design, sample, interpretation, analysis and results of a qualitative study. Checklists are tools that can serve as metapositions for your own project and also for a clear and feasible critical appraisal of a scientific publication, whether you are a researcher or not. In the same way, medical researchers with a quantitative background should also be able to understand what it takes for a qualitative study to be sound and sufficiently rigorous.

A well-written qualitative article may wrongly persuade the reader that it also represents rigorous methodological craft, but this is not always the case. A convincing presentation is a necessary but not sufficient condition for scientific quality. Several *checklists* have therefore been developed for quality assessment of qualitative studies (Giacomini, Cook, et al. 2000a, 2000b, Tong, Sainsbury, et al. 2007, Cohen & Crabtree 2008, Stige, Malterud, et al. 2009, Santiago-Delefosse, Gavin, et al. 2016).

The checklists are structured to lead the reader through a systematic review of methodological details that might otherwise be overshadowed by the article's readability and topicality. A checklist can therefore be a useful starting point for those who want to learn to distinguish between strong and weak. Checklists are also used for critical appraisal in qualitative metasynthesis (see Chapter 18). However, to fulfil this purpose, the checklists must convey values, criteria and concepts that appropriately reflect and operationalise different shades of what is most important, in a way that harmonises properly with the study to be evaluated. For our purpose, checklists should also attend to the Big Q/(small q issue (see Chapter 4). But such criteria can be difficult to craft and to fulfil.

Consolidated criteria for reporting qualitative research (*COREQ*) is a widely used checklist for interview studies and focus group studies, and it also serves as mandatory criteria for peer review of qualitative studies in several journals (Tong, Sainsbury, et al. 2007). This checklist was developed with an EBM strategy grounded in a systematic review where the authors identified 22 existing checklists. 76 items from the included checklists were compiled into 32 questions covering research team/reflexivity, study design and data analysis/reporting. The author provides page numbers where each question is answered.

A similar strategy was used for the development of a checklist for qualitative studies in the Critical Appraisal Skills Programme (*CASP*) series (Critical Appraisal Skills Programme). The checklist was created by an expert group and piloted and further developed it in several versions. The version from 2024 contains 10 questions about the study aim, relevance of qualitative methods, consistency between research question and design, recruitment strategy, data development, researcher/participant relationship, ethics, analysis, presentation of results and usefulness. For each of the questions, there are some supplementary questions. The questions should be answered with yes/no/do not know.

A review of 58 such checklists demonstrated many corresponding quality criteria summarised in 12 points with supplementary definitions (Santiago-Delefosse, Gavin, et al. 2016). In their article about systematic reviews of public health research, Harden, Garcia and et al. (2004) made use of four existing checklists as a starting point. They agreed on seven quality criteria used to evaluate the methodological quality of qualitative primary studies. For both checklists, the authors recommend further development for better operationalisation and consensus.

It may seem tempting to carry out a quality assessment of a scientific article by ticking off and counting yes or no answers to several questions. But it is not that simple. Checklists create the illusion that complex questions can be answered yes or no, and that quality is measurable. Now and then, the editor seems to rely on the peer's completion of the checklist for a submitted article, as if this were an unequivocal conclusion where acceptance of the article requires "yes" on all points. But methodological perfection is of little use if the article does not convey new and valuable knowledge developed in a convincing way with relevant and robust methods, congruent with the study aim.

There are many well-founded objections to the checklists (Barbour 2001, Stige, Malterud, et al. 2009, Buus & Agdal 2013, Braun & Clarke 2024a), primarily because they standardise qualitative studies into a technical format that does not respect the specificity of the various qualitative methods. While some criteria may be relevant for interview studies, the same criteria may be directly misleading for participant observation. Some checklists also invite scoring or yes/no answers for each criterion, giving a false understanding of research quality as something that can be dichotomised and quantified.

Many have warned about the risk that an excessive methodology focus—also known as methodolatry (see Chapter 11)—can contribute to the instrumentalisation of research at the expense of subjectivity, interpretation and creative knowing (Janesick 1994, Chamberlain 2000, Thorne 2014). In the worst cases, such checklists can therefore consolidate and legitimise "the instrumentalist mistake" described by Skjervheim (see Chapter 1) (Skjervheim 2002). A checklist must therefore never become a goal in itself (Barbour 2001), but can at best function as a tool—a specification of questions referring to key meta-criteria.

When checklists are based on systematic reviews of previous checklists, you look backwards, not forwards, in the question about strong or weak qualitative studies. The checklists and their summaries usually lack ideals that reflect the Big Q, i.e. methodology that are congruent with the interpretive paradigm, characterised by inductive, organic and flexible strategies open to subjectivity, diversity and movement (see Chapter 4) (Braun & Clarke 2024a). Instead, prevailing checklists often can be aligned with the small q, with standardisation of ideals that may provide legitimacy in the biomedical culture, while they correspond poorly with the assumptions underpinning qualitative research methods.

I have myself developed and published a checklist where items about the study aim, reflexivity, method/design, data development/selection, theoretical frame of reference, analysis, results, discussion, presentation and references, based on the meta-criteria of reflexivity, relevance and validity are included (Malterud 2001b). Today, I consider this checklist to be outdated, first and foremost because it also lacks a consistent focus on the Big Q. However, the meta-criteria, harmonising well with the interpretive paradigm, still stand the test of time.

Reflexivity in dialogue rather than scoring and rating

It is ultimately a matter of overall judgement when assessing the strengths and weaknesses of an article. Such appraisal requires methodological expertise and experience and must be learnt and maintained. Collaboration on methodological quality assessment occurs at best in a dynamic way, with dialogues between the author, editor and peer reviewers on a few selected main topics that may be substantial for quality, depending on what the article is about and the design used.

The acronym *EPICURE* provides an agenda for discussions on the following meta-criteria deserving attention for assessment of a qualitative study (Stige, Malterud, et al. 2009):

E—Engagement
P—Processing
I—Interpretation
C—Critique
U—Usefulness
R—Relevance
E—Ethics

Engagement concerns the extent to which the study's empirical material is firmly anchored in the field or phenomenon under investigation. What does the text communicate about access to the field or context, level of participation and interaction, sustained engagement (context sensitivity) and level of observation and reporting (content productivity)?

Processing deals with how data has been developed and processed. Is the problem clear? Are positions, analysis strategies and theoretical perspectives adequate? How are raw data handled in terms of coding, abstraction, development of interpretations and result categories? How are the interpretations and results communicated to the reader?

Interpretation focuses on the understanding of the empirical material. What does the author write specifically about awareness of interpretive challenges such as the relationship between part and whole, the impact of the researcher's preconceptions, considerations regarding the level of and strategy for abstraction in the analysis, contextualisation of the results and reflexivity in relation to the study's situatedness?

Critique has a double meaning in this context: We will consider how the author established critical metapositions related to interpretations and results, both internally in terms of academic self-critique and externally in the form of social critique.

Usefulness is about how the research process and results can be made applicable to specific, concrete matters. In what way are the results valuable for the participants, for practice and policy, and for understanding and reflection?

Relevance asks how this study contributes to the development of understanding and knowledge base in the field. How do the results correspond with relevant literature? How are the interpretations discussed as an additional contribution to the understanding of a field or a phenomenon, or to development of concepts, theory or methods?

Ethics focuses on the author's management and communication of ethical responsibility in the research process and results in relation to patients, colleagues and others involved. Do we get to know enough about procedures that safeguard privacy and informed consent, and does the text testify to respectful interaction, participation, vigilance and co-creation for the practical and political consequences of the conclusions?

These keywords can also be summarised as a discussion of whether the author presents a study that delivers credible stories (EPIC) that can make a difference (CURE). This coincides well with the criteria "relevant and robust" and "new and valuable" that I have used throughout this book. You can read more about this in the article on EPICURE (Stige, Malterud, et al. 2009).

Another recent example of a dialogue-based evaluation strategy is the *Reflexive Thematic Analysis Reporting Guidelines* (RTARG) (Braun & Clarke 2024b). This checklist may be criticised for being too detailed, but it represents an open and nuanced approach to what might be meaningful to a specific qualitative study. This allows the evaluation to respect the uniqueness of the study, while putting key challenges on the agenda with questions and recommendations. With RTARG, basic methodological assumptions for qualitative research methods, with explicit reference to the Big Q, are conveyed.

Through reflexive dialogue with yourself and others during the project and in the final report, you can also make progress by using the meta-criteria discussed throughout this book to ask and answer the following question:

> How and why can my study offer new and valuable knowledge developed with relevant and robust methods, congruent with the assumptions underpinning the methodology?

CHAPTER 25

Recognising vulnerability as ethical responsibility

Medical research is governed by international ethical standards establishing respect for persons and patients and protecting their health and rights when participating in scientific projects. Research involving human subjects can only be conducted if the purpose outweighs the risks and burdens that the project may entail for the individual. In addition, research is regulated by national laws and regulations. In qualitative studies, encounters and relationships are invariably value-laden and implicate different aspects of vulnerability incorporated in the process of knowing. Hence, you need to be familiar with and attend to the specific ethical challenges arising in qualitative studies. You must also comply with the regulations governing medical and health research.

Trust, safety and security in qualitative studies

In 1964, the World Medical Association (2025) first presented the *Declaration of Helsinki*, summarising ethical principles for medical research involving human subjects. The establishment of *research ethics committees*, preapproving all medical and health research, follows from the Declaration of Helsinki. However, not all matters of research ethics significance are explicitly mentioned in regulations. Data protection and digital handling of research data are also important matters reviewed below.

In qualitative research, close interaction with participants creates unique ethical challenges. Richards and Schwartz list four types of potential strain in this setting, namely psychological distress, abuse, distortion and recognition (Richards & Schwartz 2002). In data development and interaction, participants allow the researcher access to their knowledge and experiences, often regarding sensitive and confidential matters. This is particularly pertinent when conducting research on delicate topics and with vulnerable groups (Øye, Bjelland, et al. 2007, Duncan, Drew, et al. 2009, Werner & Malterud 2016a). For example, an interview about the pelvic examination can easily bring the conversation to questions about sexuality, intimate relationships or abuse (Larsen, Oldeide, et al. 1997).

DOI: 10.4324/9781003786016-30

The co-creation of qualitative data always is an inherently subjective context. The dialogue between participant and researcher requires mutual trust and respect, and a reluctant participant may choose to withhold information that may be perceived as disadvantageous. Proximity that enhances information power places particular demands on sound research ethics. Participants need to feel safe, without experiencing pressure or intrusion (Øye, Bjelland, et al. 2007).

Research with participants who are seriously ill or particularly vulnerable places especially high demands on ethical consideration. Several details in the implementation of the project can make a big difference in relation to the participants' integrity, for example when the participants are seriously ill patients in a risk situation where trust in healthcare professionals is key (Gjengedal 1994).

Once the researcher has established a justifiable and trustworthy relationship in the co-creating of data, this relationship needs to be sustained with due care. It is essential that the participant feels confident that the trust will not be abused, and the researcher therefore assumes responsibility for handling what is said in a way that best corresponds to how it was intended. Still, participants are not necessarily entitled to review and accept the researcher's interpretations or summaries, although some choose to include member check in the research process (Goldblatt, Karnieli-Miller, et al. 2011) (see Chapter 21).

Nor is it a given that the researcher will share the participant's perception of reality, for example in a project interviewing abusers to understand how sexual abuse can come into being. However, particularly in projects dealing with controversial issues, the researcher is expected to show loyalty to participant's intention behind sharing the story (Hjorleifsson & Schei 2006). A crucial criterion is that the participant understands how the information will be used.

The intimacy of the data interaction also demands emotional sobriety from the researcher. When facing knowledge that is emotionally or politically charged, the researcher may forget the clear-headedness necessary to handle such knowledge in a considerate and reflexive manner. They may become upset or carried away by the stories they hear, so that alternative versions or interpretations are not considered, or they may forget their mission of research. There are also situations where we may feel the need to intervene or sort things out because of the information we receive. In an action research project (see Chapter 17), this can even be part of the study aim.

Under special circumstances, there may be good reasons to follow one's intuition to act adequately. The researcher is not exempt from the obligations we all have as citizens in the face of distress or injustice. But precisely because qualitative data may convey powerful imprints, the researcher carries a responsibility to safeguard these dimensions of subjectivity and humanity in a serious manner (Morse 2007).

Dialogue and awareness raising

A conversation about crucial life issues can evoke considerations and reflections that have previously been suppressed or unconscious for the participant. Questions about health and illness may trigger anxiety about issues that have previously been taken for granted. Participants may also be prompted to recall experiences that they would rather have left unremembered. For example, women with chronic muscular pain may start reflecting on their own situation when interviewed, and by telling the whole story, they may see connections they had not seen before. It may then become a challenge for the researcher to fulfil their responsibility so that the participants do not feel abused. One solution is to return the results to the women for further exchange of experience.

A participatory action research study may explicitly aim to create processes that foster increased awareness and subsequent action (see Chapter 17) (Thesen & Kuzel 1999). However, it can also be a legitimate objective to develop knowledge about a phenomenon as it is experienced by the participant here and now, without necessarily proceeding with wide-ranging change. In such situations, we need to reflect upon what is needed to ensure that the research process does not mess up the participants' agenda, and perhaps rather take steps to reduce the intervention effect of the data interaction.

However, data interaction and co-creation constitute an intervention that may potentially initiate processes and evoke anxiety (Øye, Bjelland, et al. 2007). Choosing between different designs, we can decide whether an intervention effect is intentional, or the opposite—something we want to reduce. It is therefore important to contemplate the potential consequences of the study aim already in the planning phase, particularly in contexts of vulnerability and suffering. The project's design must therefore take such considerations into account. In projects that may nonetheless pose a risk of triggering undesirable reactions, there is a responsibility to prepare a satisfactory plan for professional follow-up of participants in need of support, if needed.

On the other hand, an exaggerated fear of serious consequences of interpersonal processes may lead to excessive and adverse safety measures. It is important to ensure that participants do not mistake the interview situation for a clinical or therapeutic interview. Practising respectful interaction, we can usually rely on participants to maintain their self-understanding and inner balance (Reventlow & Tulinius 2005).

As a rule, participants who are patients are also quite robust. Many participants describe the value in being able to talk about their experiences with an interested listener. Personally, I have never experienced that contingency plans for follow-up have been exercised, even in projects comprising sensitive topics. The researcher is responsible for assessing the impact of different strategies for data interaction and co-creation, and for using the experience gained along the way to reflect upon how the dialogue works. This makes it possible to steer clear of dialogues activating painful experiences.

It is not merely a methodological obligation, but also a research ethics prerequisite that the researcher clarifies their own role in the project, both for themselves and for the participants. In a health research project, the researcher will easily be perceived as a person who has and will take medical responsibility (Richards & Schwartz 2002, Reventlow & Tulinius 2005). Such expectations may lead to conflicting anticipations, which can be mitigated by ensuring that any need for medical follow-up is handled by someone else than the researcher and that participants are informed of this in advance.

Free and informed consent

Qualitative data are texts articulating people's subjective life experiences and thoughts. The linguistic expression often bestows the material with a particularly sensitive and personal character (Synnes, Råheim, et al. 2021). In medical and health research, qualitative methods are well-suited for the exploration of matters carrying a personal, existential significance. Substantive knowing may take root in safe spaces where participants are willing to present themselves openly and honestly, even when doing so is personally unflattering (Malterud & Thesen 2008, Aase, Nordrehaug, et al. 2008, Malterud, Fredriksen, et al. 2009).

This entails particularly stringent requirements for *informed consent*. Consent may be regarded as free and informed when it is provided voluntarily and with sufficient knowledge of the purpose and procedures of the study. Participants therefore need to be notified of their right to raise questions about the researcher or the study and, if necessary, to withdraw or otherwise act on these concerns at any stage of the research. At the same time, it is ultimately the researcher's responsibility to safeguard research ethics and privacy, regardless of what the participants have consented to.

In advance, the participant needs to receive sufficient information about how data will be developed and handled to make it possible to say no without setting up a difficult situation (Øye, Bjelland, et al. 2007). Written information constitutes a prerequisite for free and informed consent and sound research ethics, though presuming literacy (World Medical Association 2025). Along the way, situations may arise where the participant regrets what has been said or senses that things are evolving differently than intended. The project outline and the documents regarding research ethics must therefore make explicit the conditions that enable the participant to stop the recording or delete the material.

Anonymity, confidentiality and recognition

Researchers must establish conditions under which participation does not carry a risk of recognition and personal exposure. This is especially imperative when the participant discloses matters that are normally subject to confidentiality.

When the person you are talking to is a patient, you are also required to comply with formally correct procedures for clinical practice. Patients generally expect *confidentiality* to apply in medical consultations and interactions with other healthcare professionals. Yet, the research interview is an entirely different situation, demanding that the participant is always thoroughly informed about how the data will be used and who will have access to what has been said. If the analysis is carried out by more people than the person conducting the interview or observations, the participants need to be informed of this. The participant may have a relative or neighbour on the research team who ought not be involved in the matters under discussion.

Challenges related to *recognition* arise predominantly at the reporting stage, when documentation, quotes and demographic information are communicated. Even if I know that the participant very unlikely will read a scientific article in a foreign language, I still have a responsibility to write as if the article will end up with the participants' friends and colleagues. Distance in terms of geography, language and culture is not sufficient to ensure privacy. Dialect expressions in quotes, the participant's age or profession, information about where the project was carried out, and stories that tell about a specific and exceptional event exemplify issues that can increase the risk of recognition. If we exaggerate a personal description to bring out a group-based characteristic, for example by using ideal types, participants may feel stereotyped and disrespected.

When presenting the demographic characteristics of a small sample, privacy may be better protected by reporting this information briefly in the text rather than in a table, where curious and locally knowledgeable readers might infer or guess individual identities. In particular, it is advisable to avoid tables that link personal data at the individual level. In some cases, privacy can be strengthened by changing selected information in the presentation (Malterud 1990). The prerequisite is that this can be done without distorting the basic assumptions framing the study aim. Distorted documentation always risks undermining trustworthiness.

Occasionally, the most gorgeous quotes or stories contain so many identifiable details that they cannot be used in presentations. If then the results become too weakly substantiated in the article, it may be tempting to make compromises. But compromises that threaten the participant's privacy are never ethically acceptable. Even if the participant consents to the publication of data that might communicate recognisability, the researcher retains an independent responsibility to consider whether this may harm the participant in any way. If in doubt, it is preferable to refrain from using this part of the material.

Safe handling of sensitive digital data

The day-to-day handling of qualitative data must be governed by respect for those who have disclosed themselves, irrespective of whether the researcher considers the study aim or the data to be sensitive. Remember that the participant may think differently about this than you do. In several European countries, the collection and use of personal data is regulated by national laws and the EU *General Data Protection Regulation*. These rules are designed to prevent files or transcripts from sensitive conversations going astray. Under data protection rules, all kinds of research data are expected to be secured against access by outsiders.

Early in the process of data development and co-creating, it is useful to establish a physical separation between text for analysis and personal data about the participants. This can be done already in the transcription step by assigning pseudonyms to participants that can later be linked to personal data in a safe situation when the texts are recontextualised. In the results section, there should be some traces that lead to links between result categories and individual participants, such as introducing a quote with "A middle aged woman with Parkinsons disease said…", and after the quote, a pseudonym (Mary). *Encryption* of audio files and text files with password protection and firm access control presupposes the use of an encryption programme approved and administered by your research institution or health trust.

Sensitive digital research data (text, audio, video) are normally stored on a dedicated *research server* with authorised access control. Research data should not be stored on your own computer. Procedures for application and access vary across nations and organisation. It therefore follows that you need to learn the rules that apply at your academic institution. In qualitative studies, the analysis is often carried out by more than one researcher collaborating in dialogue with the data and each other, partly individually and partly concurrently. The former often takes place directly from the research server, while the latter can come about in secure, access-controlled team directories with limited access, specially assigned for such circumstances.

Yet, development and analysis of qualitative data do not take place inside a filing cabinet, and theft of material data can occur during lunch breaks and in the car. Transporting files and printouts between workplaces poses a risk of loss or confusion, and any printouts used during interim phases of analysis should be securely destroyed. Keep in mind the risk of unauthorised access if you read sensitive texts on paper or tablet on the bus or in a café.

Researching colleagues

Consultation research from healthcare is often drawn from observational data from everyday practice (see Chapter 16). Studies in which doctors explore material developed and co-created from colleagues' practice present distinct challenges (Nessa & Malterud 1998a, 1998b, Aase, Nordrehaug, et al. 2008, Schaufel, Nordrehaug, et al. 2009, Guassora, Johansen, et al. 2021). The same applies to nurses studying activities in a hospital ward (Gjengedal 1994). The Declaration of Helsinki covers patients and citizens in medical research, but does not provide the same protection for healthcare professionals being researched. In such projects, we are called upon to use our best wisdom to exercise appropriate research ethics in the face of colleagues who entrust us with their knowing and professional lives. Granting others insight into one's consultations or everyday practice requires a high level of trust (Davidsen 2011). It may be hard (although also a relief) to share experiences about difficult professional dilemmas that sometimes have a less ideal solution (Coar & Sim 2006). Remember also that data from the health services may contain sensitive information about third parties (patients), even if your study aim deals with healthcare professionals.

When confronted with accounts or observations that cast a colleague under study in an unflattering light, it may be tempting to invoke academic freedom and present one's interpretations and results without hesitation. In that case, we fail to act in accordance with free and informed consent. The participant would have been unlikely to make themselves available if they had anticipated this kind of negative exposure, especially if there is any possibility of recognition. Try to imagine how you would react if it were you. Sometimes, data that could have given the issue an extra boost simply needs to be put aside. We have no right to ostracise those who have shown us trust in the name of research. It may be helpful to discuss such challenges with your supervisor or research colleagues.

On the other hand, a great deal of research is driven by highly respectable motives, for example to improve healthcare quality. Such considerations also have to be weighed in the balance, and the researcher must sometimes endure negative reactions from environments where unfavourable or inappropriate practices are exposed (Malterud & Thesen 2008). However, if this is repeated in project after project, the researcher will soon encounter problems gaining access to the research field. Qualitative studies insist on mutual trust.

CHAPTER 26

Negotiating paradigms in the face of medical research traditions

Qualitative methods are gradually becoming established in medical research. Still, objections persist due to a limited understanding of qualitative methodology and the underpinning epistemological assumptions, even within leading academic medical communities. Confidence in established natural science approaches, as well as in criteria situated in biomedicine and epidemiology, is often equally strong. Therefore, reluctance—and at times outright dismissal—of the scientific validity and trustworthiness of qualitative methods may arise when they are used in medical and health research. Such disputes may be theoretically productive, yet we may also meet a knowledge climate that resists forms of knowledge development other than "its own", despite limited methodological insight. Such attitudes can be challenging and exhausting, but the following advice may help strengthen dialogues in encounters of this type.

No shortcut—learn the craft

If you want to use qualitative research methods, you need to take the time and effort to learn the basics of the assumptions and the approaches. In this respect, there is no difference between qualitative and quantitative methods. We would hardly embark on a randomised-controlled study without first finding out how to do it. We read textbooks, attend courses and receive supervision. Qualitative methods are not common-sense skills to be used without training, but practices we must engage with properly if they are to function as research methods. This book is only a beginning.

Admittedly, many of us are trained and experienced in talking to people in clinical practice and health services management. And, as people who live in the world, we are constantly organising our impressions and observations into interpretive frameworks that provide meaning and context. Qualitative research methods have much in common with everyday clinical work and may therefore seem obvious as strategies for developing everyday medical knowledge (Malterud 2001b). However, such professional skills should not be confused with the craftsmanship we must master when developing,

DOI: 10.4324/9781003786016-31

processing and communicating qualitative data as scientific knowing. Insight into and systematic consideration of meta-criteria such as reflexivity, relevance and validity can help distinguish between opinion and scientific knowledge (see Chapter 3). Qualitative methods and craft can be learnt and are, in principle, no more difficult to acquire than statistics. Nor do they offer an easier path to the goal.

Qualitative inquiry should not be used as an excuse to eschew fundamental scientific considerations in the research process, for example by dismissing validity considerations (see Chapter 21). Instead, you need to remain attentive and ready to challenge epistemologically incongruent expectations, such as treating validity assessment as correspondence validity, calculating the concordance with a gold standard (see Chapters 4 and 21) (Kvale 1996). However, even if we do not find conceptual beliefs from the natural sciences appropriate to our purpose, we cannot dismiss considerations about the validity of the approach and results in our study. Admittedly, occasional claims appear that qualitative research methods in themselves constitute a guarantee of validity, because the method is supposed to provide proximity to the reality to be explored. Such a statement represents a naïve perception of scientific rigour, demonstrating that the researcher has neglected the impact of reflexivity (see Chapter 3). Intimacy in no way protects against uncritical misinterpretations, rather the opposite.

Another shortcut that I do not recommend is to rise above sample discussions and take the excellence of your own data sample for granted. Certainly, in a qualitative study, we can rightly reject a demand for a representative sample and control group (see Chapter 7). This does not mean that any other sample is relevant and robust for our purpose. As a reader, I expect a sample that is logically consistent with our study aim. Nor is it adequate to claim that we employed a purposive sample or that the Information Power was good—we must also be able to explain why and how. The fact that several procedures from the quantitative research tradition are directly unsuitable does not give the researcher a free pass to cheap solutions in a qualitative study. On the contrary, we should employ the situations that confront traditional research strategies as an opportunity for educational self-critical reflection on the assumptions and intersubjectivity of our own approach.

Utilising qualitative methods in medical research, you must be prepared to explain your assumptions and approaches more extensively than is expected if you use traditional medical research methods (Malterud 1993). The burden of proof lies with those who do not follow the beaten track. In discussions with researcher colleagues, we must therefore be prepared to spend more time and effort legitimising a qualitative study than if we had chosen a quantitative method (Yamazaki, Slingsby, et al. 2009, Greenhalgh, Annandale, et al. 2016, Loder, Groves, et al. 2016). But this should not steer us towards small q strategies based on post-positivist ideals (see Chapter 4) to defend our project (Clarke, Braun, et al. 2024). Doing so, we lose sight of the foundations of qualitative methods.

Basic knowledge of the philosophy of science is a necessary starting point when arguing that qualitative methods can lead to scientific knowledge. In this book, I have tried to open a window onto the epistemological assumptions that underpin qualitative methods. The view from this window is only a beginning, yet it may offer a useful orientation for the analytical journey ahead. This does not take much, but we must understand and be able to explain what we are trying to convince others of. This does not mean that every presentation should provide general, textbook basic arguments about the differences between qualitative and quantitative approaches. For those who do not want to spend time investing in such knowledge, choosing a quantitative approach may be a better alternative.

Active and well-founded arguments

There is no need to apologise when you use qualitative methods (Clarke, Braun, et al. 2024). Clear assumptions should underpin the choices we make in the research process, with a clear common thread between the study aim, design, method, material, analysis and results. Our argument in favour of using data based on interviews with nine participants is rather that this implies a well-founded purposive selection, not that we unfortunately did not have more material available (Carlsen & Glenton 2011, Werner & Malterud 2003). Recognising that some readers may have expected a control-group design, we nevertheless refrain from spending space and effort justifying its absence (Clarke, Braun, et al. 2024). Rather, we should make sure that we present our study aim in such a way that comparison using a control group does not appear appropriate to answer our study aim. It helps if we avoid trying to show that something is bigger or better than something else. Stay away from matters of causality and amounts.

More than a few of our colleagues in medicine and health sciences lack knowledge of qualitative methods. Still, we should not be expected to make every methodological finesse explicit. If we read an article where statistical methods have been used to calculate confidence intervals, we do not anticipate an explanation of what confidence intervals are or how they can be calculated. However, we would like to know what technique was used in this case to accomplish such an analysis. In an article based on qualitative interview data, it must be enough to refer to the literature where specific assumptions and procedures are explained in more detail.

Still, we must adhere to the qualitative methods' requirements for involvement and transparency throughout the research process. Intersubjectivity is crucial for credibility (Malterud 1993, 2001b). We have to exhibit what we have done in a way that invites the reader to follow the path we have taken. We lose contact with the reader if we write so succinctly that only those who know the internal codes can keep up. However, we must also assume that our readers and peer reviewers who assess the article hold some basic knowledge, and that they have the ability and willingness to follow the tracks suggested by our literature references (Clarke, Braun, et al. 2024).

Dialogue and the rhetoric of philosophical assumptions

Knowledge about medicine and health attains validity only when expressed in forms that enable effective dialogue with research communities. We must keep this in mind throughout the research process, especially in the stage when interpretations and conclusions are articulated for reporting and wider dissemination. Defiant positions that reinforce contradictions and tensions between qualitative and quantitative methods without explanation do not promote communicative validity (see Chapter 21). The substantial differences between different methodologies are better communicated with calm arguments than with exclamation marks and capital letters. Attitudes communicating a lack of respect for strategies other than those we personally have chosen do not contribute to the expansion of the medical knowledge base (Greenhalgh, Annandale, et al. 2016, Loder, Groves, et al. 2016, Clarke et, Braun, et al. 2024).

Medical and health researchers increasingly use qualitative methods (Yamazaki, Slingsby, et al. 2009, Maragh-Bass, Appelson, et al. 2016). When submitting your article, you ought to choose a journal with extensive experience in publishing qualitative studies. This increases the likelihood that you will receive fair and instructive editorial treatment of your manuscript, and that competent peer reviewers will provide helpful feedback to improve your article. A competent and respectful editorial dialogue entails valuable learning (Stige, Malterud, et al. 2009). Conversely, you can lose a lot of self-esteem in the face of an arrogant and incompetent peer. Unfortunately, with qualitative studies, the latter is not uncommon.

When encountering such peers, we can actively argue that our choices are deliberate, grounding them in the interpretive paradigm and in Big Q as a valuable alternative to post-positivism and small q, and as an asset for knowledge development in domains of subjectivity (see Chapter 4) (Clarke, Braun, et al. 2024). In such cases, the supervisor and senior colleague must assist the novice. If the arguments fail, we should rather send the article to another journal with better editorial expertise. Do not hesitate to advance well-founded arguments when you disagree with your peers' assessments. If you accept a poor compromise, you as the author are still responsible for what is published. However, you should also demonstrate that you are open to good advice, even when you do not immediately see why your own text may fall short.

Thoughtful communication and dialogue with traditional medical research culture does not imply giving in to the small q or overlooking the particular value of qualitative methods. Although there are commonalities between quantitative and qualitative research methods, it does not make sense to translate all concepts and procedures into quantitative tradition and terminology. Working with qualitative methods in medical research requires methodological bilingualism and the ability to communicate both common ground and divergence. A helpful investment of time and effort is to learn a language that enables rewarding communication about your research, even with sceptics. Rhetoric is an important skill in this field, as is basic knowledge of the philosophy of science.

Repeated experiences of having manuscripts rejected on the basis of poorly informed peer or editorial comments can easily lead to frustration (Clarke, Braun, et al. 2024). At certain points, it can be tempting to opt out of the medical research culture and continue researching independently in peace, perhaps linking with allies from other academic disciplines, without being suspected or ridiculed. But self-perpetuating separatism does not promote dialogue and is not beneficial to the dissemination of medical and healthcare knowledge developed with qualitative methods. Instead, focus your efforts on providing knowledge that others recognise as new and valuable, grounded in relevant and robust methods.

I wish you well with your own project!

References

Abrahamsen C, Lindbæk M, Werner EL. Experiences with a structured conversation tool: a qualitative study on feasibility in general practice in Norway. *Scand J Prim Health Care.* 2022;40(2):190–6.

Alderson P. The importance of theories in health care. *BMJ.* 1998;317(7164):1007–10.

Alowais SA, Alghamdi SS, Alsuhebany N, Alqahtani T, Alshaya AI, Almohareb SN, et al. Revolutionizing healthcare: the role of artificial intelligence in clinical practice. *BMC Med Educ.* 2023;23(1):689.

Alræk T, Malterud K. Acupuncture for menopausal hot flashes: a qualitative study about patient experiences. *J Altern Complement Med.* 2009;15(2):153–8.

Alvesson M, Sandberg J. The art of phenomena construction: a framework for coming up with research phenomena beyond 'the usual suspects'. *J Manag Stud.* 2024;61(5):1737–65.

Alvesson M, Sköldberg K. *Reflexive methodology - New vistas for qualitative research.* 3rd ed. London: Sage; 2018.

Andersen T. The reflecting team: dialogue and meta-dialogue in clinical work. *Fam Process.* 1987;26(4):415–28.

Anderssen N, Malterud K. Oversampling as a methodological strategy for the study of self-reported health among lesbian, gay and bisexual populations. *Scand J Public Health.* 2017;45(6):637–46.

Antonovsky A. *Health, stress and coping. New perspective on mental and physical well-being.* San Francisco, CA: Jossey-Bass; 1979.

Arborelius E, Timpka T, Nyce JM. Patients comment on video-recorded consultations--the "good" GP and the "bad". *Scand J Soc Med.* 1992;20(4):213–6.

Argyris C, Putnam R, Smith DM. *Action science.* San Francisco, CA: Jossey-Bass; 1985.

Arksey H, O'Malley L. Scoping studies: towards a methodological framework. *Int J Soc Res Meth.* 2005;8(1):19–32.

Atkins S, Lewin S, Smith H, Engel M, Fretheim A, Volmink J. Conducting a meta-ethnography of qualitative literature: lessons learnt. *BMC Med Res Methodol.* 2008;8:21.

Atkinson P, Hammersley M. Ethnography and participant observation. In: Denzin NK, Lincoln YS, eds. *Handbook of qualitative research.* Thousand Oaks, CA: Sage; 1994. p. 248–61.

Austin JL. *How to do things with words: the William James lectures delivered at Harvard University in 1955*. Cambridge, MA: Harvard University Press; 1962.

Bach Nielsen KD, Dyhr L, Lauritzen T, Malterud K. Long-term impact of elevated cardiovascular risk detected by screening. A qualitative interview study. *Scand J Prim Health Care*. 2005;23(4):233–8.

Bakken AK, Mengshoel AM, Synnes O, Strand EB. Acquiring a new understanding of illness and agency: a narrative study of recovering from chronic fatigue syndrome. *Int J Qual Stud Health Well-being*. 2023;18(1):2223420.

Barbour RS. Checklists for improving rigour in qualitative research: a case of the tail wagging the dog? *BMJ*. 2001;322:1115–7.

Barnett-Page E, Thomas J. Methods for the synthesis of qualitative research: a critical review. *BMC Med Res Methodol*. 2009;9(1):1–11.

Beich A, Gannik D, Malterud K. Screening and brief intervention for excessive alcohol use: qualitative interview study of the experiences of general practitioners. *BMJ*. 2002; 325(7369):870.

Berge SD, Brekke M, Meland E, Mildestvedt T. How patients experience discussing couple relationship problems with GPs: an interview study. *BJGP Open*. 2024;8(4):BJGPO.2024.0044.

Berger PL, Luckmann T. *The social construction of reality: a treatise in the sociology of knowledge*. London: Penguin; 1967.

Bjørkman M, Malterud K. Being lesbian - does the doctor need to know? *Scand J Prim Health Care*. 2007;25(1):58–62.

Bjørkman M, Malterud K. Lesbian women's experiences with health care: a qualitative study. *Scand J Prim Health Care*. 2009;27(4):238–43.

Bjørkman M, Malterud K. Lesbian women coping with challenges of minority stress: a qualitative study. *Scand J Publ Health*. 2012;40(3):239–44.

Black N. Evidence based policy: proceed with care. *BMJ*. 2001;323(7307):275–9.

Blumer H. *Symbolic interactionism: perspective and method*. Englewood Cliffs, NJ: Prentice-Hall; 1969.

Blystad A. *Precarious procreation: Datoga pastoralists at the late 20th century*. Bergen: University of Bergen; 2000.

Bondas T, Hall EO. Challenges in approaching metasynthesis research. *Qual Health Res*. 2007a;17(1):113–21.

Bondas T, Hall EOC. A decade of metasynthesis research in health sciences: a meta-method study. *Int J Qual Stud Health Well-being*. 2007b;2(2):101–13.

Booth A. Searching for qualitative research for inclusion in systematic reviews: a structured methodological review. *Syst Rev*. 2016;5:74.

Boss M. *Existential foundations of medicine and psychology*. New York: Jason Aronson; 1979.

Bradbury-Jones C, Breckenridge J, Clark MT, Herber OR, Wagstaff C, Taylor J. The state of qualitative research in health and social science literature: a focused mapping review and synthesis. *Int J Soc Res Methodol*. 2017;20(6):627–45.

Bradley CP. Turning anecdotes into data--the critical incident technique. *Fam Pract*. 1992;9(1):98–103.

Braun V, Clarke V. Reflecting on reflexive thematic analysis. *Qual Res Sport Exerc Health*. 2019;11(4):589–97.

Braun V, Clarke V. *Thematic analysis: a practical guide*. Los Angeles, CA: Sage; 2022.

Braun V, Clarke V. How do you solve a problem like COREQ? A critique of Tong et al.'s (2007) Consolidated Criteria for Reporting Qualitative Research. *Methods Psychol*. 2024a;11:100155.

Braun V, Clarke V. Reflexive Thematic Analysis Reporting Guidelines (RTARG). *Palliat Med*. 2024b;38(6):608–16.

Braun V, Clarke V. Reporting guidelines for qualitative research: a values-based approach. *Qual Res Psychol*. 2024c;22(6):1–40.

Braun V, Clarke V. Supporting best practice in reflexive thematic analysis reporting in Palliative Medicine: a review of published research and introduction to the Reflexive Thematic Analysis Reporting Guidelines (RTARG). *Palliat Med.* 2024d;38(6):608–16.

Britten N, Campbell R, Pope C, Donovan J, Morgan M, Pill R. Using meta ethnography to synthesise qualitative research: a worked example. *J Health Serv Res Pol.* 2002;7:209–15.

Britten N, Garside R, Pope C, Dip JF, Cooper C. Asking more of qualitative synthesis: a response to Sally Thorne. *Qual Health Res.* 2017;27(9):1370–6.

Brubaker MY, Bell JN, Berner JE, Warren JA. Climate change health assessment: a novel approach for Alaska Native communities. *Int J Circumpolar Health.* 2011; 70(3):266–73.

Butler J. Performative acts and gender constitution: an essay in phenomenology and feminist theory. *Theatre J.* 1988;40(4): 519–31.

Butler J. *Gender trouble.* New York: Routledge; 1990.

Buus N, Agdal R. Can the use of reporting guidelines in peer-review damage the quality and contribution of qualitative health care research? *Int J Nurs Stud.* 2013;50(10):1289–91.

Canadian Task Force on the Periodic Health Examination. The periodic health examination. *Can Med Assoc J.* 1979;121(9):1193–254.

Carlsen B, Glenton C. What about N? A methodological study of sample-size reporting in focus group studies. *BMC Med Res Methodol.* 2011;11:26.

Carter SM, Little M. Justifying knowledge, justifying method, taking action: epistemologies, methodologies, and methods in qualitative research. *Qual Health Res.* 2007;17(10):1316–28.

Centre for Reviews and Dissemination. *PRISMA – Preferred Reporting Items for Systematic Reviews and Meta-Analyses.* York: University of York; 2020. https://www.prisma-statement.org (17 Jan 2026).

Centre for Reviews and Dissemination. *Systematic Reviews: a Practical Guide York: Centre for Reviews and Dissemination*, University of York; 2025. https://subjectguides.york.ac.uk/systematic-review/next-steps (17 Jan 2026).

Chalmers I. The Cochrane collaboration: preparing, maintaining, and disseminating systematic reviews of the effects of health care. *Ann N Y Acad Sci.* 1993;703:156–63; discussion 63–5.

Chamberlain K. Methodolatry and qualitative health research. *J Health Psychol.* 2000;5(3): 285–96.

Charmaz K. *Constructing grounded theory: a practical guide through qualitative analysis.* 3rd ed. London: Sage; 2024.

Charon R. Narrative and medicine. *N Engl J Med.* 2004;350(9):862–4.

Clarke V, Braun V, Adams J, Callaghan JEM, LaMarre A, Semlyen J. "Being really confidently wrong": Qualitative researchers' experiences of methodologically incongruent peer review feedback. *Qual Psychol.* 2024;12(1):7–24.

Coar L, Sim J. Interviewing one's peers: methodological issues in a study of health professionals. *Scand J Prim Health Care.* 2006;24(4):251–6.

Cochrane AL. Archie Cochrane in his own words. Selections arranged from his 1972 introduction to "Effectiveness and efficiency: random reflections on the health services" 1972. *Control Clin Trials.* 1989;10(4):428–33.

Cohen DJ, Crabtree BF. Evaluative criteria for qualitative research in health care: controversies and recommendations. *Ann Fam Med.* 2008;6(4):331–9.

Craig P, Dieppe P, Macintyre S, Michie S, Nazareth I, Petticrew M. Developing and evaluating complex interventions: the new medical research council guidance. *BMJ.* 2008;337:a1655.

Creswell JW, Poth CN. *Qualitative inquiry and research design: choosing among five approaches.* 5th ed. Thousand Oaks, CA: Sage; 2024.

Creswell JW. *A concise introduction to mixed methods research.* Thousand Oaks, CA: Sage 2022.

Critical Appraisal Skills Programme. CASP Qualitative Research Checklist 2023. https://casp-uk.net/casp-tools-checklists/qualitative-studies-checklist (17 Jan 2026).

Crotty M. *The foundations of social research. Meaning and perspective in the research process.* London/Thousand Oaks, CA/New Delhi: Sage; 2003.

Dahl B, Fylkesnes AM, Sørlie V, Malterud K. Lesbian women's experiences with healthcare providers in the birthing context: a meta-ethnography. *Midwifery*. 2013;29(6):674–81.

Dahl B, Malterud K. Neither father nor biological mother. A qualitative study about lesbian co-mothers' maternity care experiences. *Sex Reprod Health*. 2015;6(3):169–73.

Daniel SL. The patient as text: a model of clinical hermeneutics. *Theor Med*. 1986;7(2):195–210.

Danielsson U, Johansson EE. Beyond weeping and crying: a gender analysis of expressions of depression. *Scand J Prim Health Care*. 2005;23(3):171–7.

Davidsen AS. And then one day he'd shot himself. Then I was really shocked': General practitioners' reaction to patient suicide. *Patient Educ Couns*. 2011;85(1):113–8.

DePaulo P. Sample size for qualitative research. The risk of missing something important. *Quirk's Marketing Res Rev*. 2000;14(11):22–7.

Denzin NK, Lincoln YS. *The Sage Handbook of qualitative research*. 6th ed. Thousand Oaks, CA: Sage; 2023.

Diaz E, Hjorleifsson S. Immigrant general practitioners in Norway: a special resource? A qualitative study. *Scand J Public Health*. 2011;39(3):239–44.

Dixon-Woods M, Agarwal S, Jones D, Young B, Sutton A. Synthesising qualitative and quantitative evidence: a review of possible methods. *J Health Serv Res Policy*. 2005;10(1):45–53.

Dixon-Woods M, Cavers D, Agarwal S, Annandale E, Arthur A, Harvey J, et al. Conducting a critical interpretive synthesis of the literature on access to healthcare by vulnerable groups. *BMC Med Res Methodol*. 2006;6:35.

Dixon-Woods M, Shaw RL, Agarwal S, Smith JA. The problem of appraising qualitative research. *Qual Saf Health Care*. 2004;13(3):223–5.

Duncan RE, Drew SE, Hodgson J, Sawyer SM. Is my mum going to hear this? Methodological and ethical challenges in qualitative health research with young people. *Soc Sci Med*. 2009;69(11):1691–9.

Eagleton T. *Literary theory. An introduction*. 2nd ed. Chicester: Wiley; 2011.

Eakin JM, Mykhalovskiy E. Reframing the evaluation of qualitative health research: reflections on a review of appraisal guidelines in the health sciences. *J Eval Clin Pract*. 2003;9(2):187–94.

Editorial Lancet. Aspirin after myocardial infarction. *Lancet*. 1980;315(8179):1172–3.

Ehrenreich B, Hilden J, Malterud K. Patients' written life stories: a gateway for understanding. *Scand J Prim Health Care*. 2007;25(1):33–7.

Elder-Vass D. *The reality of social construction*. Cambridge: Cambridge University Press; 2012.

Elmore JG, Wells CK, Lee CH, Howard DH, Feinstein AR. Variability in radiologists' interpretations of mammograms. *N Engl J Med*. 1994;331(22):1493–9.

Engebretsen E, Vollestad NK, Wahl AK, Robinson HS, Heggen K. Unpacking the process of interpretation in evidence-based decision making. *J Eval Clin Pract*. 2015;21(3):529–31.

Eriksson K, Martinsen K. The hidden and forgotten evidence. *Scand J Caring Sci*. 2012;26(4):625–6.

Eriksson L, Lindström B, Ekenberg L. Patients' experiences of telerehabilitation at home after shoulder joint replacement. *J Telemed Telecare*. 2011;17(1):25–30.

Ertmann RK, Söderström M, Reventlow S. Parents' motivation for seeing a physician. *Scand J Prim Health Care*. 2005;23(3):154–8.

Fixsen DL, Naaom SF, Blase KA, Friedman RM, Wallace F. *Implementation research: A synthesis of the literature*. Tampa: University of South Florida; 2005.

Flanagan JC. The critical incident technique. *Psychol Bull*. 1954;51(4):327–58.

Flyvbjerg B. Five misunderstandings about case-study research. *Qual Inquiry*. 2006;12(2):219–45.

Forssen A, Carlstedt G. Work, health and ill health. New research makes women's experiences visible. *Scand J Prim Health Care*. 2001;19(3):154–7.

Fosse A, Schaufel MA, Ruths S, Malterud K. End-of-life expectations and experiences among nursing home patients and their relatives--a synthesis of qualitative studies. *Patient Educ Couns*. 2014;97(1):3–9.

Foucault M. *The order of things: an archaeology of the human sciences*. London: Tavistock Publications; 1970.

France EF, Ring N, Thomas R, Noyes J, Maxwell M, Jepson R. A methodological systematic review of what's wrong with meta-ethnography reporting. *BMC Med Res Methodol.* 2014;14(1):1–16.

Frank AW. *The wounded storyteller: body, illness, and ethics.* Chicago, IL: University of Chicago Press; 1995.

Frank AW. Practicing dialogical narrative analysis. In: Holstein JA, Gubrium JF, eds. *Varieties of narrative analysis.* Los Angeles, CA: Sage; 2012. p. 33–52

Freire P. *Pedagogy of the oppressed.* New York: Seabury Press 1970.

Frich JC, Ose L, Malterud K, Fugelli P. Perceived vulnerability to heart disease in patients with familial hypercholesterolemia: a qualitative interview study. *Ann Fam Med.* 2006;4(3): 198–204.

Frodeman R. *Sustainable knowledge: a theory of interdisciplinarity.* Basingstoke: Palgrave; 2014.

Gadamer H-G. *Truth and method.* 2nd ed. London: Continuum; 2004.

Garfinkel H. *Studies in ethnomethodology.* Englewood Cliffs, NJ: Prentice-Hall; 1967.

Gatens-Robinson E. Clinical judgment and the rationality of the human sciences. *J Med Philos.* 1986;11(2):167–78.

Genette G. *Narrative discourse.* Oxford: Basil Blackwell; 1980.

Giacomini MK, Cook DJ, for the Evidence-Based Medicine Working Group. Users' guides to the medical literature. *XXIII. Qualitative Research in Health Care. A. Are the Results of the Study Valid? JAMA.* 2000a;284(3):357–62.

Giacomini MK, Cook DJ, for the Evidence-Based Medicine Working Group. Users' guides to the medical literature. *XXIII. Qualitative Research in Health Care. B. What Are the Results and How Do They Help Me Care for My Patients? JAMA.* 2000b;284(4):478–82.

Giorgi A. Sketch of a psychological phenomenological method. In: Giorgi A, ed. *Phenomenology and psychological research.* Pittsburg, PA: Duquesne University Press; 1985. p. 8–22.

Giorgi A. *The descriptive phenomenological method in psychology: a modified Husserlian approach.* Pittsburgh, PA.: Duquesne University Press; 2009.

Gjengedal E. *Understanding a world of critical illness. A phenomenological study of the experiences of respirator patients and their caregivers.* Bergen: University of Bergen; 1994.

Glaser B, Strauss A. *The discovery of Grounded Theory: strategies for qualitative research.* London: Weidenfeld and Nicholson; 1967.

Glasziou P, Meats E, Heneghan C, Shepperd S. What is missing from descriptions of treatment in trials and reviews? *BMJ.* 2008;336(7659):1472–4.

Glenton C, Carlsen B. When "normal" becomes normative: a case study of researchers' quotation errors when referring to a focus group sample size study. *Int J Qual Methods.* 2019; 18:1–6.

Goffman E. *The presentation of self in everyday life.* Garden City, NY: Doubleday Anchor Books; 1959.

Goldblatt H, Karnieli-Miller O, Neumann M. Sharing qualitative research findings with participants: study experiences of methodological and ethical dilemmas. *Patient Educ Couns.* 2011;82(3):389–95.

Good BJ. *Medicine, rationality, and experience: an anthropological perspective.* Cambridge, MA: Cambridge University Press; 1994.

Gough D, Oliver S, Thomas J. Introducing systematic reviews. In: Gough D, Oliver S, Thomas J, eds. *An introduction to systematic reviews.* 2nd ed. London: Sage; 2017a. p. 1–17.

Gough D, Oliver S, Thomas J, editors. *An introduction to systematic reviews.* 2nd ed. London: Sage; 2017b.

Graham H. Women's smoking and family health. *Soc Sci Med.* 1987;25(1):47–56.

Graham R, Mancher M, Wolman DM, Greenfield S, Steinberg E. *Clinical practice guidelines we can trust.* Washington, DC: Institute of medicine, The National Academies Press; 2011.

Graneheim UH, Lundman B. Qualitative content analysis in nursing research: concepts, procedures and measures to achieve trustworthiness. *Nurse Educ Today.* 2004;24(2):105–12.

Grant MJ. How does your searching grow? A survey of search preferences and the use of optimal search strategies in the identification of qualitative research. *Health Inform Libraries J*. 2004;21(1):21–32.

Greenhalgh T. Papers that summarise other papers (systematic reviews and meta-analyses). *BMJ*. 1997;315(7109):672–5.

Greenhalgh T, Annandale E, Ashcroft R, Barlow J, Black N, Bleakley A, et al. An open letter to The BMJ editors on qualitative research. *BMJ*. 2016;352:i563.

Greenhalgh T, Malterud K. Systematic reviews for policymaking: muddling through. *Am J Public Health*. 2018;107(1):97–9.

Greenhalgh T, Thorne S, Malterud K. Time to challenge the spurious hierarchy of systematic over narrative reviews? *Eur J Clin Invest*. 2018;48:e12931.

Grol R, Wensing M, Eccles M. *Improving patient care. The implementation of change in clinical practice*. Hoboken: Wiley 2005.

Grønseth IM, Malterud K, Nilsen S. Why do doctors in Norway choose general practice and remain there? A qualitative study about motivational experiences. *Scand J Prim Health Care*. 2020;38(2):184–91.

Guassora AD, Baarts C. Smoking cessation advice in consultations with health problems not related to smoking? Relevance criteria in Danish general practice consultations. *Scand J Prim Health Care*. 2010;28(4):221–8.

Guassora AD, Johansen M-L, Malterud K. Agenda navigation in consultations covering multiple topics. A qualitative case study from general practice. *Scand J Prim Health Care*. 2021;39(3):339–47.

Guassora AD, Reventlow S, Malterud K. Shame, honor and responsibility in clinical dialog about lifestyle issues: a qualitative study about patients' presentations of self. *Patient Educ Couns*. 2014;97(2):195–9.

Guassora AD, Reventlow S, Malterud K. *22 temateorier til kvalitativ forskning* (22 substantive theories for qualitative research). København: FADL's Forlag; 2022. (In Danish).

Guest G, Bunce A, Johnson L. How many interviews are enough? An experiment with data saturation and variability. *Field Methods*. 2006;18(1):59–82.

Gullbrå F, Smith-Sivertsen T, Rørtveit G, Anderssen N, Hafting M. To give the invisible child priority: children as next of kin in general practice. *Scand J Prim Health Care*. 2014;32(1):17–23.

Gullbrå F, Smith-Sivertsen T, Graungaard AH, Rørtveit G, Hafting M. How can the general practitioner support adolescent children of ill or substance-abusing parents? A qualitative study among adolescents. *Scand J Prim Health Care*. 2016;34(4):360–7.

Gullestad M. *Kitchen-table society: a case study of the family life and friendships of young working-class mothers in urban Norway*. Oslo: Universitetsforlaget; 1984.

Guyatt G, Oxman AD, Akl EA, Kunz R, Vist G, Brozek J, et al. GRADE guidelines: 1. Introduction—GRADE evidence profiles and summary of findings tables. *J Clin Epidemiol*. 2011;64(4):383–94.

Guyatt G, Oxman AD, Vist GE, Kunz R, Falck-Ytter Y, Alonso-Coello P, et al. GRADE: an emerging consensus on rating quality of evidence and strength of recommendations. *BMJ*. 2008;336(7650):924–6.

Haas LF. Phineas Gage and the science of brain localisation. *J Neurol Neurosurg Psychiatry Res*. 2001;71(6):761.

Habermas J. *The theory of communicative action*. Boston, MA: Beacon Press; 1984.

Halcomb EJ, Davidson PM. Is verbatim transcription of interview data always necessary? *Appl Nurs Res*. 2006;19(1):38–42.

Hamberg K, Johansson E, Lindgren G, Westman G. Scientific rigour in qualitative research--examples from a study of women's health in family practice. *Fam Pract*. 1994;11(2):176–81.

Hammersley M. *Reading ethnographic research: a critical guide*. 2nd ed. London: Longman; 1998.

Hana J, Rudebeck CE. Leadership in rural medicine: the organization on thin ice? *Scand J Prim Health Care*. 2011;29(2):122–8.

Hannes K, Booth A, Harris J, Noyes J. Celebrating methodological challenges and changes: reflecting on the emergence and importance of the role of qualitative evidence in Cochrane reviews. *Syst Rev.* 2013;2(1):84.
Hannes K, Macaitis K. A move to more transparent and systematic approaches of qualitative evidence synthesis: update of a review on published papers. *Qual Res.* 2012;12(4):402–42.
Haraway D. Situated knowledges; the science question in feminism and the privilege of partial perspective. In: Haraway D, ed. *Simians, cyborgs, and women: the reinvention of nature.* New York: Routledge; 1991. p. 183–201.
Harden A, Garcia J, Oliver S, Rees R, Shepherd J, Brunton G, et al. Applying systematic review methods to studies of people's views: an example from public health research. *J Epidemiol Community Health.* 2004;58(9):794–800.
Have PT. *Doing conversation analysis.* London: Sage; 2007.
Hedlund L, Gyllensten AL. The experiences of basic body awareness therapy in patients with schizophrenia. *J Body Mov Ther.* 2010;14(3):245–54.
Helsebiblioteket (2021). Modell for kunnskapsbasert praksis (Model for knowledge based practice). Oslo: Helsebiblioteket; 2021. https://www.helsebiblioteket.no/innhold/artikler/kunnskapsbasert–praksis/kunnskapsbasertpraksis.no (17 Jan 2026).
Hjorleifsson S, Schei E. Scientific rationality, uncertainty and the governance of human genetics: an interview study with researchers at deCODE genetics. *EJHG.* 2006;14(7):802–8.
Høyer K. What is theory, and how does theory relate to method? In: Vallgarda S, Koch L, eds. *Forskningsmetoder i folkesundhedsvidenskab.* København: Gyldendal Akademisk; 2008. p. 17–41.
Hunter KM. *Doctors' stories: the narrative structure of medical knowledge.* Princeton, NJ: Princeton University Press; 1991.
Hurwitz B, Greenhalgh T. *Narrative based medicine: Dialogue and discourse in clinical practice.* London: BMJ Books; 1998.
Hvas L. Positive aspects of menopause: a qualitative study. *Maturitas.* 2001;39(1):11–7.
Hvas L, Gannik DE. Discourses on menopause--Part I: menopause described in texts addressed to Danish women 1996-2004. *Health (London).* 2008;12(2):157–75.
Iden KR, Ruths S, Hjorleifsson S. Residents' perceptions of their own sadness--a qualitative study in Norwegian nursing homes. *BMC Geriatrics.* 2015;15:21.
Idland S, Iversen E, Brattebø G, Kramer-Johansen J, Hjortdahl M. From hearing to seeing: medical dispatchers' experience with use of video streaming in medical emergency calls – a qualitative study. *BMJ Open.* 2022;12(12):e063395.
Iser W. *The act of reading: a theory of aesthetic response.* Baltimore, MD: Johns Hopkins University Press; 1978.
Janesick VJ. The dance of qualitative research design: metaphor, methodolatry, and meaning. In: Denzin NK, Lincoln YS, eds. *Handbook of qualitative research.* Thousand Oaks, CA: Sage; 1994. p. 209–19.
Jangland E, Larsson J, Gunningberg L. Surgical nurses' different understandings of their interactions with patients: a phenomenographic study. *Scand J Caring Sci.* 2010;25(3):533–41.
Jansen K, Ruths S, Malterud K, Schaufel MA. The impact of existential vulnerability for nursing home doctors in end-of-life care: a focus group study. *Patient Educ Couns.* 2016;99(12):2043–8.
Johansen ML, Holtedahl KA, Davidsen AS, Rudebeck CE. 'I deal with the small things': the doctor–patient relationship and professional identity in GPs' stories of cancer care. *Health.* 2012a;16(6):569–84.
Johansen ML, Holtedahl KA, Rudebeck CE. How does the thought of cancer arise in a general practice consultation? Interviews with GPs. *Scand J Prim Health Care.* 2012b;30(3):135–40.
Johansson EE, Hamberg K, Westman G, Lindgren G. The meanings of pain: an exploration of women's descriptions of symptoms. *Soc Sci Med.* 1999;48(12):1791–802.
Josselson R. Narrative research. Constructing, deconstructing, and reconstructing story. In: Wertz FJ, Ed. *Five ways of doing qualitative analysis Phenomenological psychology,*

grounded theory, discourse analysis, narrative research, and intuitive inquiry. New York: Guilford Press; 2011. p. 224–42.
Khalil H, Tricco AC. Differentiating between mapping reviews and scoping reviews in the evidence synthesis ecosystem. *J Clin Epidemiol*. 2022;149:175–82.
Kidder LH, Fine M. Qualitative and quantitative methods - When stories converge. In: Mark MM, Shotland RL, eds. *Multiple methods in program evaluation: new directions for program evaluation*. San Francisco, CA: Jossey-Bass; 1987. p. 57–75.
Kirkengen AL. *Inscribed bodies: health impact of childhood sexual abuse*. Dordrecht: Kluwer; 2001.
Kleinman A. *Patients and healers in the context of culture: an exploration of the borderland between anthropology, medicine, and psychiatry*. Berkeley: University of California Press; 1980.
Kleinman A. *Writing at the margin: discourse between anthropology and medicine*. Berkeley: University of California Press; 1995.
Koch T. Establishing rigour in qualitative research: the decision trail. *J Adv Nurs*. 1994; 19(5):976–86.
Kohak E. *Idea & experience - Edmund Husserl's project of phenomenology in IDEAS I*. Chicago, IL & London: The University of Chicago Press; 1978.
Krueger RA, Casey MA. *Focus groups: a practical guide for applied research*. 3rd ed. Thousand Oaks, CA: SAGE; 2000.
Kuhn TS. *The structure of scientific revolutions*. Chicago, IL: University of Chicago Press; 1962.
Kumar V, Mohanty S, Kumar A, Misra RP, Santosham M, Awasthi S, et al. Effect of community-based behaviour change management on neonatal mortality in Shivgarh, Uttar Pradesh, India: a cluster-randomised controlled trial. *Lancet*. 2008;372(9644):1151–62.
Kuzel A. Sampling in qualitative inquiry. In: Miller W, Crabtree B, eds. *Doing qualitative research*. 2nd ed. Thousand Oaks, CA: Sage; 1999. p. 33–45.
Kvale S. InterViews. *An introduction to qualitative research interviewing*. Thousand Oaks, CA: Sage; 1996.
Labov W. *Language in the inner city: studies in the black English vernacular*. Philadelphia: University of Pennsylvania Press; 1972.
Lakoff G, Johnson M. *Metaphors we live by*. Chicago, IL: University of Chicago Press; 1980.
Lapadat JC, Lindsay AC. Transcription in research and practice: from standardization of technique to interpretive positionings. *Qual Inq*. 1999;5(1):64–86.
Larsen M, Oldeide CC, Malterud K. Not so bad after all..., Women's experiences of pelvic examinations. *Fam Pract*. 1997;14(2):148–52.
Larun L, Malterud K. Identity and coping experiences in Chronic Fatigue Syndrome: a synthesis of qualitative studies. *Patient Educ Couns*. 2007;69(1–3):20–8.
Larun L, Malterud K. Finding the right balance of physical activity: a focus group study about experiences among patients with chronic fatigue syndrome. *Patient Educ Couns*. 2011a;83(2):222–6.
Larun L, Malterud K. Treningsbehandling ved kronisk utmattelsessyndrom (Graded Exercise Therapy in Chronic Fatigue Syndrome). *Tidsskr Nor Legeforen*. 2011b;131(3):231–6. (In Norwegian, English summary).
Latour B, Woolgar S. *Laboratory life: the construction of scientific facts*. Princeton, NJ: Princeton University Press; 1986.
Launer J. *Narrative-based primary care: a practical guide*. Oxford: Radcliffe; 2003.
Lave J, Wenger E. *Situated learning - legitimate peripheral participation*. Cambridge: Cambridge University Press; 1991.
Lavis J, Davies H, Oxman A, Denis JL, Golden-Biddle K, Ferlie E. Towards systematic reviews that inform health care management and policy-making. *J Health Serv Res Policy*. 2005;10 Suppl 1:35–48.
Leder D. Clinical interpretation: the hermeneutics of medicine. *Theor Med*. 1990;11(1):9–24.

Levenstein JH, McCracken EC, McWhinney IR, Stewart MA, Brown JB. The patient-centred clinical method. 1. A model for the doctor-patient interaction in family medicine. *Fam Pract.* 1986;3(1):24–30.

Lévinas E, Hand S. *The Levinas reader.* Oxford: B. Blackwell; 1989.

Lewin K. Action research and minority problems. In: Lewin GW, ed. *Resolving social conflicts: selected papers on group dynamics.* New York: Harper & Brothers; 1948. p. 201–216.

Lewin S, Glenton C, Munthe-Kaas H, Carlsen B, Colvin CJ, Gülmezoglu M, et al. Using qualitative evidence in decision making for health and social Interventions: an approach to assess confidence in findings from qualitative evidence syntheses (GRADE-CERQual). *PLoS Med.* 2015;12(10):e1001895.

Lewin S, Glenton C, Noyes J, Hendry M, Rashidian A. *CerQual approach: assessing how much certainty to place in findings from qualitative evidence syntheses.* Quebec, Canada: 21st Cochrane Colloquium; 2013.

Li H, Zhang R, Lee YC, Kraut RE, Mohr DC. Systematic review and meta-analysis of AI-based conversational agents for promoting mental health and well-being. *NPJ Digit Med.* 2023;6(1):236.

Liberati A, Altman DG, Tetzlaff J, Mulrow C, Gotzsche PC, Ioannidis JP, et al. The PRISMA statement for reporting systematic reviews and meta-analyses of studies that evaluate health care interventions: explanation and elaboration. *J Clin Epidemiol.* 2009;62(10):e1–34.

Lid TG, Eraker R, Malterud K. "I recognise myself in that situation..." Using photographs to encourage reflection in general practitioners. *BMJ.* 2004;329(7480):1488–90.

Lid TG, Malterud K. General practitioners' strategies to identify alcohol problems: a focus group study. *Scand J Prim Health Care.* 2012;30(2):64–9.

Lid TG, Oppedal K, Pedersen B, Malterud K. Alcohol-related hospital admissions: missed opportunities for follow up? A focus group study about general practitioners' experiences. *Scand J Public Health.* 2012;40(6):531–6.

Lincoln YS, Guba EG. *Naturalistic inquiry.* Newbury Park, CA: Sage; 1985.

Lingiardi V, Capozzi P. Psychoanalytic attitudes towards homosexuality: an empirical research. *Int J Psychoanal.* 2004;85(Pt 1):137–57.

Lipsky M. *Street-level bureaucracy: Dilemmas of the individual in public services.* 30th anniversary expanded edition. New York: Russell Sage Foundation; 1980/2010.

Lock A, Strong T. *Social constructionism: sources and stirrings in theory and practice.* Cambridge: Cambridge University Press; 2010.

Loder E, Groves T, Schroter S, Merino JG, Weber W. Qualitative research and the BMJ. *BMJ.* 2016;352.

Lonergan BHR. *Insight. A study of human understanding.* Toronto: University of Toronto Press; 1992.

Lykkeslet E, Gjengedal E, Skrondal T, Storjord MB. 'On one's own strength' Healthcare providers' experience with introducing Marte Meo Counselling in dementia care. *Int J Older Peopl Nurs.* 2016;11(1):24–31.

Major CH, Savin-Baden M. *An introduction to qualitative research synthesis. Managing the information explosion in social science research.* London/New York: Routledge; 2010.

Malinowski B. *A scientific theory of culture.* Chapel Hill, NC: The University of North Carolina Press; 1944.

Malpass A, Shaw A, Sharp D, Walter F, Feder G, Ridd M, et al. "Medication career" or "Moral career"? The two sides of managing antidepressants: a meta-ethnography of patients' experience of antidepressants. *Soc Sci Med.* 2009;68(1):154–68.

Malterud K. *Almenpraktikerens møte med kvinnelige pasienter. (The general practitioner encountering female patients).* Oslo: Tano; 1990. (In Norwegian, English summary).

Malterud K. Shared understanding of the qualitative research process. Guidelines for the medical researcher. *Fam Pract.* 1993;10(2):201–6.

Malterud K. Action research--a strategy for evaluation of medical interventions. *Fam Pract.* 1995a;12(4):476–81.
Malterud K. The legitimacy of clinical knowledge: towards a medical epistemology embracing the art of medicine. *Theor Med.* 1995b;16(2):183–98.
Malterud K. Making changes with key questions in medical practices: studying what makes a difference. In: Miller WL, Crabtree BF, eds. *Doing qualitative research.* 2nd ed. Thousand Oaks, CA: Sage; 1999. p. 313–30.
Malterud K. The art and science of clinical knowledge: evidence beyond measures and numbers. *Lancet.* 2001a;358(9279):397–400.
Malterud K. Qualitative research: standards, challenges, and guidelines. *Lancet.* 2001b; 358(9280):483–8.
Malterud K. Reflexivity and metapositions: strategies for appraisal of clinical evidence. *J Eval Clin Pract.* 2002;8(2):121–6.
Malterud K. *Fokusgrupper som forskningsmetode for medisin og helsefag (Focus groups as research methods for medicine and health research).* Oslo: Universitetsforlaget; 2012a. (In Norwegian).
Malterud K. Systematic text condensation: a strategy for qualitative analysis. *Scand J Public Health.* 2012b;40(8):795–805.
Malterud K. Theory and interpretation in qualitative studies from general practice: why and how? *Scand J Public Health.* 2016;44:120–9.
Malterud K. The impact of evidence-based medicine on qualitative metasynthesis: benefits to be harvested and warnings to be given. *Qual Health Res.* 2019a;21(1):7–17.
Malterud K. *Qualitative metasynthesis: a research method for medicine and health sciences.* Abingdon: Routledge; 2019b.
Malterud K. Systematisk tekstkondensering. (Systematic Text Condensation). In: Lorås L, Ness O, eds. *Håndbok i kvalitativ forskning for psykologi, helsefag og sosialfag.* Bergen: Fagbokforlaget; 2024. p. 273–87. (In Norwegian)
Malterud K, Bærheim A. Peeing barbed wire. Symptom experiences in women with lower urinary tract infection. *Scand J Prim Health Care.* 1999;17(1):49–53.
Malterud K, Bjelland AK, Elvbakken KT. Evidence-based medicine - an appropriate tool for evidence-based health policy? A case study from Norway. *Health Res Policy Syst.* 2016;14:15.
Malterud K, Bjørkman M. The invisible work of closeting: a qualitative study about strategies used by lesbian and gay persons to conceal their sexual orientation. *J Homosex.* 2016;63(10):1339–54.
Malterud K, Bjørkman M, Flatval M, Ohnstad A, Thesen J, Rørtveit G. Epidemiological research on marginalized groups implies major validity challenges: lesbian health as an example. *J Clin Epidemiol.* 2009;62(7):703–10.
Malterud K, Elvbakken KT. Patients participating as co-researchers in health research: a systematic review of outcomes and experiences. *Scand J Publ Health.* 2020;48(6):617–28.
Malterud K, Fredriksen L, Gjerde MH. When doctors experience their vulnerability as beneficial for the patients: a focus-group study from general practice. *Scand J Prim Health Care.* 2009;27(2):85–90.
Malterud K, Guassora AD, Graungaard AH, Reventlow S. Understanding medical symptoms: a conceptual review and analysis. *Theor Med Bioeth.* 2015;36(6):411–24.
Malterud K, Guassora AD, Reventlow S, Jutel A. Embracing uncertainty to advance diagnosis in general practice. *Br J Gen Pract.* 2017;67(659):244–5.
Malterud K, Hamberg K, Reventlow S. Qualitative methods in PhD theses from general practice in Scandinavia. *Scand J Prim Health Care.* 2017;35(4):309–12.
Malterud K, Hollnagel H. Women's self-assessed personal health resources. *Scand J Prim Health Care.* 1997;15(4):163–8.
Malterud K, Hollnagel H. Talking with women about personal health resources in general practice. Key questions about salutogenesis. *Scand J Prim Health Care.* 1998;16(2):66–71.

Malterud K, Hollnagel H. Avoiding humiliations in the clinical encounter. *Scand J Prim Health Care.* 2007;25(2):69–74.
Malterud K, Kamps H. General practice – a fertile lagoon in the ocean of medical knowledge. *Scand J Prim Health Care.* 2021;39(4):515–8.
Malterud K, Reventlow S, Guassora AD. Diagnostic knowing in general practice: interpretative action and reflexivity. *Scand J Prim Health Care.* 2019:37(4):393–401.
Malterud K, Reventlow S, Guassora AD. Clinical practice enhanced by interdisciplinary theoretical perspectives. *Scand J Prim Health Care.* 2024;42(4):602–8.
Malterud K, Siersma V, Guassora AD. Information power - Sample content and size in qualitative studies. In: Camic PM, ed. *Qual Res Psychol. Expanding perspectives in methodology and design.* Washington, DC: American Psychological Association; 2021. p. 67–81.
Malterud K, Siersma VD, Guassora AD. Sample size in qualitative interview studies: guided by information power. *Qual Health Res.* 2016;26(13):1753–60.
Malterud K, Thesen J. When the helper humiliates the patient: a qualitative study about unintended intimidations. *Scand J Public Health.* 2008;36(1):92–8.
Malterud K, Ulriksen K. "Norwegians fear fatness more than anything else"--a qualitative study of normative newspaper messages on obesity and health. *Patient Educ Couns.* 2010a;81(1):47–52.
Malterud K, Ulriksen K. Obesity in general practice: a focus group study on patient experiences. *Scand J Prim Health Care.* 2010b;28(4):205–10.
Malterud K, Ulriksen K. Obesity, stigma, and responsibility in health care: a synthesis of qualitative studies. *Int J Qual Stud Health Well-being.* 2011;6(4):8404.
Malterud K, Aamland A, Fosse A. How can task shifting put patient safety at risk? A qualitative study of experiences among general practitioners in Norway. *Scand J Prim Health Care.* 2020;38(1):24–32.
Malterud K, Aamland A, Iden KR. Small-scale implementation with pragmatic process evaluation: a model developed in primary health care. *BMC Fam Pract.* 2018;19(1):93.
Maragh-Bass AC, Appelson JR, Changoor NR, Davis WA, Haider AH, Morris MA. Prioritizing qualitative research in surgery: a synthesis and analysis of publication trends. *Surgery.* 2016:160(6):1447–55.
Marshall MN. Sampling for qualitative research. *Fam Pract.* 1996;13:522–5.
Mason M. Sample size and saturation in PhD studies using qualitative interviews. *Forum Qual Soc Res.* 2010;11(3).
Mattingly C. *Healing dramas and clinical plots: the narrative structure of experience.* Cambridge: Cambridge University Press; 1998.
Mays N, Pope C. Qualitative research: observational methods in health care settings. *BMJ.* 1995a;311(6998):182–4.
Mays N, Pope C. Rigour and qualitative research. *BMJ.* 1995b;311(6997):109–12.
McWhinney IR. Changing models: the impact of Kuhn's theory on medicine. *Fam Pract.* 1984;1(1):3–8.
McWhinney IR. "An acquaintance with particulars…". *Fam Med.* 1989;21:296–8.
Mengshoel AM. Mixed methods research–so far easier said than done? *Man Ther.* 2012;17(4):373–5.
Mengshoel AM. Experiences of shifts in physiotherapy for rheumatoid arthritis over time - an autoethnography. *Physiother Theory Pract.* 2024;40(6):1372–82.
Mengshoel AM, Robinson HS. Clinical significance of specific spinal mobilization for patients with ankylosing spondylitis evaluated by quantitative assessments and patient interviews. *Disabil Rehabil.* 2008;30(5):355–64.
Menichetti J, Hillen MA, Papageorgiou A, Pieterse AH. How can ChatGPT be used to support healthcare communication research? *Patient Educ Couns.* 2023;115:107947.
Merleau-Ponty M. *Phenomenology of perception.* London: Routledge & Kegan; 1962.
Migiro SO, Magangi BA. Mixed methods: a review of literature and the future of the new research paradigm. *African J Business Management.* 2011;5(10):3757–64.

Miles MB, Huberman AM, Saldaña J. *Qualitative data analysis: a methods sourcebook*. 4th ed. Thousand Oaks, CA: Sage; 2018.
Miller WL, Crabtree BJ. Clinical Research. A multimethod typology and qualitative roadmap. In: Crabtree B, Miller WL, eds. *Doing qualitative research*. 2nd ed. Thousand Oaks, CA: Sage; 1999. p. 20–4.
Mishler EG. *The discourse of medicine. Dialectics of medical interviews*. Norwood, NJ: Ablex Publishing Company; 1984.
Mjølstad BP, Kirkengen AL, Getz L, Hetlevik I. Standardization meets stories: contrasting perspectives on the needs of frail individuals at a rehabilitation unit. *Int J Qual Stud Health Well-being*. 2013;8:21498.
Modin S, Törnkvist L, Furhoff A-K, Hylander I. Family physician' experiences when collaborating with district nurses in home care-based medical treatment. A grounded theory study. *BMC Fam Pract*. 2010;11(1):82.
Morgan DL, ed. *Successful focus groups*. Newbury Park/London/New Dehli: Sage; 1993.
Morgan D. *Focus groups as qualitative research*. Thousand Oaks, CA: Sage; 1997.
Morse JM. Going in "blind". *Qual Health Res*. 1994;4:3–5.
Morse JM. Theory innocent or theory smart? *Qual Health Res*. 2002;12(3):295–6.
Morse JM. Diagramming qualitative theories. *Qual Health Res*. 2006;16(9):1163–4.
Morse JM. Ethics in action: ethical principles for doing qualitative health research. *Qual Health Res*. 2007;17(8):1003–5.
Munn Z, Pollock D, Khalil H, Alexander L, McLnerney P, Godfrey CM, et al. What are scoping reviews? Providing a formal definition of scoping reviews as a type of evidence synthesis. *JBI Evid Synth*. 2022;20(4):950–2.
Murray C, Turpin M, Edwards I, Jones M. A qualitative meta-synthesis about challenges experienced in occupational therapy practice. *Br J Occup Ther*. 2015;78(9):534–46.
Mæland S, Magnussen LH, Eriksen HR, Malterud K. Why are general practitioners reluctant to enrol patients into a RCT on sick leave? A qualitative study. *Scand J Public Health*. 2011;39(8):888–93.
Nagel T. *The view from nowhere*. New York: Oxford University Press; 1986.
Natvik E, Råheim M, Andersen JR, Moltu C. An experientially derived model of flexible and intentional actions for weight loss maintenance after severe obesity. *Front Psychol*. 2019;10:2503.
Nelson PA. Exploring new worlds: expanding the reach of qualitative research in dermatology. *Br J Dermatol*. 2016;174(5):951–2.
Nessa J. From a medical consultation to a written text. 1. Transcribing the doctor-patient dialogue. *Scand J Prim Health Care*. 1995a;13(2):83–8.
Nessa J. From a medical consultation to a written text. 2. Pragmatics and textlinguistics applied to medicine. *Scand J Prim Health Care*. 1995b;13(2):89–92.
Nessa J, Malterud K. Discourse analysis in general practice: a sociolinguistic approach. *Fam Pract*. 1990;7(2):77–83.
Nessa J, Malterud K. "Feeling your large intestines a bit bound": clinical interaction - talk and gaze. *Scand J Prim Health Care*. 1998a;16(4):211–5.
Nessa J, Malterud K. Tell me what's wrong with me: a discourse analysis approach to the concept of patient autonomy. *J Medical Ethics*. 1998b;24(6):394–400.
Nilsen S, Malterud K, Werner EL, Mæland S, Magnussen LH. GPs' negotiation strategies regarding sick leave for subjective health complaints. *Scand J Prim Health Care*. 2015;33(1):40–6.
Nilsen S, Werner EL, Mæland S, Eriksen HR, Magnussen LH. Considerations made by the general practitioner when dealing with sick-listing of patients suffering from subjective and composite health complaints. *Scand J Prim Health Care*. 2011;29(1):7–12.
Njeru MK, Blystad A, Shayo EH, Nyamongo IK, Fylkesnes K. Practicing provider-initiated HIV testing in high prevalence settings: consent concerns and missed preventive opportunities. *BMC Health Serv Res*. 2011:11:87. Epub 21 April 2011.

Noblit GW, Hare RD. *Meta-ethnography: synthesizing qualitative studies.* Newbury Park, CA: Sage; 1988.
Noyes J, Booth A, Cargo M, Flemming K, Harden A, Harris J, et al. Chapter 21: Qualitative evidence. Cochrane handbook for systematic reviews of interventions. https://training.cochrane.org/handbook/current/chapter-21 (17 Jan 2026).
Ochberg RL. Life stories and storied lives. In: Lieblich A, Josselson R, eds. *Exploring identity and gender: the narrative study of lives.* Thousand Oaks, CA: Sage; 1994. p. 113–44.
Ohnstad A. If I am not straight or gay, who am I? *Clin Soc Work J.* 2011;37(4):357–67.
Oliver K, Lorenc T, Innvær S. New directions in evidence-based policy research: a critical analysis of the literature. *Health Res Policy Syst.* 2014;12:34.
Orton L, Lloyd-Williams F, Taylor-Robinson D, O'Flaherty M, Capewell S. The use of research evidence in public health decision making processes: systematic review. *Plos One.* 2011;6(7):e21704.
Oxman A, Guyatt GH. The science of reviewing research. *Ann N Y Acad Sci.* 1993;703:125–33; discussion 33–4.
Patton MQ. *Utilization-focused evaluation.* Thousand Oaks, CA: Sage; 2008.
Patton MQ. *Qualitative research & evaluation methods: integrating theory and practice.* 4th ed. Thousand Oaks, CA: Sage; 2015.
Pawson R, Greenhalgh T, Harvey G, Walshe K. Realist review--a new method of systematic review designed for complex policy interventions. *J Health Serv Res Policy.* 2005;10 Suppl 1:21–34.
Pearson A. Balancing the evidence: incorporating the synthesis of qualitative data into systematic reviews. *JBI Reports.* 2004;2(2):45–64.
Peters DH, Adam T, Alonge O, Agyepong IA, Tran N. Implementation research: what it is and how to do it. *BMJ.* 2013;347:f6753.
Peters DH, Tran NT, Adam T. *Implementation research in health: a practical guide.* Geneva: Alliance for Health Policy and Systems Research, World Health Organization; 2013. https://apps.who.int/iris/bitstream/handle/10665/91758/9789241506212_eng.pdf. (17 Jan 2026).
Peters M, Robinson V. The origins and status of action research. *J Appl Behav Sci.* 1984; 20(2):113–24.
Petticrew M. Time to rethink the systematic review catechism? Moving from 'what works' to 'what happens'. *Syst Rev.* 2015;4:36.
Polanyi M. *The tacit dimension.* Gloucester, MA: Peter Smith; 1983.
Popay J, Rogers A, Williams G. Rationale and standards for the systematic review of qualitative literature in health services research. *Qual Health Res.* 1998;8(3):341–51.
Pope C, Mays N, ed. *Qualitative research in health care.* 4th ed. Chichester: John Wiley & Sons/Wiley-Blackwell; 2020.
Porrit P, Evans C, Bennett C, Loveday H, Bjerrum M, Salmond S, et al. Systematic reviews of qualitative evidence: Joanna Briggs Institute; 2024. https://jbi-global-wiki.refined.site/space/MANUAL/355860482 (17 Jan 2026).
Potter J, Wetherell M. *Discourse and social psychology: beyond attitudes and behaviour.* London: SAGE; 1987.
Potthoff S, O'Donnell AJ, Karlsen AT, Brendryen H, Lid TG. Pragmatic approaches for addressing alcohol in general practice: development of a tailored implementation intervention. *Front Health Serv.* 2022;2:940383.
Ree E, Harris A, Indahl A, Tveito TH, Malterud K. How can a brief intervention contribute to coping with back pain? A focus group study about participants' experiences. *Scand J Public Health.* 2014;42(8):821–6.
Ree E, Lie SA, Eriksen HR, Malterud K, Indahl A, Samdal O, et al. Reduction in sick leave by a workplace educational low back pain intervention: a cluster randomized controlled trial. *Scand J Publ Health.* 2016;44(6):571–9.
Reeves S, Albert M, Kuper A, Hodges BD. Why use theories in qualitative research? *BMJ.* 2008;337:a949.

Reventlow SD. Perceived risk of osteoporosis: restricted physical activities? *Scand J Prim Health Care*. 2007;25(3):160–5.
Reventlow S, Hvas AC, Tulinius C. "In really great danger..." The concept of risk in general practice. *Scand J Prim Health Care*. 2001;19(2):71–5.
Reventlow SD, Overgaard IS, Hvas L, Malterud K. Metaphorical mediation in women's perceptions of risk related to osteoporosis: a qualitative interview study. *Health Risk Soc*. 2008;10(2):103–15.
Reventlow S, Tulinius C. The doctor as focus group moderator--shifting roles and negotiating positions in health research. *Fam Pract*. 2005;22(3):335–40.
Richards HM, Schwartz LJ. Ethics of qualitative research: are there special issues for health services research? *Fam Pract*. 2002;19(2):135–9.
Ricoeur P. *Interpretation theory: discourse and the surplus of meaning*. Fort Worth: Texas Christian University Press; 1976.
Ricoeur P. *Oneself as another*. Chicago, IL: University of Chicago Press; 1992.
Riessman CK. *Narrative methods for the human sciences*. Los Angeles, CA: Sage; 2008.
Rudebeck CE. What is general clinical competence? Facing the theoretical challenge to general practice. *Scand J Prim Health Care Suppl*. 1992;10 Suppl 1:61–82.
Rudebeck CE. The doctor, the patient and the body. *Scand J Prim Health Care*. 2000;18(1):4–8.
Røthing M, Malterud K, Frich JC. Caregiver roles in families affected by Huntington's disease: a qualitative interview study. *Scand J Caring Sci*. 2014;28(4):700–5.
Røthing M, Malterud K, Frich JC. Balancing needs as a family caregiver in Huntington's disease: a qualitative interview study. *Health Soc Care Community*. 2015;23(5):569–76.
Råheim M, Håland W. Lived experience of chronic pain and fibromyalgia: women's stories from daily life. *Qual Health Res*. 2006;16(6):741–61.
Sackett DL. *Evidence-based medicine: how to practice & teach EBM*. New York: Churchill Livingstone; 1997.
Sackett DL, Rosenberg WM, Gray JA, Haynes RB, Richardson WS. Evidence based medicine: what it is and what it isn't. *BMJ*. 1996;312(7023):71–2.
Saini M, Shlonsky A. *Systematic synthesis of qualitative research*. Oxford: Oxford University Press; 2012.
Sandelowski M. Theory unmasked: the uses and guises of theory in qualitative research. *Res Nurs Health*. 1993;16(3):213–8.
Sandelowski M. Sample size in qualitative research. *Res Nurs Health*. 1995;18(2):179–83.
Sandelowski M. One is the liveliest number: the case orientation of qualitative research. *Res Nurs Health*. 1996;19(6):525–9.
Sandelowski M. Metasynthesis of qualitative research. In: Cooper H, Camic PM, Long DL, Panter AT, Rindskopf D, Sher KJ, eds. *APA handbook of research methods in psychology, Vol 2: Research designs: quantitative, qualitative, neuropsychological, and biological*. Washington, DC: American Psychological Association; 2012. p. 19–36.
Sandelowski M, Barroso J. *Handbook of synthesizing qualitative research*. New York: Springer Publishing Company; 2007.
Santiago-Delefosse M, Gavin A, Bruchez C, Roux P, Stephen SL. Quality of qualitative research in the health sciences: analysis of the common criteria present in 58 assessment guidelines by expert users. *Soc Sci Med*. 2016;148:142–51.
Savage J. Participative observation: standing in the shoes of others? *Qual Health Res*. 2000; 10(3):324–39.
Schaufel MA, Nordrehaug JE, Malterud K. "So you think I'll survive?": a qualitative study about doctor-patient dialogues preceding high-risk cardiac surgery or intervention. *Heart*. 2009;95(15):1245–9.
Schaufel MA, Nordrehaug JE, Malterud K. Hope in action-facing cardiac death: a qualitative study of patients with life-threatening disease. *Int J Qual Stud Health Well-being*. 2011;6(1):5917.

Schibbye A-LL. The role of "acknowledgement" in the resolution of a specific interpersonal dilemma. *J Phenomenol Psychol.* 1993;24(2):175–89.
Schutz A. *Collected papers.* Nijhoff: The Hague; 1962.
Schwartz N. Self-reports - How the questions shape the answers. *American Psychologist.* 1999;54(2):93–105.
Schön DA. *The reflective practitioner: how professionals think in action.* Aldershot: Avebury; 1991.
Sebeok T, Sebeok JU. "You know my method": A juxtaposition of Charles S. Peirce and Sherlock Holmes. In: Sebeok T, ed. *The play of musement.* Bloomington, IA: Gaslight Publications; 1981. p. 17–52.
Seidman I. *Interviewing as qualitative research: A guide for researchers in education and the social sciences.* 5th ed. New York: Teachers College Press; 2019.
Skagestad P. *The road of inquiry. Charles Peirce's pragmatic realism.* New York: Columbia University Press; 1981.
Skjervheim H. *Objectivism and the study of man.* Oslo: Universitetsforlaget; 1959.
Skjervheim H. *Mennesket (Being Human).* Oslo: Universitetsforlaget; 2002. (In Norwegian).
Slåtten H, Malterud K. Boys perpetrating sexual harassment on peer girls in secondary school: a focus group study about pupils' experiences. *Scand J Public Health.* 2024;52:582–289.
Smart C. Families, secrets and memories. *Sociology.* 2011;45(4):539–53.
Smith C. *What is a person?* Chicago, IL: University of Chicago Press; 2010.
Smith JA, Jarman M, Osborn M. Doing interpretative phenomenological analysis. In: Murray M, Chamberlain K, eds. *Qualitative health psychology - theories & methods.* London: Sage; 1999. p. 218–40.
Smith LH, Holm L. Obesity in a life-course perspective: an exploration of lay explanations of weight gain. *Scand J Public Health.* 2011;39(4):396–402.
Snow CP. *The two cultures and the scientific revolution.* New York: Cambridge University Press; 1959.
Sollaci LB, Pereira MG. The introduction, methods, results, and discussion (IMRAD) structure: a fifty-year survey. *J Med Libr Assoc.* 2004;92(3):364–7.
Steier F. Reflexivity and methodology: an ecological constructionism. In: Steier F, ed. *Research and reflexivity.* London/Thousand Oaks, CA/New Delhi: Sage; 1991. p. 163–85.
Steihaug S, Ahlsen B, Malterud K. From exercise and education to movement and interaction. Treatment groups in primary care for women with chronic muscular pain. *Scand J Prim Health Care.* 2001;19(4):249–54.
Steihaug S, Ahlsen B, Malterud K. "I am allowed to be myself": women with chronic muscular pain being recognized. *Scand J Public Health.* 2002;30(4):281–7.
Steihaug S, Malterud K. Recognition and reciprocity in encounters with women with chronic muscular pain. *Scand J Prim Health Care.* 2002;20(3):151–6.
Steihaug S, Malterud K. Stories about bodies: a narrative study on self-understanding and chronic pain. *Scand J Prim Health Care.* 2008;26(3):188–92.
Stensland P. Action research on own practice. Methodological challenges. *Scand J Prim Health Care.* 2003;21(2):77–82.
Stensland P, Malterud K. New gateways to dialogue in general practice. Development of an illness diary to expand communication. *Scand J Prim Health Care.* 1997;15(4):175–9.
Stensland P, Malterud K. Approaching the locked dialogues of the body. Communicating symptoms through illness diaries. *Scand J Prim Health Care.* 1999;17(2):75–80.
Stensland P, Malterud K. Unravelling empowering internal voices-a case study on the interactive use of illness diaries. *Fam Pract.* 2001;18(4):425–9.
Stern PN, Harris CC. Women's health and the self-care paradox: a model to guide self-care readiness. *Health Care Women Int.* 1985;6(1–3):151–63.
Stige B, Malterud K, Midtgarden T. Toward an agenda for evaluation of qualitative research. *Qual Health Res.* 2009;19(10):1504–16.

Strauss A, Corbin J. *Basics of qualitative research: grounded theory procedures and techniques*. London: Sage; 1990.

Sviland R, Martinsen K, Råheim M. Towards living within my body and accepting the past: a case study of embodied narrative identity. *Med Health Care Philos*. 2018;21(3):363–74.

Synnes O. Narratives of nostalgia in the face of death: the importance of lighter stories of the past in palliative care. *J Aging Stud*. 2015;34:169–76.

Synnes O, Malterud K. Queer narratives and minority stress: stories from lesbian, gay and bisexual individuals in Norway. *Scand J Publ Health*. 2018;47(2):105–14.

Synnes O, Råheim M, Lykkeslet E, Gjengedal E. A complex reminding: the ethics of poetry writing in dementia care. *Dementia*. 2021;20(3):1025–43.

Søderlund A, Skoge AM, Malterud K. "I could not lift my arm holding the fork…". Living with chronic fatigue syndrome. *Scand J Prim Health Care*. 2000;18(3):165–9.

Teddlie C, Tashakkori A. *Foundations of mixed methods research. Integrating quantitative and qualitative approaches in the social and behavioral sciences*. Thousand Oaks, CA: Sage; 2009.

Tesch R. *Qualitative research: analysis types and software tools*. London: Falmer Press; 1990.

Thaulow J, Eide TB, Høye S, Skjeie H. Decisions regarding antibiotic prescribing for acute sinusitis in Norwegian general practice. A qualitative focus group study. *Scand J Prim Health Care*. 2023;41(4):469–77.

Thesen J. Being a psychiatric patient in the community--reclassified as the stigmatized "other". *Scand J Public Health*. 2001;29(4):248–55.

Thesen J, Kuzel AJ. Participatory Inquiry. In: Crabtree B, Miller W, eds. *Doing qualitative research. Research methods for primary care*. Thousand Oaks, CA; London: Sage; 1999. p. 269–90.

Thomas J, Harden A. Methods for the thematic synthesis of qualitative research in systematic reviews. *BMC Med Res Methodol*. 2008;8:45.

Thorne SE. Is the story enough? *Qual Health Res*. 2009;19(9):1183–5.

Thorne SE. Toward methodological emancipation in applied health research. *Qual Health Res*. 2011;21(4):443–53.

Thorne SE. The science and art of theoretical location. *Evid Based Nurs*. 2014;17(2):31.

Thorne S. Qualitative metasynthesis: a technical exercise or a source of new knowledge? *Psychooncology*. 2015:24(11):1347–8.

Thorne S. Metasynthetic madness: what kind of monster have we created? *Qual Health Res*. 2017;27(1):3–12.

Thorne S. Interpretive Description. *Qualitative research for applied practice*. 3rd ed. New York/Abingdon: Routledge; 2025.

Thorne S, Jensen L, Kearney MH, Noblit G, Sandelowski M. Qualitative metasynthesis: reflections on methodological orientation and ideological agenda. *Qual Health Res*. 2004;14(10):1342–65.

Thornquist E. Face-to-face and hands-on: assumptions and assessments in the physiotherapy clinic. *Med Anthropol*. 2006;25(1):65–97.

Tollefsrud I, Mengshoel AM. A fragile normality - illness experiences of working-age individuals with osteoarthritis in knees or hips. *Disabil Rehabil*. 2020;42(18):2593–9.

Tong A, Flemming K, McInnes E, Oliver S, Craig J. Enhancing transparency in reporting the synthesis of qualitative research: ENTREQ. *BMC Med Res Methodol*. 2012;12:181.

Tong A, Sainsbury P, Craig J. Consolidated criteria for reporting qualitative research (COREQ): a 32-item checklist for interviews and focus groups. *Int J Qual Health Care*. 2007;19:349–57.

Undeland M, Malterud K. Diagnostic work in general practice: more than naming a disease. *Scand J Prim Health Care*. 2002;20(3):145–50.

Undeland M, Malterud K. The fibromyalgia diagnosis: hardly helpful for the patients? A qualitative focus group study. *Scand J Prim Health Care*. 2007;25(4):250–5.

Undeland M, Malterud K. Diagnostic interaction: the patient as a source of knowledge? *Scand J Prim Health Care*. 2008;26(4):222–7.
van Maanen J. *Tales of the field. On writing ethnography*. Chicago, IL: University of Chicago Press; 2011.
van Manen M. *Phenomenology of practice: meaning-giving methods in phenomenological research and writing*. London: Routledge; 2023.
Varpio L, Ajjawi R, Monrouxe LV, O'Brien BC, Rees CE. Shedding the cobra effect: problematising thematic emergence, triangulation, saturation and member checking. *Med Educ*. 2017;51(1):40–50.
Varpio L, O'Brien B, Rees CE, Monrouxe L, Ajjawi R, Paradis E. The applicability of generalisability and bias to health professions education's research. *Med Educ*. 2021;55(2):167–73.
Vedung E. *Process evaluation and implementation theory. Public policy and program evaluation*. Piscataway, NJ and London: Transaction; 1997. p. 209–45.
Viney W, Callard F, Woods A. Critical medical humanities: embracing entanglement, taking risks. *Med Humanit*. 2015;41(1):2–7.
Waldorff FB, Bulow LB, Malterud K, Waldemar G. Management of dementia in primary health care: the experiences of collaboration between the GP and the district nurse. *Fam Pract*. 2001;18(5):549–52.
Walseth LT, Abildsnes E, Schei E. Lifestyle, health and the ethics of good living. Health behaviour counselling in general practice. *Patient Educ Couns*. 2011;83(2):180–4.
Walsh D, Downe S. Meta-synthesis method for qualitative research: a literature review. *J Adv Nurs*. 2005;50(2):204–11.
Weiss CH. The many meanings of research utilization. *Public Adm*. 1979;39(5):426–31.
Werner A, Isaksen LW, Malterud K. 'I am not the kind of woman who complains of everything': illness stories on self and shame in women with chronic pain. *Soc Sci Med*. 2004;59(5):1035–45.
Werner A, Malterud K. It is hard work behaving as a credible patient: encounters between women with chronic pain and their doctors. *Soc Sci Med*. 2003;57(8):1409–19.
Werner A, Malterud K. Children of parents with alcohol problems performing normality: a qualitative interview study about unmet needs for professional support. *Int J Qual Stud Health Well-being*. 2016a;11:30673.
Werner A, Malterud K. Encounters with service professionals experienced by children from families with alcohol problems: a qualitative interview study. *Scand J Publ Health*. 2016b;44(7):663–70.
Whyte WF. *Participatory action research*. Newbury Park, CA: Sage; 1991.
Wilson HS, Hutchinson SA. Methodologic mistakes in grounded theory. *Nurs Res*. 1996;45(2):122–4.
Winter R. *Learning from experience: principles and practice in action-research*. London; New York: Falmer Press; 1989.
Wong G. Knowledge synthesis approaches - spoilt for choice? *J Clin Epidemiol*. 2016;73:8–10.
World Health Organization. *Using evidence from qualitative research to develop WHO guidelines (Chapter 15). WHO handbook for guideline development*, 2nd ed. Geneva: WHO; 2014. https://apps.who.int/iris/bitstream/handle/10665/145714/9789241548960_chap15_eng.pdf (17 Jan 2027).
World Medical Association. *WMA Declaration of Helsinki - Ethical Principles for Medical Research Involving Human Participants*; 2025. https://www.wma.net/policies-post/wma-declaration-of-helsinki/ (17 Jan 2026).
Yamazaki H, Slingsby BT, Takahashi M, Hayashi Y, Sugimori H, Nakayama T. Characteristics of qualitative studies in influential journals of general medicine: a critical review. *Biosci Trends*. 2009;3(6):202–9.
Yin RK. *Case study research: design and methods*. 4th ed. Los Angeles, CA: Sage; 2009.
Ytterhus B, Hafting M, Vallesverd VU, Wiig EM, Kallander EK, Trondsen MV. Children as next of kin's experiences, practices, and voice in everyday life: a systematic review of studies with Norwegian data (2010–2022). *Scand J Publ Health*. 2024; 53:14034948241232040.

Yu KH, Healey E, Leong TY, Kohane IS, Manrai AK. Medical artificial intelligence and human values. *N Engl J Med.* 2024;390(20):1895–904.

Øien AM, Solheim IJ. Supervision of professionals: interdependency between embodied experiences and professional knowledge. *Int J Qual Stud Health Well-being.* 2015;10:28432.

Øien AM, Steihaug S, Iversen S, Råheim M. Communication as negotiation processes in long-term physiotherapy: a qualitative study. *Scand J Caring Sci.* 2011;25(1):53–61.

Östlund U, Kidd L, Wengström Y, Rowa-Dewar N. Combining qualitative and quantitative research within mixed method research designs: a methodological review. *Int J Nurs Stud.* 2011;48(3):369–83.

Øye C, Bjelland AK, Skorpen A. Doing participant observation in a psychiatric hospital--research ethics resumed. *Soc Sci Med.* 2007;65(11):2296–306.

Aamland A, Malterud K, Werner EL. Patients with persistent medically unexplained physical symptoms: a descriptive study from Norwegian general practice. *BMC Fam Pract.* 2014;15(1):107.

Aamland A, Werner EL, Malterud K. Sickness absence, marginality, and medically unexplained physical symptoms: a focus-group study of patients' experiences. *Scand J Prim Health Care.* 2013;31(2):95–100.

Aarseth G, Natvig B, Engebretsen E, Lie AK. 'Working is out of the question': a qualitative text analysis of medical certificates of disability. *BMC Fam Pract.* 2017;18(1):55.

Aarseth G, Natvig B, Engebretsen E, Maagerø E, Lie AH. Writing the patient down and out: the construal of the patient in medical certificates of disability. *Sociol Health Illn.* 2016;38(8):1379–95.

Aase M, Nordrehaug JE, Malterud K. "If you cannot tolerate that risk, you should never become a physician": a qualitative study about existential experiences among physicians. *J Med Ethics.* 2008;34(11):767–71.

Index

For Product Safety Concerns and Information please contact our EU representative GPSR@taylorandfrancis.com
Taylor & Francis Verlag GmbH, Kaufingerstraße 24, 80331 München, Germany

www.ingramcontent.com/pod-product-compliance
Ingram Content Group UK Ltd.
Pitfield, Milton Keynes, MK11 3LW, UK
UKHW050758180926
475701UK00008B/1112

* 9 7 8 1 0 4 1 3 3 0 7 9 0 *